Fundamentals of U.S. Health Care

T0314383

All health care students must be familiar with the basic concepts of health care in the United States. This introductory textbook presents vital information on health care careers and legal, ethical, financial, and policy issues that will help their future practice. It includes chapters on:

- careers in the health care profession;
- the complexity of health care;
- the Patient Protection and Affordable Care Act;
- professionalism in health;
- health care for special populations;
- the Occupational Safety and Health Administration (OSHA) standards;
- research and advancements in health care;
- the future of health care.

Fundamentals of U.S. Health Care is unique in the way it highlights the important elements of each health career, including job requirements, length of study, and salaries. With the student in mind, this book is accompanied by a website that features detailed PowerPoints and test banks with more than 1,000 review questions.

Well-organized and easily understood, this overview provides a reliable, relevant resource and up-to-date reference. It is essential reading for all allied health students, including nurses, surgical technicians, dental hygienists, radiology technicians, medical assistants, pharmacy technicians, physician assistants, and more.

Jahangir Moini is Professor of Science and Health at Eastern Florida State College, USA.

Morvarid Moini is a Pediatric Dentistry Resident at Tufts University, USA.

Fundamentals of U.S. Health Care

An Introduction for Health Professionals

Jahangir Moini
and
Morvarid Moini

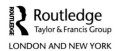

Routledge
Taylor & Francis Group

LONDON AND NEW YORK

First published 2017
by Routledge
2 Park Square, Milton Park, Abingdon, Oxon OX14 4RN

and by Routledge
711 Third Avenue, New York, NY 10017

Routledge is an imprint of the Taylor & Francis Group, an informa business

British Library Cataloguing-in-Publication Data
A catalogue record for this book is available from the British Library

Library of Congress Cataloging-in-Publication Data
Names: Moini, Jahangir, 1942– author. | Moini, Morvarid, author.
Title: Fundamentals of US health care: an introduction for health professionals / Jahangir Moini and Morvarid Moini.
Description: Abingdon, Oxon; New York, NY: Routledge, 2017. | Includes bibliographical references.
Identifiers: LCCN 2016047797 | ISBN 9781138659216 (hbk) | ISBN 9781138659223 (pbk) | ISBN 9781315620374 (ebk)
Subjects: | MESH: Delivery of Health Care | Health Policy | United States
Classification: LCC RA418.3.U6 | NLM W 84 AA1 | DDC 362.10973–dc23
LC record available at https://lccn.loc.gov/2016047797

Visit the companion website: www.routledge.com/cw/moini

ISBN: 978-1-138-65921-6 (hbk)
ISBN: 978-1-138-65922-3 (pbk)
ISBN: 978-1-315-62037-4 (ebk)

Typeset in Sabon and Frutiger
by Wearset Ltd, Boldon, Tyne and Wear

Dedication (from Dr. Jahangir Moini)

This book is dedicated to the memory of my mother, my wife Hengameh, my daughters, and my precious granddaughters Laila and Anabelle.

Dedication (from Dr. Morvarid Moini)

This book is dedicated to my father Jahangir, my mother Hengameh, my sister Mahkameh, and my nieces Laila and Anabelle.

Contents

List of tables   xv
About the authors   xvii
Preface   xviii
Acknowledgments   xx

Unit I   Health care today   1

1   The complexity of health care   3

Overview   3
U.S. health care   4
Health care industry   5
Health care services   12
Challenges facing health care systems   23
Case study   29
Chapter highlights   29
Summary   31
Review questions   31
Bibliography   31

2   The Patient Protection and Affordable Care Act   35

Overview   35
National Health Expenditure   36
Health care reform   37
Implementation of the PPACA   38
Legal challenges to the Act   40
Supreme Court modifications   41
State coverage   42
Minimum essential coverage   42
Costs of premiums and implementation   42
Medicaid expansion   45
Advantages and disadvantages of the PPACA   46
Case study   50
Chapter highlights   51

Summary   53
Review questions   53
Bibliography   54

3   Legal and ethical aspects of health care   56

Overview   56
Law   57
Classifications of law   57
Tort liability   58
Respondeat superior   60
Contract law   60
Professional liability and medical malpractice   62
Provider's rights and responsibilities   65
Privacy law and HIPAA   65
Ethics and health care   66
Professional ethics   68
Patient's rights and responsibilities   68
Biomedical concerns   68
Special considerations   69
End-of-life issues   71
Case study   73
Chapter highlights   74
Summary   75
Review questions   76
Bibliography   76

Unit II   Financial management   79

4   Health care financing and payment for services   81

Overview   81
Reimbursement for health care services   82
Government-funded health care   82
Privately funded health care   87
Insurance and managed care   91
Direct payments from patients   93
Comparisons of U.S. health care with other countries   94
Case study   95
Chapter highlights   95
Summary   97
Review questions   98
Bibliography   98

5   Customer service   **100**

Overview   100
Quality of care   101
Dimensions of quality   101
Quality assurance   103
Quality improvement   106
Quality improvement organizations   107
Customer satisfaction   107
Case study   111
Chapter highlights   111
Summary   113
Review questions   114
Bibliography   114

Unit III   Professionals and professional practice   117

6   Careers in the health care profession   **119**

Overview   119
Therapeutic divisions of the health care system   120
Diagnostic divisions of the health care system   150
Health care management   157
Health care education   157
Case study   158
Chapter highlights   158
Summary   160
Review questions   160
Bibliography   161

7   Professionalism in health care   **165**

Overview   165
Professionalism   166
Professional behavior   167
Stress management   175
Personal health   178
Personal hygiene   180
Case study   181
Chapter highlights   181
Summary   183
Review questions   183
Bibliography   184

Unit IV Patient populations   187

8 Health care for special populations   189

Overview   189
Children   190
Women   191
Ethnic minorities   193
Elderly   196
People with disabilities   199
HIV and AIDS   200
Chronically ill   202
Homeless   202
Uninsured   203
Illegal immigrants   204
Case study   205
Chapter highlights   205
Summary   207
Review questions   207
Bibliography   207

9 Introduction to global health issues   210

Overview   210
Concepts of global health   211
Concepts of public health and community-based care   211
Smallpox eradication   212
The effects of disease on life expectancy   213
Risk factors for disease   214
Ethical and human rights concerns   216
Universal health coverage   216
Culture and health   217
Nutrition and global health   220
Case study   225
Chapter highlights   225
Summary   227
Review questions   228
Bibliography   228

10 Global health: communicable and non-communicable
diseases   230

Overview   230
Communicable diseases   231
Non-communicable diseases   241
Case study   251
Chapter highlights   251

Summary 253
Review questions 253
Bibliography 254

11 Emergencies 256

Overview 256
Emergency and urgent care 257
Triage 258
Natural and man-made disasters 258
Health care during natural disasters 261
Emergency procedures 263
Case study 276
Chapter highlights 276
Summary 278
Review questions 278
Bibliography 278

Unit V   Safety in the workplace 281

12 Infection control 283

Overview 283
Classification of microorganisms 284
Infectious disease process 288
Chain of infection 288
Hand hygiene 293
Microorganism control 294
Personal protective equipment 295
Antiseptics, disinfectants, and sterilization 296
Surgical asepsis 299
Case study 299
Chapter highlights 299
Summary 301
Review questions 301
Bibliography 301

13 Occupational Safety and Health Administration (OSHA) standards 303

Overview 303
OSHA Bloodborne Pathogens Standard 304
Components of the OSHA Standard 311
OSHA Hazard Communication 315
Fire safety and emergency plan 318
Chemical hazards and safety 322
Physical safety 324

Contents

Latex allergy   325
Ergonomics   325
Radiation hazards   328
Workplace violence   328
Employee responsibilities   328
Case study   329
Chapter highlights   329
Summary   331
Review questions   332
Bibliography   332

Unit VI Communication in the health care profession   335

14   The communication process   337

Overview   337
Maslow's hierarchy of human needs   338
Steps of the communication process   339
Types of communication   340
Improving your communication skills   343
Therapeutic communication   345
Interprofessional communication   347
Methods of communication   347
Barriers to communication   349
Written communication   350
Defense mechanisms   351
Dealing with conflict   353
Case study   353
Chapter highlights   354
Summary   355
Review questions   356
Bibliography   356

15   Computers and technology in health care   358

Overview   358
Types of computer   359
Computers in health care   362
Computer security   371
Case study   372
Chapter highlights   372
Summary   374
Review questions   374
Bibliography   375

16   Record-keeping   377

  Overview   377
  Contents of the medical record   378
  Types of medical records   379
  Electronic health records   381
  Personal health records   382
  Medical documentation   383
  HIPAA and the medical record   384
  Case study   386
  Chapter highlights   386
  Summary   388
  Review questions   389
  Bibliography   389

Unit VII Predictions for health care in the United States   391

17   Research and advancements in health care   393

  Overview   393
  Types of research   394
  Research ethics and conflicts of interest   401
  Patient satisfaction   403
  Future challenges   403
  Case study   405
  Chapter highlights   405
  Summary   407
  Review questions   407
  Bibliography   407

18   The future of health care   409

  Overview   409
  Essentials of reform   410
  Clinical advancements   410
  Increasing ambulatory, outpatient, and home care   412
  Predictions for long-term care   413
  Increasing populations   414
  Increasing obesity   415
  Case study   417
  Chapter highlights   418
  Summary   419
  Review questions   420
  Bibliography   420

Appendices

Appendix A: A chemical safety data sheet   **422**

Appendix B: HIPAA complaint form   **427**

Appendix C: Glossary   **428**

Index   **451**

List of tables

1.1	Fastest-growing segments of the health care industry	5
1.2	Examples of medical technologies	7
1.3	The 15 highest paying medical specialties	8
1.4	Life expectancy in the United States based on birth year	11
1.5	Hospitals in the United States	14
1.6	Long-term care services	19
1.7	Breakdown of patients seeking addiction rehabilitation	20
1.8	U.S. mental health statistics	21
2.1	Required essential health benefits (by all qualified plans)	45
2.2	Advantages and disadvantages of the Affordable Care Act	48
3.1	Types of torts	58
4.1	Medicaid enrollment and payouts	84
5.1	Quality improvement organizations	108
5.2	Methods to provide better customer satisfaction	110
6.1	Types of physician specialties	121
6.2	Types of dental specialties	127
6.3	Types of dietitian specialties	143
6.4	Types of psychologist specialties	148
6.5	Types of laboratory technologist specialties	153
7.1	Steps used in maintaining professional distance	169
7.2	Steps used in health care problem solving	171
8.1	Percentages of larger minority groups in the USA	193
8.2	Levels of disability	200
8.3	Reported AIDS cases in various groups, in the United States	201
8.4	Uninsured percentages of various Americans	204
9.1	Life expectancy at birth and health-adjusted life expectancy (HALE) for various countries	213
9.2	Top 10 risk factors for deaths in various types of countries	214
9.3	Conditions and treatments based on theories of "hot" and "cold"	218
9.4	Examples of health care providers in various cultures	219
9.5	Rates of U.S. obesity in individual populations	224
10.1	Methods of spreading communicable disease	231
10.2	Methods of controlling communicable diseases	233

10.3	Prevalence of deaths from communicable diseases	233
10.4	Causes of disability	241
10.5	Most commonly diagnosed types of cancer and prevalence of cancer deaths	244
10.6	Risk factors for cancer	245
10.7	Deaths from diabetes	246
10.8	Prevalence of mental disorders in adults	248
10.9	Percentages of adolescents who smoke	249
10.10	Alcohol consumption in adolescents	250
11.1	The five levels of the Emergency Severity Index (ESI)	257
11.2	Examples of man-made and natural disasters	260
11.3	Types of fractures	270
12.1	Modes of transmission	291
12.2	Control of microorganisms	295
13.1	Viral hepatitis	307
14.1	Defense mechanisms	352
15.1	Benefits of computer use in health care systems	363
16.1	Advantages of electronic health records	383
16.2	The four areas of compliance under the HIPAA Security Rule	385
17.1	Overview of advances due to medical research	395
18.1	Long-term care statistics	413

About the authors

Jahangir Moini, MD, MPH, graduated from the medical school at Tehran University and also from Tulane University. He was assistant professor at Tehran University School of Medicine for nine years, teaching preventive medicine and epidemiology for medical and allied health students. The author is a professor and former director (for 15 years) of health science programs at Everest University. In total, he has been a physician and professor for the past 38 years. Also, Dr. Moini was an epidemiologist with the Brevard County Health Department in Florida for 18 years. Dr. Moini is currently a professor of science and health at Eastern Florida State College. He has been an internationally published author of various health science books since 1999.

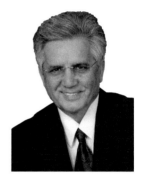

Morvarid Moini, DMD, MPH, received her Bachelor of Arts in Architecture from Florida International University, and her Bachelor of Science in Biology from the University of Central Florida. Additionally, she received her Doctor of Dental Medicine degree and Master's of Public Health from Nova Southeastern University. Currently, she is a pediatric dentistry resident at Tufts University.

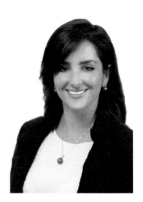

Preface

Introduction

Fundamentals of U.S. Health Care: An Introduction for Health Professionals is written for all health care professionals. Its main purpose is to present information on the current problems and complexities of the health care system in the United States. This book is written in a direct, easy-to-comprehend style suitable for all types of health care students and practitioners. It is a strong reference source for individuals who intend to continue their studies further.

Organization of content

This book is organized into seven units comprising 18 chapters that focus on various aspects of health care in the United States. Unit I, "Health Care Today," includes chapters on the complexity of health care, the Patient Protection and Affordable Care Act, and the legal and ethical aspects of health care. Unit II, "Financial Management," focuses on health care financing and payment for services and customer service. Unit III, "Professionals and Professional Practice," discusses careers in the health care profession, and professionalism in health care. Unit IV, "Patient Populations," covers health care for special populations, an introduction to global health issues, communicable and non-communicable diseases, and emergencies.

Unit V, "Safety in the Workplace," discusses infection control and standards put forth by the Occupational Safety and Health Administration, or OSHA. Unit VI, "Communication in the Health Care Profession," features vital information about the communication process, computers and technology in health care, and record-keeping. The final unit, Unit VII, "Predictions for Health Care in the United States," explores research and advancements in health care, as well as the future of health care.

Following the actual chapters are three Appendices with many unique areas of information. They include a chemical safety data sheet, privacy violation complaint form, and the glossary. Also, the accompanying website contains additional Appendices. These include: reference laboratory values, normal vital signs, American sign language and manual communication, health promotion, an overview of medical terminology, an overview of math in medicine, and an answer key.

Features

Each chapter contains a list of objectives, an overview, bolded terms throughout the text, which correspond to the Glossary, a case study, chapter highlights, a summary, review questions, and a bibliography. Figures serve to accurately illustrate chapter principles. Numerous helpful and accurate tables are included to highlight key components of information. In each chapter, the **case study** includes critical thinking questions for students to explore information in greater depth. The **chapter highlights** correspond to the **objectives** that appear early in each chapter, and provide responses to them. Each chapter features ten **review questions** that students should be able to answer after reading the text. The **bibliography** leads students to other books and articles that will deepen their understanding of the subject matter, along with Internet links to websites with additional information (all links correct at the time of writing in August 2016).

Note on the text

Key terms can be found highlighted in blue throughout the book. These are listed in full in the Glossary, found at the end of the book.

Ancillary materials

www.routledge.com/cw/moini

Acknowledgments

The authors would like to acknowledge all their colleagues, students, and friends who have allowed themselves to be photographed for the figures appearing in this book. Additional thanks go to Dr. Christopher Prusinski, Mabry Dental Care, Dr. Mohammad Moini, Medical Associates of Brevard LLC, Dr. Manohar Reddy, and Eau Gallie Discount Pharmacy for providing photographic locations and equipment. The authors would also like to especially thank their assistant, Greg Vadimsky, and Grace McInnes, Carolina Antunes, and Christina O'Brien at Routledge.

Reviewers

We would also like to acknowledge R. Christopher Harvey and all of the reviewers who have dedicated their time to helping us improve this book.

Health care today

Contents

1 The complexity of health care   3

Overview   3
U.S. health care   4
Health care industry   5
Health care services   12
Challenges facing health care systems   23
Case study   29
Chapter highlights   29
Summary   31
Review questions   31
Bibliography   31

2 The Patient Protection and Affordable Care Act   33

Overview   33
National Health Expenditure   34
Health care reform   35
Implementation of the PPACA   36
Legal challenges to the Act   38
Supreme Court modifications   39
State coverage   40
Minimum essential coverage   40
Costs of premiums and implementation   40
Medicaid expansion   43
Advantages and disadvantages of the PPACA   44
Case study   48
Chapter highlights   49
Summary   51
Review questions   51
Bibliography   52

3 Legal and ethical aspects of health care   54

Overview	54
Law	55
Classifications of law	55
Tort liability	56
Respondeat superior	58
Contract law	58
Professional liability and medical malpractice	60
Provider's rights and responsibilities	63
Privacy law and HIPAA	63
Ethics and health care	64
Professional ethics	66
Patient's rights and responsibilities	66
Biomedical concerns	66
Special considerations	67
End-of-life issues	69
Case study	71
Chapter highlights	72
Summary	73
Review questions	74
Bibliography	76

Chapter 1

The complexity of health care

After study of the chapter, readers should be able to:

1 Discuss factors concerning older people that affect the health care industry.
2 Explain ambulatory centers and rehabilitation hospitals.
3 Discuss hospice.
4 Describe the effects of the aging population.
5 Classify the various types of hospital.
6 Discuss how habits and behaviors may affect health care.
7 List public health issues of today.
8 Discuss the three levels of preventive medicine.

Overview

Today, health care is becoming more complex, in every area, and in every country. There have been many changes in health care resulting from advancements in technology, medical studies, cultural values, the understanding of genetics, lifestyle choices, and the impact of the environment. In earlier times, most patients were treated by a single practitioner acting as their *physician*. Today, most patients have a *primary care physician*, who then refers them to a variety of specialists as needed. There are more areas of specialization than ever before. Likewise, there are more types of health care treatment facility, offering patients increased opportunities for larger varieties of care. Yet, many people cannot access these opportunities. This is perhaps the central factor related to the complexity of health care today.

U.S. health care

In the United States, the majority of diseases are now related to a person's lifestyle. Diet, exercise, hygiene, and habits such as smoking cigarettes or drinking alcoholic beverages influence the status of public health. Chronic illnesses such as hypertension and diabetes are more common than communicable illnesses, which had been more prevalent in earlier history. Disease is also caused by genetic and environmental factors. Air pollution, ultraviolet radiation, and contaminated water or food are some environmental factors linked to disease.

Almost 200 years ago, infectious disease was the most common cause of death because of lack of sanitation and clean water, and contaminated foods. Even 100 years ago, the most common cause of death still was infectious disease. After 1938, with the development of antibiotics and the discovery of various vaccinations, infectious diseases in the United States began to be controlled, decreasing their prevalence. Improvements in general hygiene, available clean water, and food preparation greatly reduced deaths from infectious diseases as well. Another factor was improved nutrition, particularly for children, which increased resistance to infection and boosted immunity. The discoveries of new medicines, medical techniques, and methods of diagnosis resulted in people living longer.

With increased aging, non-communicable diseases became more prevalent, such as cardiovascular disorders, cancer, diabetes, Alzheimer's disease, and degenerative diseases. With chronic illness, the disease process usually begins a long time before symptoms appear. Health care is affected by this fact, and therefore the focus of today's health care is on *disease prevention*. However, the public must be educated about the fact that personal lifestyle choices greatly influence overall health outcomes. For chronic diseases, the best methods of treatment continue over a long period of time – yet most health care involves short-term treatment.

Drugs and surgery are widely believed to be the "core" of today's health care, yet most poor health is caused by behavioral and environmental factors. In the United States, health insurance pays for acute disease treatments and hospitalization, yet most insurers emphasize coverage for specialized services such as cardiac care or surgery, which are short-term services. Resources must be redistributed to focus on disease prevention, then the provision of immediate care for those with acute diseases, and finally, continuous care for chronic diseases.

Preventive efforts help protect against, reduce the severity of, and detect diseases earlier. Still, utilization is often inadequate, such as when younger children do not receive adequate vaccinations, and remain not fully protected against common childhood infectious diseases. Another example of the lack of preventive efforts exists in poorer people, such as the lack of mammography screening, Pap smears, and pneumococcal vaccinations.

The leading causes of death in the United States include heart disease, cancer, stroke, chronic lower respiratory disease, and Alzheimer's disease. This is different than in earlier times, when communicable diseases included tuberculosis and smallpox. Life expectancy today is at its highest level in history in the United States. Americans have the ability to greatly control their own health, since more than half of all causes of disease are linked to their behaviors and lifestyle. Individuals of lower socioeconomic status have higher disease rates, linked to poorer nutrition, housing, environmental hazard exposure, unhealthy lifestyles, and less access to health care services. People who cannot speak English may have reduced access to health care services. The lack of health insurance coverage is the most important factor in receiving needed care.

Health care industry

Today's health care industry includes many different individuals and organizations, and is experiencing tremendous growth. According to the U.S. Department of Labor, health care employment growth accounted for more than 3.5 million new jobs over the last decade, and is projected to increase in the future.

Members of the health care industry include physicians' offices, hospitals, nursing homes, assisted-living organizations, pharmaceutical companies, medical equipment manufacturers, and insurance companies. As the population ages, increased amounts of money are spent on health care. Older individuals statistically require more health care. For example, in the United States, in adults over age 80, three out of four people have more than one chronic disease. Of those between ages 65 and 80, two out of three have more than one chronic disease.

Medical costs are continually rising faster than overall economic growth. This also means that the employment outlook for the health care industry is growing quickly, and offers many opportunities for employment. The fastest-growing segments of the health care industry are summarized in Table 1.1.

In the United States alone, health care is the largest service industry. According to the U.S. Census Bureau, prior to the passage of the Patient Protection and Affordable Care Act (ACA), there were 42 million people who were uninsured, which makes up 13.4% of the total population. Of the 42 million uninsured people, 19.7% (or 8,274,000) were non-citizens. The ACA was intended to reduce the huge health care costs in the nation. If the Act is successful in its goals, health care coverage will be extended to more than 32 million people who currently have no health insurance, by the year 2019. The projected cost of the implementation of the Act was $1.1 trillion. As of July 1, 2015, approximately 15 million Americans became insured under the ACA.

As of 2015, medical care cost a total of $3.8 trillion in the United States. Given the fact that the United States has such large health care costs, the country ranks only eighth in life expectancy at birth, and also ranks number one in infant mortality rate and in the likelihood of individuals dying between the ages of 15 and 60. While the United States spends more than three times the amount of money on health care than Japan, it attains nowhere near the same successes in health outcomes.

Table 1.1 Fastest-growing segments of the health care industry

Segment	Growth (%)
Home health aids	56
Medical assistants	52
Physician assistants	50
Physical therapist assistants	44

Source: https://doleta.gov/brg/indprof/healthcare_profile.cfm (U.S. Bureau of Labor Statistics, 2006–07 Career Guide to Industries).

Technological advancements

Medical technology is the application of scientific knowledge to improve health and to deliver health care more efficiently. Today, technological advancements have improved infection control, aided in human reproduction, provided less-invasive surgical techniques, and created more effective cancer therapies. As a result, people live longer, recover from serious diseases, and survive excessive trauma. Laser surgery, magnetic resonance imaging (MRI), computed axial tomography (CAT), and organ transplants are commonly performed. Technology has also provided e-prescribing, electronic medical records, telemedicine, and robotic surgery.

Since technology can actually sustain life artificially, however, expenses regarding patients who will probably never recover have risen. Mechanical ventilation, parenteral feeding, and kidney dialysis can all prolong life without providing any improvement in a patient's condition, yet remain expensive technologies. The U.S. health care system has been affected by these expenses, resulting in higher costs of insurance, more expensive hospitalization, higher medical bills, and increased government reimbursements. Also, due to limits in funding, not every citizen can receive advanced-level treatments, meaning some people die because of lack of access to the health care they require. The federal government, therefore, has become more powerful in regard to providing health care.

The advance of medical technology has increased in the last 20 years more than ever before. Nanomedicine utilizes nanotechnology for medical needs, manipulating atoms and molecules for diagnostic and therapeutic procedures. For example, *nanoparticles* are being manipulated to carry drugs to specific body regions in the fight against cancer. Additional developments include the areas of gene therapy, robotic and microscopic surgery, and targeted drug therapy. *Information technology* has changed in revolutionary ways, and the manipulation of intensive data for medical use is faster and more efficient than ever before.

The 21st century will probably outpace the 20th century, which saw more technological advancements in the health care professions than ever before. New vaccines, cures, treatments, and procedures such as cloning of organs for transplantation are on the horizon. With all of these advancements, the lifespan of humans may be able to exceed an average of 100 years. Table 1.2 lists examples of medical technologies, all of which are continually developing and advancing.

Specialization

In the last 30 years, more areas of specialization in medicine have developed than throughout history. In fact, the Association of American Medical Colleges lists more than 120 specialties and subspecialties. Practitioners are focusing on specific areas of expertise, which improves diagnosis and treatment. However, many health care professionals treat only one aspect of a patient's condition, and not the patient as a whole. Other negative factors of

Table 1.2 Examples of medical technologies

Area	Technology
Curative	Hip joint replacement
	Lithotripsy
	Organ transplantation
Diagnostic	Automated clinical laboratory
	Blood pressure monitors
	CAT scans
	Computerized electrocardiography
	Fetal monitors
	Magnetic resonance imaging
Disease management	Pacemakers
	Percutaneous transluminal coronary angioplasty (PTCA)
	Renal dialysis
	Stereotactic cingulotomy or psychosurgery
Facilities and clinics	Clinical laboratories
	Hospital "satellite" centers
	Modern home health care
	Subacute care units
Life-saving measures	Autologous bone marrow transplantation
	Bone marrow transplantation (traditional)
	Cardiopulmonary resuscitation (CPR)
	Intensive care units (ICUs)
	Liver transplantation
Organizational delivery	Integrated delivery networks
	Managed care
Preventative	Diet control (for phenylketonuria)
	Implantable automatic cardioverter defibrillators
	Pediatric orthopedic repair
	Vaccines and immunizations
System management	Health information systems
	Telemedicine

specialization include increased costs and poorer relationships between patients and primary care physicians, since today there are more specialists involved in a single patient's care. As a result of specialization, employment opportunities are increasing.

According to the American Medical Association (AMA), there are eight major medical specialization areas in today's health care. These include:

- Emergency medicine
- Family practice
- Internal medicine
- Obstetrics-gynecology
- Orthopedic surgery
- Pediatrics
- Psychiatry
- General surgery.

Medical specialists are not distributed equally throughout the country, with more specialists practicing in major cities than in rural areas. Today, 42% of physicians are considered primary care, and 58% are considered specialists. The proportion of primary care providers has been declining continually for more than 70 years. The increasing number of medical specialists may be linked to the growth of new medical technology, as well as higher income potential. Imbalances between primary and specialty care have caused more serious medical interventions to occur earlier in patient treatment timelines, resulting in higher costs. The highest-paying medical specialties are listed in Table 1.3.

Table 1.3 The 15 highest paying medical specialties

Specialty	Average base salary
Invasive cardiologists	$525,000
Orthopedic surgeons	$497,000
Gastroenterologists	$455,000
Urologists	$412,000
Dermatologists	$398,000
Emergency physicians	$345,000
General surgeons	$339,000
Otolaryngologists	$334,000
Pulmonologists	$331,000
Non-invasive cardiologists	$291,000
Neurologists	$277,000
Obstetricians/gynecologists	$276,000
Physiatrists	$244,000
Hospitalists	$232,000
Psychiatrists	$226,000

Source: www.forbes.com/pictures/fjle45mdhk/no-1-cardiology-invasive/#1ab539567182.

Costs

Health care costs have risen dramatically over the last few decades, and more than 50% of uninsured people say that *cost* is the primary factor in their lack of coverage. The reasons for rising health care costs include general inflation, which includes the need for higher wages and supply costs. Additional costs are related to third-party payers, fraud and abuse, defensive medicine, technology advancements, increases in the elderly population, the imperfectness of the market, the medical model of how health care is delivered, administrative costs and the multi-payer system, and variations in medical practices. Medical equipment and supplies, as well as pharmaceutical products, are often extremely expensive. Costs may also increase because of the larger number of available diagnostic tests and treatments.

Another important factor is the effect of medical malpractice lawsuits. According to the Congressional Budget Office, total direct costs to health care providers resulting from medical malpractice liability averages $35 billion per year. These lawsuits result in increased liability insurance costs paid by practitioners. Because of this, practitioners increase the rates of their services. The term **defensive medicine** refers to medical procedures that are performed to reduce the likelihood of legal outcomes. A lack of competition for many practitioners also allows higher fees to be charged. To better understand the distribution of health care costs, see Figures 1.1a and 1.1b.

Fraud and abuse includes illegal billing claims or cost reports, as well as **upcoding**, which is the practice of billing for higher-priced services when lower-priced services were actually

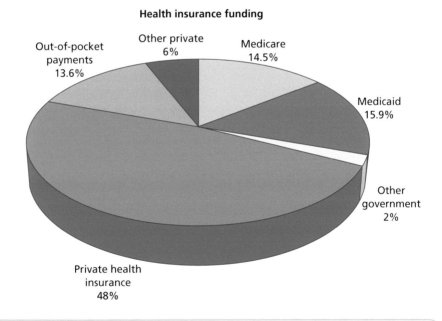

Health insurance funding

Out-of-pocket payments 13.6%
Other private 6%
Medicare 14.5%
Medicaid 15.9%
Other government 2%
Private health insurance 48%

Figure 1.1a Health insurance funding.

Sources: http://dpeaflcio.org/programs-publications/issue-fact-sheets/the-u-s-health-care-system-an-international-perspective/; www.center-forward.org/wp-content/uploads/2012/04/Medicare-Medicaid-and-the-Military-04-12-update-2.pdf; www.bls.gov/opub/mlr/2003/03/art3full.pdf.

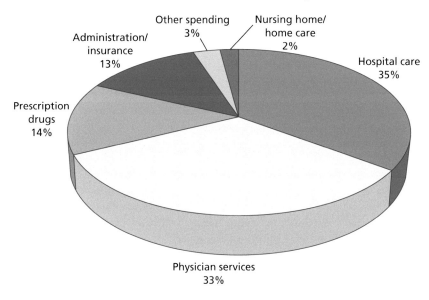

Figure 1.1b Where health care dollars are spent.

Sources: www.hcsc.com/pdf/economics_health_care2.pdf; www.mcgohanbrabender. com/our-approach/the-entire-health-care-dollar.

provided. The *medical model* of health care delivery means that medical interventions are emphasized after patients become sick, and does not put equal focus on prevention or behavioral changes that could promote health. *Practice variations* mean that physicians may have widely differing treatment patterns for similar patients, which may be based on location, demographics, fluctuating prices, and many other reasons.

Focus on increased health expenditures

As of 2013, national health expenditures grew 3.6% to $2.9 trillion. This is equivalent to $9,255 per person living in the United States. Medicare spending grew 3.4% to $585.7 billion, and Medicaid spending grew 6.1% to $449.4 billion.

Source: www.cms.gov/Newsroom/MediaReleaseDatabase/Press-releases/2014-Press-releases-items/2014-12-03-2.html

The aging population

Advances in health care have contributed to the fact that Americans are living longer. Table 1.4 lists life expectancies for people born in 1900, 2000, and 2010.

With a longer life expectancy, an elderly person can also expect to spend more years in declining health, needing more medical care than all other age groups. Living longer causes

Table 1.4 Life expectancy in the United States based on birth year

	Males	Females	Average
1900 – Average	40	41.5	40.7
White	47	49	48
Black	33	34	33.5
2000 – Average	71.5	77.5	74.5
White	75	80	77.5
Black	68	75	71.5
2010 – Average	76.4	81.1	78.8
White	78.5	83.8	81.2
Black	71.4	77.7	74.7

Sources: www.elderweb.com/book/appendix/1900-2000-changes-life-expectancy-united-states; www.cdc.gov/nchs/
data/databriefs/db99.pdf.

an increase in many chronic and degenerative diseases, such as Alzheimer's disease, diabetes, hypertension, cancers, and osteoporosis. Hearing and visual impairments are also more common. Elderly people are at higher risk for dementia, hip fractures, and stroke. As a result, the elderly spend more time in hospitals, nursing homes, long-term care facilities, and adult family care.

In the United States, the elderly population now totals more than 44.7 million (which is 14.1% of the population), with people over age 85 making up the age group with the most rapid growth.

The *baby boom generation* has begun reaching the age of 65. Therefore, the elderly will make up more than 26% of the population in less than two decades. The people referred to as **baby boomers** signify the extremely large number of births in the period following the end of World War II, beginning in 1946 and ending in 1964. As these people reach their later years, their need for health care is having a large impact upon available resources. The increasing elderly population is resulting in an unbalanced financial situation, pulling resources away from the working population, which is shrinking.

As a result of the increased elderly population and the chronic illnesses that they have, there has been significant growth in the treatment facilities and services they need. These include long-term care, home health care, and **adult day care**. Also known as *adult day service*, adult day care provides help to the elderly so that their adult children who are still in the working population can maintain their careers. Senior citizens with physical or mental impairments are supervised in a safe environment while their children are working or otherwise unable to supervise them. The majority of adult day care services focus on patients with dementia, and related nursing care, psychosocial therapy, and rehabilitation. Most are funded by Medicaid and private funding.

> ### You should remember
>
> The Administration on Aging predicts that by 2060, there will be about 98 million elderly persons in the United States, which is more than twice their number in 2013.
>
> *Source:* https://aoa.acl.gov/aging_statistics/index.aspx.

Health care services

Today's health care market offers a larger variety of organizations than in previous years. Patients may receive services at inpatient hospitals, post-acute brain injury facilities, outpatient or ambulatory care hospitals, long-term care facilities, rehabilitation hospitals, mental health facilities, hospice, government health services, and even in their own homes. Various health care professionals are employed at these different types of facility (see Figure 1.2).

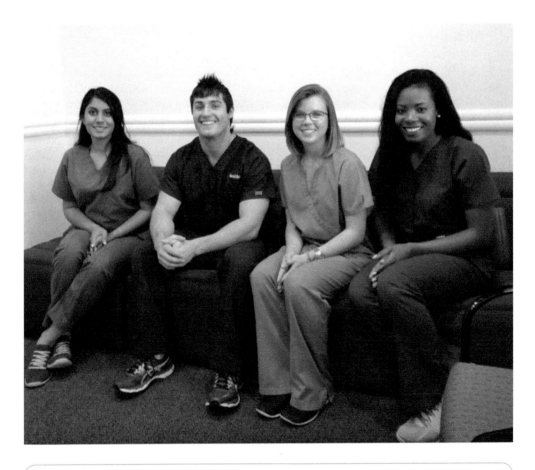

Figure 1.2 Various health care professionals employed in different types of facilities.

Hospitals

Today, inpatient hospital services make up the largest share of this country's total health care expenditures. In the 1980s and 1990s, as costs increased, the length of inpatient stays began to be reduced as part of aggressive utilization reviews as well as prospective, capitated payment methods. The majority of hospitals had many empty beds because of the reduced use of acute care beds. Hospitals had to change their business practices as acute inpatient care became less profitable. This resulted in multi-hospital systems, diversification into non-acute services, and affiliation with hospital networks. The non-acute services that many hospitals diversified into include home health care, outpatient centers, long-term care, and subacute care. The process of hospital consolidation in the 1990s resulted in increased costs, by approximately 5%, due to the lack of competition that these changes caused.

Still, hospital employment is continually increasing. Today, patient hospitalizations are carefully monitored so that they occur less often, and for shorter periods of time. Instead, other health care facilities are often used to reduce costs. The average hospital stay is now approximately 4.8 days, and measures are always being undertaken to reduce this figure. A total of about 51.4 million procedures are performed in hospitals annually.

There are just fewer than 6,000 registered hospitals of all types in the United States. The breakdown of types of hospital is dominated by private non-profit hospitals (nearly 3,000), followed by state and local government hospitals, and private for-profit hospitals (see Table 1.5).

Less common types include psychiatric hospitals, federal hospitals, and non-federal long-term hospitals. Psychiatric hospitals also treat behavioral disorders and monitor daily living activities, while providing medication management, counseling, and crisis assistance. Psychiatric patients may be treated in inpatient or outpatient facilities, based on needs.

Hospitals are also subdivided into teaching and nonteaching hospitals. A teaching hospital is one affiliated with a medical school that provides clinical education for medical and dental residents, as well as medical students. They may also provide clinical education for allied health personnel, nurses, and many different technical specialists. Approximately 341 hospitals (which is 6%) in the United States are teaching hospitals, and are usually not-for-profit or government-sponsored, either at the state or federal level. Only 2,904 (which is slightly more than 50%) of all U.S. hospitals are not-for-profit hospitals that are sponsored by community-based organizations, which include religious groups such as Catholic hospitals.

Of all hospitalization costs, Medicare and Medicaid pay for the majority of bills. The majority of hospitals are classified as private, non-profit, general hospitals in which patients stay for only a relatively short time. Unfortunately, the overall number of hospitals is on the decline, even though private, for-profit hospitals are one type that are increasing in number. Hospitals attempt to control costs by offering diverse services, eliminating services that are offered by nearby hospitals, merging with other hospitals, joining larger health care networks, or becoming a part of national corporations that manage a variety of hospitals.

General hospitals are those that provide varied services. These include general and specialized medicine and surgery, as well as obstetrics. Diagnostic and treatment-related services are included. The majority of hospitals in the United States are general hospitals. The most common conditions for which people are hospitalized include: heart problems, cancer, mental illness, stroke, respiratory conditions, and fractures related to osteoporosis.

To maintain quality of care, many hospitals seek voluntary accreditation through The Joint Commission, which is a private, non-profit organization that establishes high standards of hospital operation. It also accredits other types of health care institution. Accreditation by The Joint Commission is important, since Medicare and Medicaid will not pay for services received from non-accredited facilities.

Table 1.5 Hospitals in the United States

Type of hospital	Number
Total of all registered hospitals	**5,686**
Community hospitals	4,974
Non-government, not-for-profit community hospitals	2,904
Investor-owned, for-profit community hospitals	1,060
State and local government community hospitals	1,010
Non-federal psychiatric hospitals	406
Federal government hospitals	213
Non-federal long-term care hospitals	81
Hospital units of institutions (colleges, prisons, etc.)	12
Total urban community hospitals	**3,003**
Total rural community hospitals	**1,971**
Community hospitals in "systems"	**3,144**
Community hospitals in "networks"	**1,582**
Total staffed beds in all registered hospitals	914,513
Staffed beds in community hospitals	795,603
Total admissions in all registered hospitals	35,416,020
Admissions in community hospitals	33,609,083
Total expenses for all registered hospitals	$859,419,233,000
Expenses for community hospitals	$782,035,350,000

Source: www.aha.org/research/rc/stat-studies/fast-facts.shtml.

There are various types of care offered by hospitals. *Emergency departments* treat conditions needing immediate attention, such as accident or heart attack victims. A significant cost factor arises when a patient goes to an emergency department for a condition that could have been treated elsewhere with less expense. Often, patients who have worsening conditions do not seek treatment until these have become severe. They go to an emergency department, which is usually required by law to treat them, and then the hospital is not reimbursed for their services. As a result, many hospitals have closed their emergency departments or set up hospital clinics offering basic care to "walk-in" patients.

Trauma centers focus on life-threatening injuries, offering specific, high-level diagnostic equipment and surgery. *Cardiac care units (CCUs)* care for patients with serious heart conditions, and have the specific equipment and staff needed for this type of care. An *intensive care unit (ICU)* offers specific equipment and care for patients with serious injuries or illnesses. *Transitional care units (TCUs)* provide care of a lower level and assess patient needs, while making arrangements to send patients to other care facilities or allow them to return home. *General care units (GCUs)* treat seriously ill patients who do not require highly specialized equipment or continuous nursing care.

You should remember

The cost of excess capacity in hospitals, which is measured by the inpatient hospital bed occupancy rate, has declined over the past ten years. It now stands at about 65%.

Source: www.nber.org/papers/w3872.

Post-acute brain injury facilities

After a brain injury, there are basically three steps involved in recovery. In the first step, the patient is hospitalized and efforts are focused on preserving life and managing acute medical issues that are immediately secondary to the injury. The second step involves acute rehabilitation and the beginning of skilled therapy (usually 1–4 hours per day), while carefully managing the secondary injuries. The final step is post-acute rehabilitation, in which brain injury rehabilitation continues as attention is paid to adjusting to long-term injury-related symptoms as strategies are developed to help the patient cope with permanent deficits that may remain.

In general, the total combined rates for traumatic brain-injury-related emergency department visits, hospitalizations, and deaths have increased in past decades. About 824 out of 100,000 U.S. residents experience a traumatic brain injury every year. Although deaths from traumatic brain injuries have been declining, the overall amount of these injuries has increased in occurrence.

The term "post-acute" describes care required following a patient being hospitalized. An "acute" hospital provides emergency, neurosurgical, and medical stabilization as well as early treatment and attempts to minimize future complications. With advanced medical treatments and technology, brain-injured patients may receive post-acute care in specialized facilities that is extremely successful. For the severely brain-injured, care is available that can prolong their lives even if there is no promise of functional survival.

Post-acute brain injury facilities may help patients to recover from their injuries, or at least be able to cope with day-to-day living once they no longer require continued hospitalization. Patients are taught how to compensate for injury-related behavioral, cognitive, and emotional problems. Post-acute facilities are staffed by teams of medical professionals who have expertise in management of *traumatic brain injuries*.

Post-acute rehabilitation for brain injuries may also involve physical therapy, psychotherapy, speech therapy, home care, residential apartment centers offering therapy, outpatient programs, skilled nursing facilities, intermittent respite care, and assisted-living facilities.

Ambulatory centers

Ambulatory care is also known as outpatient care. Ambulatory centers handle health services that do not require overnight hospital stays. While previously, certain conditions required hospitalization, today these same conditions are often provided by ambulatory care facilities. Same-day surgeries may be performed in either *ambulatory surgical units* or separate facilities called *ambulatory surgical centers* (see Figure 1.3). Patients are routinely discharged in as little as one to three hours following surgery. Ambulatory care includes physician offices, dentist offices, other health practitioners, outpatient care centers, medical laboratories, diagnostic laboratories, home health care services, and other ambulatory health care services.

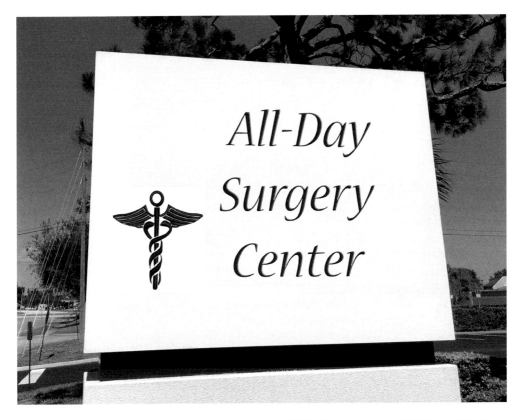

Figure 1.3 Ambulatory surgical center.

The various forms of ambulatory care facility have expanded as either hospital-based or non-hospital-based. Many hospitals still offer ambulatory surgical services inside their main facilities. However, there has been a shift to ambulatory surgical services and various ambulatory procedures within hospitals, and physician offices are still where most ambulatory services occur. The trend for more free-standing ambulatory facilities, outside of hospitals, grew from customer demand for facilities and services that were closer to them and easier to access. Many surgeries are more conveniently performed outside of the actual hospital setting, simplifying scheduling and other areas of complexity.

Physicians have developed outpatient diagnostic, treatment, and surgical facilities, including those specializing in ophthalmologic, gynecologic, gastrointestinal, chemotherapy, dialysis, and various imaging disciplines. Other ambulatory care practitioners include dentists, optometrists, physical therapists, podiatrists, psychologists, and social workers. Other facilities that may be considered ambulatory include adult day care, emergency and urgent care centers, and the health care services provided within companies, prisons, and schools. Laboratories often offer ambulatory services such as collection of body fluid and other samples, various testing services, and dental services. Another type of ambulatory facility is the *wellness center*, which provides routine physicals, immunizations, other preventive measures, and educational programs.

Urgent care centers provide walk-in access for acute illness or injury care that may be beyond the types of care provided by typical primary practices or retail clinics.

Appointments are not required, and even chronic illnesses and injuries may be treated. All types of medical professional may be employed at urgent care centers, which do not offer *ongoing care* for chronic conditions. Retail clinics are a new form of ambulatory care that may operate as part of pharmacies or even supermarkets (see Figure 1.4). They often have lower costs than many other facilities, yet are widely opposed by many primary care physicians.

Home health care

Home health care facilities provide certain types of services to patients in their own homes. Examples are skilled nursing care, physical therapy, speech therapy, occupational therapy, financial planning, other social assistance, and care provided by home health aides. When these services are provided in a patient's home, they are conducted by home health agencies. Home health care helps to treat patients in the least restrictive types of environments that are possible. According to the Centers for Disease Control and Prevention (CDC), there are more than 12,200 home health agencies in the United States, and nearly five million people receive or complete their home health care annually.

Many hospitals now have separate *home health departments*, focusing on rehabilitation and post-acute care. In this way, hospitals can keep discharged patients part of their systems. Nearly one in four Medicare-certified home health agencies are operated by hospitals. Under Medicare, patients are eligible for home health services if they are homebound, have their treatment plan periodically reviewed by their physician, need skilled nursing care or rehabilitation, and are expected to improve and recover. Other home health services may include meal preparation, transportation, shopping, and household maintenance and cleaning, but these are usually not covered by health insurers.

The trend for home health care grew out of the need for shorter hospital stays, technological advancements, the increasing elderly population, and the fact that most patients want to remain in their own homes in their senior years. Home health care-related jobs are increasing faster than many other areas of health care. Quality of care must be maintained, but this is difficult to monitor. Therefore, individual states now require home health

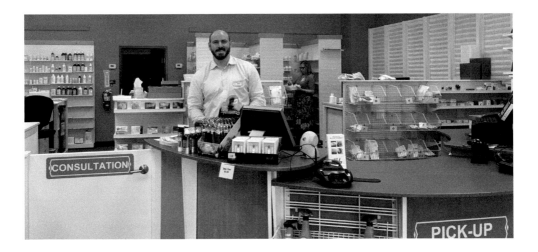

Figure 1.4 Retail pharmacy.

agencies to become licensed, and these agencies are strictly regulated by state law and insurance guidelines. Coverage by Medicare and most other insurers is approved only when services are provided by specific personnel.

> ## You should remember
>
> Medicare is the largest single payer of home health care services, accounting for more than 41% of home health expenditures. Other public funding sources include Medicaid, the Veterans' Administration, and the Civilian Health and Medical Program of the Uniformed Services (CHAMPUS).
>
> *Source:* www.nahc.org/assets/1/7/10HC-stats.pdf.

Long-term care facilities

Long-term care facilities include nursing homes and other facilities that provide custodial care for patients who have prolonged illnesses or chronic disabilities. This is a quickly growing area of health care, which is being improved upon to offer better care and a more supportive environment for patients. Long-term care is financed in different ways, but not under regular health insurance plans, or only with limited coverage. Long-term care is mostly but not exclusively used by elderly patients. It may also be used for children, adolescents, young adults, and HIV/AIDS patients.

Statistics show that nearly three in four elderly Americans will eventually need long-term care in some capacity, often occurring in their own homes. This type of care is often related to reduced functionality caused by chronic medical conditions, including cognitive impairment. According to Caregiver.org, the lifetime probability of becoming disabled in at least two daily living activities or of being cognitively impaired is 68% for people age 65 and older. It is expected that by 2050, there will be approximately 27 million individuals using paid long-term care services. This is more than double the amount that used these services in the year 2000. According to the American Association for Long-Term Care Insurance, the average need for this type of care lasts for 1,040 days (which is two years, 320 days).

Approximately two-thirds of long-term care costs are paid for by Medicaid and other public sources. Patients receive care that helps to maximize their quality of life, as much as possible, which requires use of up-to-date technology and evidence-based practices. The service provided to every patient should fit the patient's needs, be flexible enough to cover changes in his or her needs over time, and should be well-received according to personal preferences. Holistic health care is stressed, which addresses not only physical needs, but also the patient's mental, social, and even spiritual needs.

Long-term care patients often lose their self-worth over time, because of disability, and often feel that they have little hope of recovery, even when recovery is actually possible. Long-term care facilities include nursing homes, adult foster homes, assisted-living facilities, and continuing care communities.

Skilled nursing facilities provide around-the-clock nursing and rehabilitation services for patients needing regular medical care, or recovering from surgery, illness, or injury. Skilled nursing homes are relatively expensive, beginning at $4,000 per month, but may be covered by long-term care insurance, which is also expensive. *Intermediate nursing care* facilities do not provide 24-hour care, but focus on patients who cannot care for themselves, requiring regular nursing care, personal care, and social services.

Assisted-living facilities (ALFs) provide for individuals who do not need daily nursing care, but require housing, meals, and personal care according to their specific needs. Other names for these residences include *residential long-term care facilities*, *supportive housing*, *adult residential care facilities*, *board-and-care*, and *rest homes*. Continuing care communities are flexible, providing various living accommodations as residents eventually require regular medical and nursing care. Meals and daily nursing care can be contracted for if needed. Table 1.6 lists all of the types of long-term care services that may be provided for patients in need.

The newer options for the care of the elderly include adult foster care, which involves small home settings run by families who provide supervision and care. They offer a supplementary "family unit" to up to ten elderly residents at one time. This type of care is also called *adult family care*, *community residential care*, and domiciliary care. The titles and licensing standards for adult foster care settings vary from state to state. Funding comes from Medicaid, personal sources, or private insurance. While Medicare does not pay for adult foster care, Medicare Part B may cover rehabilitation.

Elderly people can also gather at *senior centers* in their communities. These centers often serve one or more meals per day, and many offer health and wellness programs, counseling, information and referrals, recreational activities, and certain health care services, such as screening for hypertension or glaucoma. They are usually supported by public funding, private donations, and the United Way.

Rehabilitation hospitals

A rehabilitation hospital is a facility that provides care for stabilized patients who still require inpatient hospital care. These patients require additional assistance to recover from injuries. This may include physical, occupational, or speech therapies, and also may require social work assistance to assist with the needs of living after the patient is released. Though patients in rehabilitation hospitals are usually more stable than those in standard hospitals, 24-hour nursing care is still available.

Certain illnesses or injuries may cause a lot of physical damage that takes time to heal. Amputation or traumatic injury usually requires significant time to regain function and adjust to the use of various support devices or even prosthetic limbs. Rehabilitation hospitals offer physical therapy and training as well as counseling for these patients. For patients who have had brain injuries, rehabilitation may focus on cognitive, speech, and physical function therapies. Family members may be invited to participate in therapies in order to

Table 1.6 Long-term care services

Medical services	Other services
Nursing	Mental health
Rehabilitation	Dementia
Prevention and therapeutic care	Social support
Informal and formal care	Short-term respite care in an facility outside the home
End-of-life care	Community-based and institutional services
	Housing

better assist patients once they go home. Rehabilitation hospitals are often the intermediary between total hospitalization and returning to a normal home life. The top diagnoses for rehabilitation hospitals in the United States include orthopedic, general rehabilitation, stroke, brain injury, amputations, and spinal cord injuries.

Rehabilitation hospitals may also focus on patients who are recovering from drug or alcohol addiction. The majority of patients seeking addiction rehabilitation were alcohol abusers (41.4%), while heroin and other opiate abusers made up 20% of admitted patients, followed by marijuana abusers at 17% (see Table 1.7). Patients may require much less care once they have gone through detoxification. Therefore, medical staff members may or may not be present on a constant basis in these facilities. Bedside care is often not required in rehabilitation hospitals that focus on substance recovery. Common names for these facilities include *rehab facilities*, or simply the word *rehab* itself.

Mental health services

Mental disorders are some of the leading types of disability in the United States. In 2015, approximately one in three Americans was suffering from a mental disorder. This means about 107 million people. Mental disorders can be either psychological or biological in nature. According to the CDC, more than 63 million people in the United States who seek medical treatment every year are primarily diagnosed with a mental disorder. A mental disorder is a risk factor for death from suicide, cancer, and cardiovascular disorder. Suicide is the 11th leading cause of death in the United States, and the 4th leading cause of death in people between the ages of 18 and 65.

Table 1.7 Breakdown of patients seeking addiction rehabilitation

Type of addiction	Percentage of patients
Alcohol	41.4 (this includes 23.1% that are alcohol-addicted only, plus 18.3% that are addicted to alcohol and another drug)
Opiates, including heroin	20 (this includes 14.1% addicted to heroin and 5.9% addicted to other opiates)
Marijuana	17
Smoked cocaine (crack)	8.1
Stimulants	6.5
Non-smoked cocaine (including powered cocaine)	3.2
Tranquilizers	0.6
PCP	0.2
Sedatives	0.2

Source: www.drugabuse.gov/publications/drugfacts/treatment-statistics.

Examples of mental disorders that are biological in nature include developmental disabilities, mental retardation, and schizophrenia. The most common mental disorders include anxiety disorders (which include phobias), mood disorders (such as depression), psychotic disorders (such as schizophrenia), eating disorders, impulse control and addiction disorders, personality disorders (such as obsessive-compulsive disorder), and post-traumatic stress disorder. Nearly one in four adults has a mental disorder that can be diagnosed. Approximately one in five children has a mental disorder, and about five million children or adolescents have a serious mental illness. Unfortunately, only about 50% of these children receive mental health services, meaning that the remainder is likely to develop more severe conditions, or to develop co-concurring conditions. Table 1.8 lists the latest statistics on mental health in the United States.

Most mental health services are not provided by specialists, but rather, by primary care settings, nursing homes, and community health centers. In both inpatient and outpatient facilities, public and private resources are used to provide these services. The majority of mental health services are provided by non-federal general hospital psychiatric divisions. In the United States, the mental health system is divided into one that is focused mostly on individuals who have insurance coverage or private funding, and another for those who do not have private coverage.

There is a definite shortage of mental health professionals and facilities. The costs of mental health services are usually quite high. Fortunately, managed care organizations have expanded to include mental health services. In managed care networks, the predominant type of professional handling these services is the psychiatric social worker, followed by mental health counselors, and then psychologists and psychiatrists.

Hospice

Hospice care focuses on terminally ill patients, which generally means those who are not expected to live longer than six months. The majority of hospice patients are those with various types of cancer. According to the National Hospice and Palliative Care Organization, as many as 1.6 million patients receive hospice services every year. Hospice provides palliative care, and also emphasizes pain management, in familiar and comfortable places, which may be the patient's home or in a special hospice facility. This type of care services

Table 1.8 U.S. mental health statistics

Factor	Statistic
Adults with serious psychological distress in the past 30 days	3.1%
Number of visits with mental disorders as primary diagnosis	63.3 million
Number of discharges with psychoses as first-listed diagnosis	1.5 million
Average length of stay for mental disorders	7.2 days
Suicide deaths per 100,000 population	13

Sources: www.healthindicators.gov/indicators/Serious-psychological-distress-adults-percent_50055/profile/classicdata; www.cdc.gov/nchs/fastats/mental-health.htm; www.sciencedirect.com/science/article/pii/s2095754816000302; http://piperreport.com/blog/2011/06/25/hospitalizations-for-mental-health-and-substance-abuse-disorders-costs-length-of-stay-patient-mix-and-payor-mix/; www.cdc.gov/nchs/fastats/suicide.htm.

not only patients, but also their families and caregivers. A hospice is not a location, but a type of care. Therefore, hospice can be a type of home health care as well as a part of nursing homes, hospitals, or retirement centers.

Hospice strives to meet the physical needs of the patient (see Figure 1.5). It focuses on quality of life and not prolonging life. It also is designed to assist with the emotional and spiritual needs of patients and family members. Hospice focuses on providing a patient's final days with as much meaning and lack of pain as possible. Support continues before and after the death of the patient. A hospice may be certified by Medicare as long as it provides 24-hour services, registered nursing services, inpatient care optional services, social services, counseling and support, pain management and palliation, therapy services if required, and both home health aide and homemaker services if required.

Focus on hospice

Hospice is paid for by Medicare, Medicaid, and most insurance plans. It serves anyone with a life-limiting illness, regardless of age or type of illness. People receiving hospice care can live longer than similar patients who do not opt for hospice.

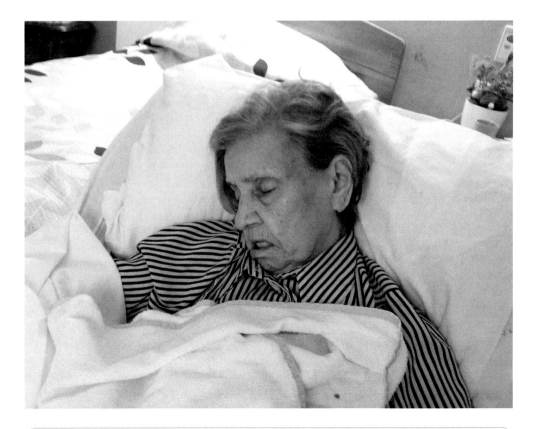

Figure 1.5 A patient in a hospice center.

Challenges facing health care systems

Challenges facing health care systems are quite diverse. They include access to health care, how habits and social conditions affect health care, the maintenance of quality of care, and common health issues that affect the public.

Access to health care

Access means the ability of an individual to obtain health care services when needed. Good access allows individuals to receive needed care in a timely manner. Care should also be affordable, acceptable, convenient, and effective. Access may refer to having a usual source of care, such as a primary care physician; reflect how acceptable services are, based on preferences and values; and indicate the individual's ability to use health care services. Good access to health care is vital in determining health along with environment, heredity, and lifestyle. Access measures the effectiveness of the health care delivery system, its fairness, its quality, and its efficiency.

Uninsured people can access health care in certain situations, but may not be able to access it for everything they need. The locations of free clinics, which provide health care to anyone regardless of whether or not they can pay, are very limited. Laws in the United States require hospital emergency departments to offer care for no charge unless they determine the patient has the ability to pay.

However, uninsured people are not usually able to access basic, routine care on a continual basis, which is also called *primary care*. People who are unemployed usually cannot afford to buy private health insurance, and yet may not qualify for Medicaid. Those called the *working poor*, while having jobs, are not offered group coverage by their employer. These people include part-time and temporary workers, who often do not earn enough money to buy their own health insurance. Also, many individuals who have pre-existing conditions are not approved by health insurers for coverage.

Access to health care involves five basic dimensions:

- *Accessibility* – locations of patients and providers
- *Acceptability* – a comparison of the attitudes concerning health care between patients and providers
- *Accommodation* – how resources are organized in regard to needed services, and how patients can utilize arrangements
- *Affordability* – patients' abilities to pay
- *Availability* – the relationship between patient requirements and service capacity.

Access to health care may differ in a variety of ways. Ideally, it should be effective as well as efficient, but other factors exist concerning individual patient needs, methods of accessing health care, and the actual compatibility of services to match consumers' needs. This may be broken down as follows:

- *Effective and efficient access to health outcomes* – relates to immunization, preventive services, and quality of care
- *Equitable or inequitable access* – equitable access concerns patient's own needs, or their evaluated needs as determined by health professionals; inequitable access is related to services distributed according to income or insurance status

- *Potential access* – characteristics of the health care system such as the physician–population ratio, managed care options, and health insurance coverage; also, enabling characteristics such as income or public transportation
- *Realized access* – type, size, and purpose of health care services.

Access to health care can be measured individually, as part of health plans, and in relation to how it may be delivered. In general, people of lower socioeconomic classes, those with lower levels of education, and those who work in potentially hazardous jobs have less access.

Focus on "cost versus care"

According to the CDC, the percentage of persons who failed to obtain needed medical care due to cost is 5.3%. The percentage of persons with a usual place to go for medical care is 87.9%.
Sources: www.cdc.gov/nchs/data/nhis/earlyrelease/earlyrelease201506_03.
pdf; www.cdc.gov/nchs/fastats/access-to-health-care.htm.

Habits and social conditions

Many different behavioral habits may be risk factors for disease and illness. The leading cause of preventable disease and death in the United States is smoking, which greatly increases the risk of heart and lung disease as well as stroke. Other poor habits include substance abuse; lack of physical exercise; diets that are high in fats, sugars, or salt; unsafe sex practices; and irresponsible driving habits. According to the National Center for Health Statistics, risk factors that are linked to disease are ranked as follows:

- Being overweight or obese – (68.5% of the population) – most commonly results in hypertension, diabetes, heart disease, high cholesterol, cancer
- Excessive alcohol use – (51.8%) – most commonly results in cirrhosis, pancreatitis, hypertension, osteoporosis, brain degeneration
- Hypertension – (31.9%) – most commonly results in heart attack, stroke, heart failure, aneurysms, peripheral artery disease
- Cigarette smoking – (19%) – most commonly results in cancer, respiratory disease, cardiovascular disease, stroke, hypertension
- High serum cholesterol – (13.6%) – most commonly causes angina, coronary artery disease, atherosclerosis, heart attack, stroke
- Marijuana use – (6.9%) – respiratory disease, cancer, psychotic conditions such as schizophrenia, cognitive problems, infertility
- Cocaine use – (2.6%) – cardiovascular disease, hypertension, respiratory disease, stroke, seizures.
  (*Sources:* www.cdc.gov/nchs/data/hus/2012/068.pdf; www.samhsa.gov/atod; http://healthyamericans.org/states/states.php?measure=hyper&sort=data; www.cdc.gov/tobacco/campaign/tips/resources/data/cigarette-smoking-in-united-states.html; wwwn.cdc.gov/nchs/nhanes/bibliography/results.aspx?catid=18&name=total cholesterol; www.cdc.gov/nchs/fastats/drug-use-illegal.htm; www.drugabuse.gov/drugs-abuse/cocaine.)

Social conditions and behavioral factors affect health care costs, as do many chronic conditions (primarily, hypertension, heart disease, diabetes, asthma, and arthritis). Many chronic diseases are related to ethnic, cultural, and behavioral factors. Those who abuse drugs or alcohol, are malnourished, or are in overall poor health are highly susceptible. According to the CDC, in 2013 there were nearly 9,600 reported tuberculosis cases in the United States, which is three out of every 100,000 people.

The significant social factor here is that people near the poverty level often need more health care services, yet cannot pay for them. These people regularly require emergency department treatment, and these facilities are not reimbursed. If preventive care had been available, these outcomes may not have occurred. Maintaining a healthy lifestyle is the key to good health. Nearly 95% of all chronic diseases or serious illnesses and body injuries are preventable. Health education and the changing of harmful habits may be the most important factor that will reduce the cost of health care.

As America becomes older, larger, and has more ethnic diversity, the ability of our health care system to meet the needs of the country is under continual change. Population shifts affect how the workforce is made up, affecting how many new health care professionals will join the workforce and where they will be located. Future immigration will also affect this. The mix of cultures will cause language and other barriers to further complicate health care delivery. Illegal immigrants also put more strain upon an already weakened health care system.

Social factors also include the breakdown of the family unit, single mothers, violence, various forms of abuse, and living alone. For single mothers, many of whom are near the poverty level, there is a lack of access to preventive measures such as immunizations and prenatal care. Also, many families and children are homeless. Violence in society causes emergency and other health care services to be used, often without reimbursement.

Substance abuse may lead to diseases as well as increased violence. Substance abusers may also be unable to care for their families or themselves. *Domestic violence* is abuse that happens in personal relationships and affects people from all groups, of all ages. Its likelihood is increased when substance abuse is present. When abuse of a spouse or child occurs, there may be a need for health and protective services as well as emergency services. For Americans who live alone, they may develop problems because of lack of emotional support, and require outside assistance if they are injured or become ill.

Maintaining the quality of care

The quality of health care concerns the degree to which desired health outcomes occur that follow the latest professional knowledge available. Quality performance may range from excellent to unacceptable. It focuses on health care delivery system services, not behaviors by individuals. Cost controls have been set up by federal, state, and local governments to reduce expenses while keeping quality at an acceptable level. Quality of care is discussed in Chapter 5 in greater detail.

Health issues and the public

Public health programs focus on providing optimum health for society through teaching and education, and utilize the combined efforts of epidemiologists, hygienists, food and drug inspectors, toxicologists, and other professionals. Public health issues include global pandemics such as influenza H1N1 (*swine flu*), influenza H5N1 (*bird flu*), and the Ebola virus. Between 151,700 and 575,400 people worldwide have died as a result of H1N1, while the H5N1 virus has been linked to just over 400 deaths worldwide thus far. Ebola has killed approximately 5,200 people worldwide. About 75% of new human diseases are caused by microbes originating in animals, including the previously mentioned diseases, as well as HIV/AIDS, influenza H7N9, Severe Acute Respiratory Syndrome (SARS), and Middle East Respiratory Syndrome-Coronavirus (MERS-CoV). Over the coming decades, population growth and increased interactions between animals, humans, and the environment are expected to increase the amount of new disease threats.

Unfortunately, the U.S. health care system is very slow to respond to outbreaks. Essential research into immunizations and treatments also occurs very slowly. Additional public health issues of today include the following:

● High infant mortality rates in the United States – linked to poverty, drug abuse, and lack of prenatal care; according to the CDC, just under six out of every 1,000 babies die at birth or during the first year of life
● Antibiotic resistance (globally) – pathogenic bacteria become modified, resulting in the drug use against them to be less effective.

Focus on the "MERS" vaccine

A new vaccine has begun to be effective against Middle East Respiratory Syndrome (MERS) in animals such as monkeys, mice, and camels. An international team of researchers is testing the vaccine for its effectiveness in humans.

Individual responsibility for health

Health conditions are often linked to poor lifestyle choices. As mentioned previously, risky habits and poor social conditions influence health outcomes. Each individual is responsible for his or her own health, and this is based on balanced choices concerning diet, alcohol use, exercise, caffeine use, sleep habits, proper immunizations, the wearing of seat belts in automobiles, and stress management. Even with today's advancements in medicine and health care, certain serious conditions may not be able to be cured or even treated. However, almost everyone can make positive choices in lifestyle that will improve general health.

According to the United States Library of Medicine, lifestyle choices play major roles in the majority of illnesses occurring in industrialized nations. Of the ten leading factors that contribute to disease, six are lifestyle related: hypertension, unsafe sex practices, alcohol use, tobacco use, high cholesterol, and obesity. For example, alcoholism in the United States is linked to annual health care costs of $22.5 billion. Obesity accounts for more than $75 billion.

Preventive medicine

Preventive medicine is a unique medical specialty that is recognized by the American Board of Medical Specialties. According to the American College of Preventive Medicine, it focuses on the health of individuals, communities, and defined populations. Preventive medicine is aimed at protecting, promoting, and maintaining health and well-being, as well as preventing disease, disability, and death. It includes three different levels, as follows:

- *Primary level* – in which the patient is at risk for a disease but is not yet affected. This identifies behavioral, environmental, genetic, and other factors that increase the patient's chance of contracting the disease. Risk factors such as smoking can be changed, while genetic factors cannot. The prepathogenesis period requires good health promotion in order to achieve primary disease prevention (health education, immunization, correction of poor habits).
- *Secondary level* – in which risk factors combine to produce a disease. It is usually not manifest, and clinically undetectable, until specific pathologic changes occur. An example of a factor that may suggest disease development is blood in the stool, a warning sign of colorectal cancer. During a disease's pathogenesis, secondary prevention may be achieved by early diagnosis and prompt treatment.
- *Tertiary level* – in which disease signs and symptoms appear. The *clinical horizon* is the point at which a particular condition can be scientifically detected. The majority of preventive health care focuses on this level. There must be disability limitation and rehabilitation, including the maximizing of remaining functional capacity. This level is the most expensive, in terms of health care.

The prevention of each succeeding level is therapeutically important, since pathologic changes may become fixed and irreversible at each level. In recent years, serious attention has been paid to refocusing health care toward health promotion and disease prevention.

Health insurance has traditionally focused on intervention after a disease is diagnosed, rather than on preventive medicine. This has resulted in the United States spending the majority of its health care expenditures on the treatment of diseases that could have been prevented. Today, with further focus on prevention of disease, successes are occurring in many areas, including prevention of childhood obesity, diabetes, cholesterol education, early cancer detection, and smoking cessation.

In the 1980s and 1990s, the lack of funding for preventive medicine resulted, in part, in increases in cases of AIDS, tuberculosis, measles, and premature births. Preventive medicine must increase in application in order to fulfill the needs of the public. The U.S. health care system can only benefit from the increased use of preventive medicine. Goals of preventive medicine should include:

- Prevention of drug abuse and excessive alcohol use
- Becoming tobacco-free
- Healthy eating
- Avoiding injuries by violence-free living
- Mental and emotional health
- Reproductive and sexual health.

The Affordable Care Act established a National Prevention, Health Promotion and Public Health Council to coordinate a *National Prevention Strategy*. This continued on from programs such as *Healthy People 2020* in the support of public health goals.

> ## You should remember
>
> The four things you can do immediately that are the basis of preventive medicine include: avoiding smoking or use of other tobacco products, and drinking only in moderation (preferably red wine); eating a proper, balanced diet; exercising at least three days per week; and seeing your doctor regularly for check-ups.

Healthy people 2020

Healthy People 2020 is the latest update of the Healthy People program, part of the Office of Disease Prevention and Health Promotion. It provides science-based, ten-year national objectives designed to improve the health of all American people. Since 2000, this program has established goals and monitored progress in order to encourage collaboration between communities, empower individuals regarding informed health decisions, and to measure the impact of prevention activities.

Healthy People 2020 has four primary goals:

- To *attain high-quality, longer lives* – free of preventable disease, disability, injury, and premature death
- To *achieve health equality* – eliminating disparities and improving the health of all groups of people
- To *create healthy social and physical environments* – promoting good health for all
- To *promote quality of life* – including healthy development and behaviors across all stages of life.

Healthy People 2020 has four health measures that serve as indicators of its successful progress: general health status, health-related quality of life and well-being, determinants of health, and disparities. Moving on from the previous *Healthy People 2010*, the new initiative added the following topic areas:

- Adolescent health
- Blood disorders and blood safety
- Dementias
- Early and middle childhood
- Genomics
- Global health
- Health-related quality of life and well-being
- Health care-associated infections
- Lesbian, gay, bisexual, and transgender health
- Older adults
- Preparedness
- Sleep health
- Social determinants of health.

Healthy People 2020 also developed a new electronic application called *My Healthy People* to track progress.

CASE STUDY

The complexity of health care is present even in the well-intentioned Affordable Care Act. There are many documented examples of individuals whose health care coverage was more affordable prior to the Act's implementation. Here are two examples. A healthy young male aged 29 was paying $121 per month prior to the Act. This changed to $230 per month afterwards. One of the owners of the facility in which the young man worked, a 62-year-old, was paying $798 per month, but is now paying $1,300 a month. The complexity issue here involves the wording of the Act, which said it would "increase access to affordable care ... and make care more affordable." In these examples, neither goal was achieved.

1 Did the *access* to health care change in these examples as a result of the Affordable Care Act?
2 Since both individuals' coverage increased dramatically, can you explain whether it could have been less expensive for them to remain uninsured and just pay the fee (as part of their tax returns) imposed by the Affordable Care Act?
3 Do you think that, for the younger man in the examples, the odds might be better if he did remain uninsured and just paid out-of-pocket for any health care services he needed, at the time they were needed?

Chapter highlights

This section answers the Objectives found at the beginning of the chapter.

1 **Discuss factors concerning older people that affect the health care industry.**

- As the population ages, increased amounts of money are spent on health care. Older individuals statistically require more health care. For example, in the United States, in adults over age 80, three out of four people have more than one chronic disease. Out of those between ages 65 and 80, two out of three have more than one chronic disease.

2 **Explain ambulatory centers and rehabilitation hospitals.**

- Ambulatory centers offer health care or acute care services on an outpatient basis that do not require overnight hospital stays. Same-day surgeries may be performed in *ambulatory surgical units* or *ambulatory surgical centers*. Ambulatory care includes physician or dentist offices, outpatient centers, medical and diagnostic laboratories, home health care services, and others.
- Rehabilitation hospitals specialize in providing restorative services to rehabilitate chronically ill and disabled individuals to their maximum level of functioning after recent disability due to illness or accidents. Physical, occupational, speech, and audiology services are offered.

3 **Discuss hospice.**

- Hospice serves dying individuals, including medical, spiritual, legal, financial, and family-support services. Care occurs in special facilities or in patients' homes. Most patients are those with cancer. Hospice provides palliative care and emphasizes pain management. It does not focus on prolonging life, but provides patients with the best end-of-life care possible.

4 **Describe the effects of the aging population.**

- Advances in health care have contributed to Americans living longer, and the elderly can expect to spend more years in declining health, needing more medical care than other age groups. There is an increase in chronic and degenerative diseases. Hearing and visual impairments are more common. Elderly people are at higher risk for dementia, hip fractures, and stroke. People over age 85 are the fastest-growing age group. Since the *baby boom generation* is reaching age 65, the elderly will make up more than 26% of the population within two decades. There is now an unbalanced financial situation, pulling resources away from the working population, which is shrinking.

5 **Classify the various types of hospitals.**

- General hospitals provide general, specialized medicine and surgery, and also obstetrics. Psychiatric hospitals treat patients affected with mental illnesses, in inpatient and outpatient capacities. Rehabilitation hospitals provide restorative services for chronically ill and disabled individuals. Teaching hospitals have approved residency programs for physicians.

6 **Discuss how habits and behaviors may affect health care.**

- Many habits and behaviors are risk factors for disease and illness. The leading cause of preventable disease and death in the United States is smoking, which increases risks of heart and lung disease as well as stroke. Other risks include substance abuse, lack of physical exercise, excessive alcohol use, unmanaged hypertension or cholesterol levels, poor diets, illegal drugs, unsafe sex, and irresponsible driving. Maintaining a healthy lifestyle is the key to good health. Nearly 95% of all chronic diseases or serious illnesses and body injuries are preventable.

7 **List public health issues of today.**

- Global pandemics – such as influenza H1N1 (swine flu), influenza H5N1 (bird flu), Ebola
- Other diseases originating in animals – HIV/AIDS, influenza H7N9, SARS, and MERS-CoV
- High infant mortality rates in the United States
- Antibiotic resistance (globally).

8 **Discuss the three levels of preventive medicine.**

- *Primary level* – the patient is at risk for diseases, but not yet affected. This identifies behavioral, environmental, genetic, and other factors that increase the chance of contracting the disease.
- *Secondary level* – risk factors combine to produce a disease. It is usually not manifest, and clinically undetectable, until specific pathologic changes occur.
- *Third level* – disease signs and symptoms appear. The *clinical horizon* is when a particular condition can be scientifically detected.

Summary

The complexity of health care in the United States today has resulted from a wide variety of individuals, organizations, and factors including tremendous growth, the aging population, and increased medical costs. Health care is the largest service industry in the country. Advances in technology, gene therapies, and drug therapies have propelled health care to its greatest advancements throughout history. Medicine has become more highly specialized, and with this specialization, costs have risen dramatically. Most Americans who lack health insurance say that cost is the primary factor. As baby boomers become elderly, this large amount of people will require more health care services than ever before, further complicating the U.S. health care system.

Review questions

1 What is the primary factor for health care costs?
2 What are the most common causes of chronic and degenerative disease in elderly people?
3 What is the largest share of health care expenditures in the United States?
4 What are the less common types of hospitals in the United States?
5 What is the advantage of ambulatory care?
6 List five examples of home health care facilities.
7 What is holistic health care?
8 List three examples of mental disorders that are biological in nature.
9 What types of patient are admitted to hospice, and what type of service are provided to them?
10 What are the five basic dimensions regarding access to health care?

Bibliography

Administration for Community Living. 2016. Administration on Aging (AoA) – Aging Statistics. Available at: https://aoa.acl.gov/aging_statistics/index.aspx. Washington, D.C.: U.S. Department of Health and Human Services.

All About Traumatic Brain Injury. 2016. Traumatic Brain Injury Treatment Centers – Types of Traumatic Brain Injury Treatment Centers. Available at: www.allabouttbi.com/centers. Birmingham: U.S. National Institute on Disability and Rehabilitation Research.

American Hospital Association. 2016. Fast Facts on US Hospitals – AHA Hospital Statistics – Fast Facts 2017. Available at: www.aha.org/research/rc/stat-studies/fast-facts.shtml. Chicago: American Hospital Associaiton.

Barr, P. 2013. Massachusetts trying to force costs lower. *Hospitals & Health Networks* 87, no. 7: 24.

Bielaszka-DuVernay, C. 2011. Vermont's blueprint for medical homes, community health teams, and better health at lower cost. *Health Affairs* 30, no. 3: 383–386.

Brabender, M. 2016. The Entire Health Care Dollar – Our Approach. Available at: www.mcgohanbrabender.com/our-approach/the-entire-health-care-dollar. Dublin, Ohio: McGohan Brabender.

Caudill, T., et al. 2011. Health care reform and primary care: Training physicians for tomorrow's challenges. *Academic Medicine* 86, no. 2: 158–160.

CDC, National Center for Injury Prevention and Control, Division of Unintentional Injury Prevention. 2016. Rates of TBI-related Emergency Department Visits, Hospitalizations, and Deaths – United States, 2001–2010. Available at: www.cdc.gov/traumaticbraininjury/data/rates.html. Atlanta: U.S. Department of Health and Human Services.

CDC. 2012. Healthy Weight, Overweight, and Obesity Among Adults Aged 20 and Over, by Selected Characterstics: United States, Selected Years 1960–1962 through 2009–2012. Available at: www.cdc.gov/nchs/data/hus/2012/068.pdf. Atlanta: U.S. Department of Health and Human Services.

CDC. 2014. Failure To Obtain Needed Medical Care – Early Release of Selected Estimates Based on Data From the National Health Interview Survey, 2014. Available at: www.cdc.gov/nchs/data/nhis/earlyrelease/earlyrelease201506_03.pdf. Atlanta: U.S. Department of Health and Human Services.

CDC. 2016. Access to Health Care – Data are for the U.S. Available at: www.cdc.gov/nchs/fastats/access-to-health-care.htm. Atlanta: U.S. Department of Health and Human Services.

CDC. 2016. Critical Issue Briefs on Healthy Aging. Available at: www.cdc.gov/nccdphp/publications/aag/pdf/healthy_aging.pdf. Atlanta: U.S. Department of Health and Human Services.

CDC. 2016. Illegal Drug Use – Data are for the U.S. Available at: www.cdc.gov/nchs/fastats/drug-use-illegal.htm. Atlanta: U.S. Department of Health and Human Services.

CDC. 2016. Know The Facts About High Cholesterol. Available at: wwwn.cdc.gov/nchs/nhanes/bibliography/results.aspx?catid=18&name=total cholesterol. Atlanta: U.S. Department of Health and Human Services.

CDC. 2016. Mental Health – Data are for the U.S. Available at: www.cdc.gov/nchs/fastats/mental-health.htm. Atlanta: U.S. Department of Health and Human Services.

CDC. 2016. Suicide and Self-Inflicted Injury – Data are for the U.S. Available at: www.cdc.gov/nchs/fastats/suicide.htm. Atlanta: U.S. Department of Health and Human Services.

CDC. 2016. Tips From Former Smokers – Burder of Tobacco Use in the U.S. Available at: www.cdc.gov/tobacco/campaign/tips/resources/data/cigarette-smoking-in-united-states.html. Atlanta: U.S. Department of Health and Human Services.

Center Forward. 2012. Medicare, Medicaid, and the Military: Update. Available at: www.center-forward.org/wp-content/uploads/2012/04/Medicare-Medicaid-and-the-Military-04-12-update-2.pdf. Washington, D.C.: Center Forward 2016.

Centers for Medicare and Medicaid Services. 2014. National Health Expenditures Continued Slow Growth in 2013. Available at: www.cms.gov/Newsroom/MediaReleaseDatabase/Press-releases/2014-Press-releases-items/2014-12-03-2.html. Baltimore: U.S. Centers for Medicare and Medicaid Services.

Chatterjee, P. 2011. Progress patchy on health-worker crisis. *Lancet* 377, no. 9764: 456.

CMS.gov. 2016. Physician Fee Schedule – CY2017 Physician Fee Schedule Final Rule. Available at: www.cms.gov/Medicare/Medicare-Fee-for-Service-Payment/PhysicianFeeSched/index.html?redirect=/physicianfeesched. Baltimore: U.S. Centers for Medicare and Medicaid Services.

Congressional Budget Office (CBO). 2012. *The Budget and Economic Outlook: Fiscal Years 2012 to 2022*. Washington, D.C.: CBO.

Cunningham, P.J. 2011. *State Variation in Primary Care Physician Supply: Implications for Health Reform Medicaid Expansions*. Research Brief No. 19. Washington, D.C.: Center for Studying Health System Change.

Department for Professional Employees AFL-CIO. 2016. The U.S. Health Care System: An

International Perspective. Available at: http://dpeaflcio.org/programs-publications/issue-fact-sheets/the-u-s-health-care-system-an-international-perspective/. Washington, D.C.: Department for Professional Employees, AFL-CIO.

Fan, J.X., Sharpe, D.L., and Hong, G.-S.. 2003. Health Care and Prescription Drug Spending by Seniors. Available at: www.bls.gov/opub/mlr/2003/03/art3full.pdf. Washington, D.C.: U.S. Bureau of Labor Statistics.

Forbes. 2016. The 15 Highest-Paying Medical Specialties. Available at: www.forbes.com/pictures/fjle45mdhk/no-1-cardiology-invasive/#1ab539567182. Jersey City: Forbes Media LLC.

Gaynor, M. and Anderson, G.F. 1991. Hospital Costs and the Cost of Empty Hospital Beds. Available at: www.nber.org/papers/w3872. Cambridge, Massachusetts: National Bureau of Economic Research.

Govette, J. 2013. Health Care Technology Innovations – 2013 Infographics. Available at: http://getreferralmd.com/2013/11/health-caretechnology-innovations-2013-infographic. San Francisco: ReferralMD.

Health Care Service Corporation. 2016. Economics of Health Care – Understanding Health Care Cost Drivers. Available at: www.hcsc.com/pdf/economics_health_care2.pdf. Chicago: Health Care Service Corporation.

Health Indicators Warehouse. 2016. Serious Psychological Distress: Adults (Percent) – Data Source: NHIS (CDC/NCHS) Percent of Adults 18 Years of Age and Over Who Have Experienced Serious Psychological Distress in the Past 30 Days. Available at: www.healthindicators.gov/indicators/Serious-psychological-distress-adults-percent_50055/profile/classicdata. Hyattsville: National Center for Health Statistics.

HealthyPeople.gov. 2016. HealthyPeople.gov – Healthy People 2020. Available at: www.healthypeople.gov. Washington, D.C.: U.S. Department of Health and Human Services.

HealthyPeople2020. 2016. About Healthy People – Introducing Healthy People 2020. Available at: www.healthypeople.gov/2020/about-healthy-people. Washington, D.C.: U.S. Department of Health and Human Services.

Kominski, G.F. 2013. *Changing the U.S. Health Care System: Key Issues in Health Services Policy and Management, 4th Edition*. San Francisco: Jossey-Bass. Print.

Lagomarsino, G., et al. 2012. Moving towards universal health coverage: Health insurance reforms in nine developing countries in Africa and Asia. *Lancet* 380, no. 9845: 933–943.

Mosquera, M. 2014. 5 Challenges Facing Health Systems – Pressures Won't Subside Until More Shift to Value-Based Payments. Available at: www.healthcarefinancenews.com/news/5-challenges-facing-health-systems. New Gloucester: HIMSS Media.

National Association for Home Care and Hospice. 2016. Home Care and Hospice Statistics. Available at: www.nahc.org/assets/1/7/10HC-stats.pdf. Washington, D.C.: National Association for Home Care and Hospice.

National Institute on Drug Abuse. 2011. Treatment Statistics – Drug Facts. Available at: www.drugabuse.gov/publications/drugfacts/treatment-statistics. Bethesda: National Institute on Drug Abuse.

National Institute on Drug Abuse. 2016. Cocaine – Brief Description – Statistics and Trends. Available at: www.drugabuse.gov/drugs-abuse/cocaine. Bethesda: National Institute on Drug Abuse.

Nickols, S. 2013. Real Life Examples of the Affordable Care Act. Available at: www.ahifw.com/real-life-examples-of-the-affordable-care-act. Fort Wayne: Health Market Group.

Owcharenko, N.. 2016. 2016: What's Next for Obamacare?. Available at: www.heritage.org/research/projects/impact-of-obamacare. Washington, D.C.: The Heritage Foundation.

Parente, S.T., and Feldman, R. 2013. Microsimulation of private health insurance and Medicaid take-up following the U.S. Supreme Court decision upholding the Affordable Care Act. *Health Services Research* 48, no. 2 Pt 2: 826–849.

Piper, K.. 2016. Hospitalizations for Mental Health and Substance Abuse Disorders: Costs,

Length of Stay, Patient Mix, and Payor Mix. Available at: http://piperreport.com/blog/2011/06/25/hospitalizations-for-mental-health-and-substance-abuse-disorders-costs-length-of-stay-patient-mix-and-payor-mix/. Washington, D.C.: Health Results Group, LLC.

Rodin, J., and de Ferranti, D. 2012. Universal health coverage: The third global health transition? *Lancet* 380, no. 9845: 861–862.

Roper St. Francis. 2016. Rehabilitation Services. Available at: www.rsfh.com/rehab-hospital/statistics. Charleston: Roper St. Francis Hospitals.

Sachs, J.D. 2012. Achieving universal health coverage in low-income settings. *Lancet* 380, no. 9845: 944–947.

Shi, L., and Singh, D.A. 2015. *Delivering Health Care in America: A Systems Approach, 6th Edition*. Burlington: Jones & Bartlett Learning. Print.

Steiner, J.E., Jr. 2013. *Problems in Health Care Law: Challenges for the 21st Century, 10th Edition*. Burlington: Jones & Bartlett Learning. Print.

Substance Abuse and Mental Health Services Administration. 2014. Alcohol, Tobacco, and Other Drugs – The misuse and abuse of alcohol, over-the-counter medications, illicit drugs, and tobacco affect the health and well-being of millions of Americans. Available at: www.samhsa.gov/atod. Rockville: Substance Abuse and Mental Health Services Administration.

Sultz, H.A., and Young, K.M. 2010. *Health Care USA: Understanding Its Organization and Delivery, 7th Edition*. Burlington: Jones & Bartlett Learning. Print.

TraumaticBrainInjury.com. 2016. Treatment Centers – Acute Hospitals – Rehabilitation Units and Hospitals. Available at: www.traumaticbraininjury.com/injury-resources/treatment-center. Philadelphia: TraumaticBrainInjury.com, LLC.

Trust for America's Health. 2009. State Data – Hypertension Rates, % Adults (2005–09 average). Available at: http://healthy americans.org/states/states.php?measure=hyper&sort=data. Washington, D.C.: Trust for America's Health.

Tzafrir Nachmani. 2015. Acupuncture Treatment of Substance-Induced Psychosis, Addiction and Pain: A Review with Case Study. Available at: www.sciencedirect.com/science/article/pii/s2095754816000302. Amsterdam: Elsevier B.V.

U.S. Bureau of Labor Statistics. 2006–2007. High Growth Industry Profile Health Care. Available at: www.doleta.gov/brg/indprof/healthcare_profile.cfm. Washington, D.C.: U.S. Department of Labor.

Wager, K.A., Lee, F.W., and Glaser, J.P. 2013. *Health Care Information Systems: A Practical Approach for Management, 3rd Edition*. San Francisco: Jossey-Bass. Print.

Chapter 2

The Patient Protection and Affordable Care Act

Objectives

After study of the chapter, readers should be able to:

1 Explain the primary reasons that influenced passage of the Patient Protection and Affordable Care Act (PPACA).
2 Describe how the PPACA impacted insurance coverage and access to care.
3 List examples of legal challenges to the PPACA.
4 Describe how the PPACA was modified because of Supreme Court decisions regarding contraceptive coverage and Medicaid expansion.
5 Discuss the minimum essential coverage requirements of the PPACA.
6 Explain the costs of premiums and implementation related to the PPACA.
7 Compare differences between insurance coverage in states that have or have not expanded Medicaid.
8 Which ethnic group is most likely to be uninsured in the United States, and why are some people in this group not eligible for coverage?
9 Explain the advantages of the PPACA during its first enrollment period.
10 Summarize the disadvantages of the PPACA.

Overview

The reform of the U.S. health care system has been a subject of contention for many years. The knowledge of the need for health care reform was based on government monitoring of statistics, which is a process that continues now that the Patient Protection and Affordable Care Act (PPACA) has been passed. This Act was the largest change to the U.S. health care system since the development of Medicare and Medicaid. The government continues to monitor the effects this Act is having upon the populace in order to determine whether the needs of the people are being met. In previous years, it became apparent that there were millions of Americans who were uninsured, with concerns about rising health care costs at the core of the problem.

National Health Expenditure

There are various indicators of health care costs in the United States. The National Health Expenditure (NHE) is one, which began in 1960. It was higher between the years 1960 and 2010, when the Affordable Care Act was passed by Congress (Figure 2.1). Between 2010 and 2014, the NHE reduced to an average annual rate of only 3.8%. In 2014, the Congressional Budget Office stated that the NHE would be even lower during 2014 to 2019. Projections for expenses related to Medicare, Medicaid, and private insurance were billions of dollars lower than the projections made previously, back in 2010.

The slowing of the NHE is also related to the 2007 recession, and to hospital prices reducing to a low of 2% in 2013. A slowed NHE is also related to:

- Increased cost sharing with higher deductibles and co-payments for physician visits and hospitalizations
- Smaller networks in private insurance plans
- Reduced usage of magnetic resonance imaging (MRI), computed tomography (CT) scans, and other expensive medical technology
- Increased use of low-cost generic drugs
- The changing of coverage from employer programs to lower-cost Medicaid programs
- Reduced Medicare reimbursement for providers
- Quality improvement programs such as Accountable Care Organizations and the Hospital Readmissions Reduction Program.

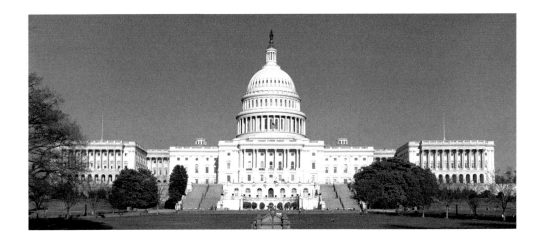

Figure 2.1 The Capitol building, where Congress is held.

Health care costs are also influenced by uncompensated care, which is non-reimbursed, charity care for people who have little or no insurance.

Focus on uncompensated care

It is estimated that in 2014, uncompensated care costs were lowered by $5.7 billion. Of this amount, $4.2 billion came from the Medicaid expansion states and $1.5 billion came from the non-expansion states.

Sources: http://kff.org/medicaid/press-release/uncompensated-hospital-care-fell-by-6-billion-nationally-in-2014-primarily-in-medicaid-expansion-states-however-many-hospitals-worry-about-future-changes-in-medicaid-supplemental-payments/; www.hcentive.com/states-without-medicaid-expansion-face-a-new-challenge-huge-unpaid-hospital-bills/.

Since newly insured people could obtain health care from primary providers, costs were much lower than when going to an emergency department for treatment. This meant fewer emergency department visits and lower uncompensated hospital admissions. In 2013, estimated costs for each person without insurance was $1,005, leading to a total of $49 billion for all uncompensated health care in the country.

Health care reform

The Patient Protection and Affordable Care Act was signed into law by President Barack Obama at the White House in 2010 (Figure 2.2). The goal of this Act was to improve health care accessibility and reduce costs for all Americans. Thus far, it has succeeded in some areas and failed in others, though we do not know what the future will bring. With the election of Donald Trump as President Obama's successor, the Affordable Care Act's future is unknown. President Trump promised during his campaign to repeal and replace the Act.

Currently, the Act requires most citizens and legal residents to have health insurance or pay a tax penalty. Those lacking coverage pay a tax penalty of the greater of $695 annually up to a maximum of $2,085 per family, or 2.5% of household income. The penalty will increase annually via cost-of-living adjustments. Exemptions will be granted for financial hardship, American Indians, religious objections, people without coverage for less than three months, incarcerated individuals, undocumented immigrants, people for whom the lowest-cost plan option exceeds 8% of income, and people with incomes below the current year's tax filing threshold.

The Act also created state-based health exchanges that offered coverage to individuals and families, created separate exchanges to allow small businesses to purchase coverage, required employers to pay penalties for employees receiving tax credits through an exchange, imposed new health plan regulations, and expanded Medicaid coverage to 133% of the Federal Poverty Level (FPL). The Act also requires employers with 50 or more full-time employees to offer health coverage, requires states to maintain current income eligibility levels for children in Medicaid and the Children's Health Insurance Program (CHIP), and offers federal premium credits and subsidies. Eligibility for premium credits and cost-sharing subsidies is limited through the exchanges to U.S. citizens and legal immigrants who meet income limits. Refundable and advanceable premium credits are provided to eligible individuals and families with

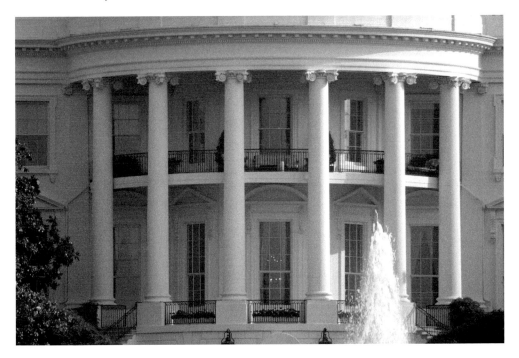

Figure 2.2 The White House.

incomes between 133% and 400% of the FPL to purchase health insurance through the exchanges. Federal premium or cost-sharing subsidies cannot be used to cover abortions if coverage extends beyond saving the life of the mother, or in cases of rape or incest.

Employers with more than 50 employees that offer coverage, but have at least one full-time employee receiving a premium tax credit, must pay $3,000 for each employee receiving the credit, or $2,000 for each full-time employee – whichever is less. Employers with 50 or fewer employees are exempted from these penalties. Small employers with no more than 25 employees and average annual wages of less than $50,000 that purchase health insurance for their employees receive tax credits of between 35% and 50%, based on employer contributions.

Employers who offer coverage to their employees must provide a free choice voucher to those with incomes less than 400% of the FPL, whose share of the premium is more than 8% but less than 9.8% of their income, and who choose to enroll in a plan in the Exchange. Employers offering free choice vouchers are not penalized because of employees receiving premium credits in the Exchange. Employers with more than 200 employees are required to enroll their employees into health insurance plans offered by the employer, but employees may opt out of coverage. The Act also imposes new taxes and tax rates as well as annual fees for a variety of health care-related businesses. The benefits and problem areas of the Affordable Care Act are discussed in detail in this chapter.

Implementation of the PPACA

The PPACA was passed in March 2010, with three main goals. These were to decrease the amount of uninsured Americans, to increase qualities and efficiencies of health care, and to slow the speed of the increase in costs of health care. In 2010, the average cost of a single American's health care was $8,402. Total costs were around $2.6 trillion, which was nearly 18% of the gross domestic product or *GDP*. This amount had increased by 7.2% from the amount it cost in 1970.

The Act was then modified by the *Health Care and Education Reconciliation Act of 2010*. Today, the PPACA and the HCERA are collectively referred to as the Affordable Care Act (ACA). The Act requires implementation through a large number of different agencies. These include the federal and state governments, private insurance companies and health care providers, hospitals, and outpatient clinics.

The ACA established the Hospital Readmissions Reduction Program, which included incentives for health care providers to improve health care quality and efficiency. Since one out of every five Medicare patients who received hospital care was then readmitted within 30 days of discharge, the result was an estimated cost of $26 million. The money received by hospitals from Medicare reimbursement was based on the readmission rate, which focuses on conditions such as heart attack, heart failure, and pneumonia. For these conditions, Medicare determined whether the hospital in question meets criteria for readmission based on a specific formula that is adjusted for wages and a base amount paid per *Diagnosis-Related Group* (which means the specific condition). If not meeting readmission requirements, reimbursements from Medicare were reduced for hospital admissions for any conditions, not just heart attack, heart failure, or pneumonia.

This resulted in losses in reimbursement between 1% and 3% of the usual reimbursement rate. Between 2010 and 2013, hospital readmission rates decreased, but then, between 2014 and 2015, a record amount of hospitals received reduced payments for Medicare patients. Today, penalties for excessive hospital readmissions are anticipated to save a substantial amount of money.

In 2013, online enrollment problems began to multiply when HealthCare.gov and the state-based marketplaces could not handle the demand of people trying to sign up for health care. The websites also could not be accessed in many cases. Most of the problems came from the information technology used in creating the websites. Applications for health care could not be verified quickly, eligibility could not always be determined, and incorrect or incomplete information provided by the enrollees complicated things further. Though individuals could still enroll over the telephone or by mail, use of the Internet was much more popular, and these problems could have been avoided by better design.

The Internet marketplaces were connected by the federal Data Services Hub to Medicaid, CHIP, and other federal data sources such as Homeland Security, the Internal Revenue Service (IRS), and the Social Security Administration. The plan was to use these connections to easily verify citizenship status, immigration status, and income in order to process health care applications as quickly as possible. However, additional breakdowns occurred in this system, complicating matters.

Though President Obama had promised the American people that they would be able to keep the insurance plans they had prior to the ACA being established, this was not the case. In reality, once the ACA came into being, many insurance plans were no longer available. Of all the aspects of the Act, the two most unpopular were the requirement for individuals without employee-covered insurance to have to purchase insurance through the marketplace, and for the states to have to expand Medicaid.

> ### You should remember
>
> Costs associated with health care rise every year. This continues to be true even after the passage of the Affordable Care Act. Rates are growing more slowly, but they are still increasing.

Legal challenges to the Act

In 2011, a lawsuit was filed in Federal District Court to challenge the constitutionality of two items: the individual mandate requiring people to have health insurance or be fined, and the Medicaid expansion in every state. The National Federation of Independent Business filed the lawsuit, in conjunction with 26 states and several individuals. It was filed as *National Federation of Independent Business v. Sebelius*. The result was the Federal District Court upholding the Medicaid expansion but not the individual mandate. The case was later taken to the U.S. Supreme Court (Figure 2.3) in 2012, where the individual mandate was upheld, but the Medicaid expansion was ruled as being in violation of the U.S. Constitution.

Regarding the Employer Shared Responsibility Payment, the IRS's ruling was challenged in federal courts because the wording in the ACA stated that the marketplace had to be established by the states. Lawsuits argued about this language and the authority of the IRS to grant premium subsidies for people who purchased plans through HealthCare.gov. The

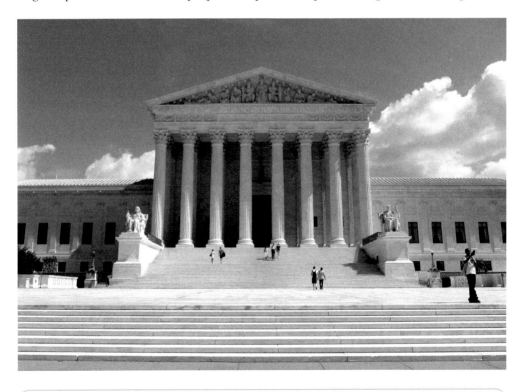

Figure 2.3 The U.S. Supreme Court.

case eventually reached the Supreme Court, where, in 2015, the court ruled in favor of the government. Approximately 6.4 million Americans who had purchased health plans from HealthCare.gov would continue to receive their premium subsidies.

In 2014, a lawsuit challenged the ACA's requirement that all health insurance policies cover women's preventive health services, including Food and Drug Administration-approved prescription contraceptives and birth control counseling. The lawsuit stemmed from employers whose religious beliefs were against a requirement that included contraception. Employers who felt this way often chose not to include contraception-related coverage in their health insurance policies. While women working for non-profit health care institutions or universities that were affiliated with religious organizations usually had access to contraceptives, their employers were not required to pay for this coverage. The women in this example could obtain coverage directly through their insurance plans.

In the case of "for-profit" employers who opposed contraceptive coverage for their female employees, stating that this interfered with religious freedom under the Religious Freedom Restoration Act of 1993, the Supreme Court heard the cases of "Hobby Lobby" and "Conestoga Wood Specialties." Though lower courts had ruled differently, the Supreme Court ruled that these two companies could not be required to cover contraceptive drugs or devices, since this was in violation of their religious beliefs. The female employees of these companies, therefore, had no coverage (or only limited coverage) for contraceptives if they continued their employment.

Though churches are exempt from providing contraceptive coverage, employers who do not wish to cover their employees in this regard must request an *accommodation* from their insurance provider or the Secretary of Health and Human Services. In these cases, the insurance provider pays for the coverage for female employees instead of the employer.

> ### Focus on legal challenges to the Affordable Care Act
>
> Regarding the ACA's birth control coverage benefit *alone*, there have been over 100 lawsuits filed in federal court. Both *for-profit* and *non-profit* organizations are involved in these lawsuits.

Supreme Court modifications

Because of the *National Federation of Independent Business v. Sebelius* case, the U.S. Supreme Court changed the ACA by allowing individual states to opt out of Medicaid expansion. It ruled that the expansion of Medicaid by the individual states was optional only. This resulted in lower enrollments by low-income adults who lived in the states that chose not to expand Medicaid.

> ### You should remember
>
> In 2015, the U.S. Supreme Court ruled that the subsidies under the ACA were legal. This means that the IRS was able to issue subsidies on behalf of those who bought a plan through the HealthCare.gov website.

State coverage

In 2010, the ACA required all states to expand Medicaid to non-pregnant adults under 65 years of age who had incomes within 138% of the Federal Poverty Level. Prior to the ACA, Medicaid coverage was different in each state, and most states did not cover adults without children.

The states do have the option to create a Basic Health Plan for uninsured individuals who have incomes between 133% and 200% of the FPL, who would otherwise be eligible for premium subsidies in the Exchange. Any state choosing to do this must contract with one or several standard plans to provide at least essential benefits, and ensure that premiums are not more than eligible individuals would have paid in the Exchange. Cost-sharing requirements cannot exceed those of the platinum plan for people who enroll and have an income of less than 150% of the FPL or the gold plan for all others. The states receive 95% of funds that would have been paid as federal premium and cost-sharing subsidies. Individuals who have incomes between 133% and 200% of the FPL in states that create Basic Health Plans are not eligible for subsidies in the exchanges.

Minimum essential coverage

Beginning in 2014, all U.S. citizens and permanent residents were required by the ACA to have minimum essential coverage or to pay a fine (tax penalty), even though not everyone is required to purchase health insurance. This is true if they have health insurance through an employer's group plan or government-sponsored programs, which include Medicare, Medicaid, CHIP, the Indian Health Service, the Department of Defense, and the Veterans' Administration. Other people who are not required to have health insurance are people in prison or undocumented immigrants. Compliance with the minimum essential coverage requirement is monitored by the IRS.

> ### Focus on minimum essential coverage
>
> The *individual shared responsibility provision* of the ACA requires each taxpayer and their family members to have qualifying health coverage known as *minimum essential coverage*, qualify for an exemption from it, or make an individual shared responsibility payment when filing a federal income tax return.

Costs of premiums and implementation

Beginning in 2014, many people in the United States were able to purchase health insurance for the first time ever in their lives, using the health exchanges, and assisted by federal subsidies to pay parts of their premiums. The ACA premium subsidies allow people to purchase affordable health insurance in several ways. For those with incomes between 100% and 400% of the FPL, they can utilize the Advance Premium Tax Credit, which is a refundable tax credit designed to help people with low or moderate income afford health insurance purchased through the Health Insurance Marketplace, also known as the "Exchange," beginning in 2014. For those with incomes between 100% and 250% of the FPL, the Cost Sharing Reduction program is used. This program offers subsidies that can greatly reduce deductibles, co-payments, co-insurance, and total out-of-pocket spending limits for qualifying individuals.

Regarding employers with 100 or more full-time employees, health insurance must be provided or financial penalties will result. These include fines or the *Employer Shared Responsibility Payment*, which will be automatically triggered if a full-time employee is receiving a marketplace premium subsidy. According to the IRS, purchasing premium subsidies through any marketplace ensures eligibility for tax credit.

The costs of premiums during 2010 varied widely across the country. Plans offered choices of different levels that were called *bronze*, *silver*, *gold*, and *platinum*. The following list summarizes the different premium costs:

- Bronze – lowest premiums, highest cost-sharing (deductibles and co-payments); individual pays 40% of medical services and insurance covers 60%
- Silver – individual pays 30% of medical services and insurance covers 70%
- Gold – individual pays 20% of medical services and insurance covers 80%
- Platinum – highest premiums, lowest cost-sharing; individual pays 10% of medical services and insurance covers 90%.

The cost of premiums was 3–4% of incomes for people with incomes at 133–150% of the FPL. Federal subsidies paid the remaining premium costs. Premiums are related to competition in the insurance markets as well as local labor costs. States with lower competition, such as Alabama, have higher premiums. States with higher competition, such as Colorado, have lower premiums. Between 2000 and 2013, average annual premium costs for small businesses (with fewer than 100 employees) increased by double digits for approximately half of the United States. However, during this period, the average increase in overall premiums had been between 3% and 7%.

The costs of implementing the Affordable Care Act were always anticipated to be significant. However, the Centers for Medicare and Medicaid (CMS) believed that the law would eventually slow the rate of growth in health care spending as time passed. The Act first intended to reduce payments to Medicare Advantage Plans and to hospitals on behalf of Medicare patients. It then established a *Center for Medicare and Medicaid Innovation* in order to study health care delivery and coordination, primarily for people who had both Medicare and Medicaid. These individuals are called *dual-eligibles*. The goal is to make future health care decisions based on the treatments and services that provide the greatest cost savings as well as the best health outcomes.

In 2011, states that took on the roles of "early innovators" in regard to operating health insurance exchanges were given cooperative agreements to assist them in their efforts. Each marketplace had to have *navigators* employed, who were specially trained to help consumers to select and enroll in Qualified Health Plans offered by various states or the federal government. Federal funds were provided to establish the information technology needed, and to assist in promotions and marketing to educate potentially eligible individuals about getting insurance through the marketplace.

Also, funding for the National Health Service Corps (NHSC) increased between 2011 and 2015 so that there were enough primary health workers available to care for newly insured people. Money was set aside for the scholarships and loan repayments to health care professionals during training as a trade-off for them working in underserved areas of the system.

Implementation of the Act is ongoing, with new parts being added every year up to a planned completion in 2018. A breakdown of the various parts that were scheduled for each year is as follows:

- 2010:

  - Adult children (under 26 years of age) covered by parents' health insurance plans
  - Clinical preventive services required in all health policies sold through health exchanges, Medicare, and Medicaid, with these services including cancer screening, contraceptives, and immunizations; this came about because preventive services are less expensive than treating serious diseases
  - Federally Qualified Health Centers expanded
  - Pre-existing conditions no longer used to exclude applicants from obtaining health insurance (example: prior to the Act, pre-existing diseases such as heart disease or diabetes meant that the patient would be denied health insurance)
  - Scholarship and loan repayments for students training to be nurses, physicians, and physician assistants.

- 2011:

  - Non-medical spending by private insurance plans limited to 15% of the cost of premiums
  - Pharmaceutical fees placed on drug manufacturers
  - Center for Medicare and Medicaid Innovation established to reward hospitals and physicians for service quality instead of volume.

- 2012:

  - Hospital Readmissions Reduction Program (HRRP), to lower Medicare payments to hospitals that fail to meet standards for readmission for heart attack, heart failure, and pneumonia; hospitals that had high readmission rates receive lower reimbursement for Medicare patients.

- 2013:

  - Electronic medical records required by private health insurers
  - Payment Reform, which concerns programs that bundle services, such as home care that follows surgical procedures.

- 2014:

  - Health exchanges (state and federal) for people with incomes between 100% and 400% of the Federal Poverty Level
  - Essential Health Benefits now required by all policies sold through state and federal health exchanges, meaning that benefits are the same for everyone regardless of the source of their coverage (see Table 2.1)
  - Medicaid Expansion for people with incomes at 138% of the Federal Poverty Level where Medicaid expansion occurred
  - Shared Responsibility, meaning that individuals must have health insurance or pay a fine, and employers, as of January 1, 2015, with at least 100 employees must offer insurance to their employees; since the employer is required to provide health insurance, if a full-time employee is receiving a marketplace premium subsidy, a fine will occur, or the *Employer Shared Responsibility Payment* will be triggered.

Table 2.1 Required essential health benefits (by all qualified plans)

Ambulatory patient services

Chronic disease management

Emergency services

Hospitalization

Maternity and newborn care

Mental health and substance use disorder services (including behavioral health treatment)

Prescription drugs

Rehabilitative services and devices

Laboratory services

Pediatric services (including oral and vision care)

Preventive and wellness services

You should remember

The cost of the Affordable Care Act is estimated to reach $1.207 trillion by the year 2025.

Source: http://obamacarefacts.com/costof-obamacare.

Medicaid expansion

The Centers for Medicare and Medicaid (CMS) originally established programs to control costs and improve health care quality. Once the ACA was established, the federal government was required to fund 100% of the cost of Medicaid expansion between 2014 and 2016. Then, funding would decrease over the following years, to 90% by the year 2020, where it would remain. Even though the federal government would fund much of this Medicaid expansion, many states did not want to add the additional costs to their already-tight budgets. According to the ACA, any state that did not comply with the Medicaid expansion would lose all federal funding for Medicaid. This resulted in legal action.

The Medicaid expansion covered all individuals under age 65 with incomes up to 133% of the FPL based on modified adjusted growth income. Undocumented immigrants are not eligible. All newly eligible adults are guaranteed coverage that provides at least *essential benefits*. Financing of the expansion meant that states would receive 100% federal funding through 2016, 95% in 2017, 94% in 2018, 93% in 2019, and 90% for all following years. States that already expanded eligibility for adults with incomes up to 100% of the FPL receive phased-in increases in federal assistance for non-pregnant childless adults. By 2019, they will receive equal federal financing as other states. States receive 100% federal financing for the increased payment rates.

By July 2015, the Medicaid expansion was utilized by 30 states as well as Washington, D.C. Alaska and Utah were considering the expansion but the other states had decided against it. In these states, approximately 10% of the population were not able to get government-sponsored health care due to income guidelines for Medicaid and the health exchanges. People falling into the coverage gap had income that was too high for Medicaid and too low for the premium subsidies obtainable through the marketplace. In the states that did expand Medicaid, people were more likely to have coverage, with the uninsured rate falling from 28% to 17% for people with incomes lower than 100% of the FPL. Comparatively, in the states that did not expand Medicaid, the uninsured rate was near 36%.

The ethnic group most likely to be uninsured in the United States consists of Latinos. Their uninsured rates exhibited very similar numbers to the remainder of the population based on the states they lived in. For example, there are more Latinos in California than in any other state. California did expand Medicaid, and today, approximately 50% of Latinos in that state who did not have health insurance are now covered. California was the first state to pass legislation to establish a health care marketplace and promoted it very well, encouraging enrollment. In Texas and Florida, which did not expand Medicaid, the largest number of uninsured Latinos are residents. Throughout the entire country, about 16% of Latinos are not eligible for coverage because they are not legal immigrants.

Eleven Southern states chose not to expand Medicaid, and about one-third of the U.S. population lives in these states – with Florida, Georgia, and Texas having the highest populations. In the South, there are higher levels of small businesses and blue-collar industries, resulting in the likelihood of more Southerners being uninsured. Health coverage is often not offered by employers and private insurance is costly. In total, approximately 3.5 million Americans living in Southern states have obtained health care through the marketplace exchanges, yet about four million are ineligible for Medicaid or premium subsidies.

Focus on Medicaid expansion under the Affordable Care Act

The ACA's Medicaid expansion for the nation's poorest people will cover nearly half of all uninsured Americans. However, changes to the law will cause millions of working families to be without coverage by 2016.

You should remember

As of the end of 2015, 50% of Americans opposed the Affordable Care Act, while 42% were in favor of it, with the remainder undecided.

Source: www.huffingtonpost.com/2015/06/21/
obamacare-approval-polls_n_7632070.html.

Advantages and disadvantages of the PPACA

Advantages of the PPACA include approximately 15 million individuals being able to obtain health coverage during its first enrollment period, which was from October 2013 to March 2015. As a result, the percentage of uninsured people in the United States went from 17% to 10%. It also gave coverage to about 12 million lower-income adults and children who were enrolled in Medicaid or CHIP. Therefore, the amount of people covered by these programs has now reached 71 million. Many of these were low- and middle-income people living in the 30 states in which Medicaid was expanded. Medicaid was also expanded in Washington, D.C. As of 2015, states received a 23% increase in the CHIP federal matching rate up to a cap of 100%.

Of younger adults (between 19 and 34), the uninsured percentage dropped from 28% to 18%. The Act also allowed young adults to remain on their parents' policies until the age of 26. Overall, the Act gave individuals increased options for obtaining insurance. Most people with health insurance continued to have it provided by their employers, with those who were self-employed purchasing insurance from private companies. The new *Small Business Health Options Program (SHOP)* provides health insurance for businesses that have up to 100 employees. People who wish to buy private plans can utilize a *State-Based Health Exchange Marketplace* or the Federally-Facilitated Marketplace. Also, states have the option to operate their own marketplaces as partnerships with the federal government.

HealthCare.gov was created as a one-stop Internet shopping website to allow people to buy non-group health plans, and also to determine eligibility for Medicaid and CHIP. It also provides resources for the SHOP program, and links to websites of the individual states that carry state-based marketplaces.

The ACA rewarded **Accountable Care Organizations** (ACOs) for providing quality care and lowering health care costs. These organizations are groups of physicians, hospitals, and other health care providers who work together to provide coordinated high-quality care to their Medicare patients. Their goal is to ensure that patients, especially the chronically ill, receive the proper care at the correct time, while avoiding unnecessary duplication of services and preventing medical errors. When an ACO succeeds in these goals, it will share in the savings it achieves for the Medicare program. Medicare offers several of these programs, including the *Medicare Shared Savings Program*, the *Advance Payment ACO Model*, and the *Pioneer ACO Model*.

One of the primary disadvantages of the Affordable Care Act is its complexity, and its need to involve so many different entities for implementation. Other disadvantages include a shortage of health care professionals and higher drug costs. As of 2012, many people who had their own private health insurance had their plans canceled because they did not meet the ACA's "essential health benefits." Often, businesses found it more cost-effective to pay the fines and allow their employees to purchase their own insurance plans on the exchanges.

The ACA favors younger people with more abundant health than older people. Uninsured individuals will pay approximately 2.5% of their income every year that they remain uninsured as the "penalty" for not participating. Taxes will also rise to cover the costs of the Act, and government costs will rise as well. Some people will find that their premiums are even higher when using the exchanges than they were with private insurance. Table 2.2 compares the advantages and disadvantages of the Affordable Care Act.

You should remember

Though millions of Americans have become insured under the Affordable Care Act, health insurance premiums average at least 14% nationally for the average American family, and this is increasing. These rising costs have consumed nearly all of the wage increases that workers have received from employers over time.

Source: http://kff.org/private-insurance/press-release/family-health-premiums-rise-4-percent-to/.

Table 2.2 Advantages and disadvantages of the Affordable Care Act

Advantages	Disadvantages
Affordability – with the use of subsidies to help cover costs, many people can get health insurance that otherwise could not afford it	**Higher costs** for certain people
80/20 Rule – Health insurance companies must spend 80% of premium dollars on patient care and quality improvement, while profits and other costs must total 20%	**Cancelations** – millions of Americans had their insurance policies canceled due to noncompliance with standards of this Act
Limited premium increases – saves money by limiting these increases from year to year using a "rate review" program	**Surprise costs** – about 39% of Americans seeking new plans under this Act ended up paying more than they did previously
Coverage cancellations and denials due to pre-existing conditions prevented – this includes those occurring from simple mistakes on insurance applications. This plan also prevented overcharging or refusing coverage for pre-existing conditions	**Coverage cancellations and denials due to pre-existing conditions can still happen if you had a "grandfathered plan,"** which is one that existed before March 23, 2010 and did not change substantially
Expansion of Medicaid – more types of individuals are now covered, including uninsured adults and people living below 138% of the federal poverty level	**States opting out of Medicaid expansion** – due to a Supreme Court ruling, certain states did not go along with the Medicaid expansion. Only 27 states and the District of Columbia decided to firmly expand coverage. Since subsidies (advanced tax credits) are only for those making between 100 and 400% of the federal poverty level, those making less than 100% of the poverty level receive no assistance in these states
Children can remain on parents' insurance until age 26	**Narrowed networks** – fewer healthcare providers are available for "in-network" coverage, meaning that while smaller networks may reduce costs, there are fewer options for consumers to choose from

Table 2.2 Continued

Advantages	Disadvantages
No annual or lifetime limits – meaning that benefits must continue to be paid as needed; however, this rule also does not apply to grandfathered plans	**The Act does not address long-term care**, meaning that those senior citizens who cannot qualify for Medicaid cannot receive the care they need. Due to costs, the initially included "Community Living Assistance Services and Supports" were scrapped
Preventive care – insurance plans must cover a long list of preventive care at no cost to the patient	**Penalties for the uninsured** – anyone without insurance who does not qualify for an exemption is subject to the "ACA Penalty," which is assessed on your taxes. This penalty will grow over time, in an attempt to persuade the uninsured to sign up

Focus on large insurance companies pulling out of the Affordable Care Act exchanges

By 2017, three of the largest insurance companies in the United States (UnitedHealthGroup, Humana, and Aetna) will stop selling health insurance through most of the exchanges created by the Affordable Care Act. Most insurers selling plans through the exchanges have been losing money because patients have been more ill than was previously forecast.

Focus on the Affordable Care Act in 2017

Rates for health insurance will increase significantly in the following states: Arizona (116%), Oklahoma (76%), Minnesota (50–67%), Tennessee (44–62%), Illinois (44%), Nebraska (35%), and Pennsylvania (33%). By October 2017, most states will see at least a 25% increase in costs. This includes the 39 states that use the federal online marketplaces. The goals of the ACA were to cover more people, improve quality of care, and reduce costs. Unfortunately, the costs have increased each year since the Act was created. Costs have affected those able to afford coverage and receive needed care.

Sources: www.healthinsurance.org/arizona/; www.healthinsurance.org/oklahoma-state-health-insurance-exchange/; www.healthinsurance.org/minnesota/; www.healthinsurance.org/tennessee/; www.healthinsurance.org/illinois/; www.healthinsurance.org/nebraska/; www.healthinsurance.org/pennsylvania/; www.forbes.com/sites/gracemarieturner/2016/10/27/middle-income-americans-take-the-biggest-hit-with-obamacare/#293831fb1393.

CASE STUDY

A Florida-based company employs 52 full-time employees and currently only offers health care benefits to ten senior managers. The Affordable Care Act now requires companies with 50 or more full-time employees to offer comprehensive health coverage to all of their full-time workers or pay a penalty. The company has five options: to insure the other employees and absorb all costs or pass some of them to the employees; lay off three workers so that they would have only 49 full-time employees; make three employees part-time; downsize the company to 25 full-time employees to collect small business tax benefits; or leave the non-management employees uninsured and just pay the tax penalties.

1 Which option do you think would be most cost-effective?
2 If the company chose to insure all of the employees, what would the employees' options be concerning premiums, seeking other insurance from the exchanges, or remaining uninsured instead?

Chapter highlights

This section answers the Objectives found at the beginning of the chapter.

1 **Explain the primary reasons that influenced passage of the Patient Protection and Affordable Care Act.**

- The PPACA was primarily influenced by millions of uninsured Americans and the rising costs of health care. Therefore, the Act attempted to decrease the number of uninsured Americans, increase qualities and efficiencies of health care, and curb the speed of the increase in costs of health care.

2 **Describe how the PPACA impacted insurance coverage and access to care.**

- The PPACA requires implementation through different agencies, such as private insurance companies and providers. It established the Hospital Readmissions Reduction Program to control Medicare costs. Reimbursements were reduced by up to 3% initially. Hospital readmissions decreased, but then a record number of hospitals received reduced payments for Medicare patients. There are now penalties for excessive hospital readmissions. Problems with the various marketplace websites resulted in lack of access to care, due to delays in verification, eligibility, and information being completed. Breakdowns in the federal Data Services Hub complicated access to coverage. The Act also caused many insurance plans to be canceled. It increased Medicaid coverage for many, improving access to health care. Today, costs continue to rise, even after passage of the Act.

3 **List examples of legal challenges to the PPACA.**

- In 2011, a federal lawsuit challenged the individual mandate requiring people to have health insurance or be fined, and the Medicaid expansion in every state. The Medicaid expansion was upheld, but not the individual mandate. Later, the U.S. Supreme Court upheld the individual mandate, but ruled the Medicaid expansion as violating the U.S. Constitution. The Employer Shared Responsibility Payment ruling was challenged, but upheld.

4 **Describe how the PPACA was modified because of Supreme Court decisions regarding contraceptive coverage and Medicaid expansion.**

- In 2014, a lawsuit challenged the requirement of all health insurance policies covering women's preventive health services, including contraceptives. Two companies stated that their religious beliefs prevented them from offering contraceptive coverage. The Supreme Court ruled that they could not, therefore, be required to cover contraceptive drugs or devices. Today, employers who do not wish to cover their employees in this regard must request an accommodation from their insurance provider or the Secretary of Health and Human Services. The provider must then pay for coverage for employees' contraceptive needs, instead of the employer.
- Regarding Medicaid expansion, the Supreme Court changed the ACA by allowing individual states to opt out. It ruled that the expansion by the individual states was optional only. This resulted in lower enrollments by low-income adults in the states that chose not to expand Medicaid.

5 **Discuss the minimum essential coverage requirements of the PPACA.**

- All U.S. citizens and permanent residents must now have minimum essential coverage or pay a tax penalty, even though not everyone is required to purchase health insurance. This is true if they have health insurance through an employer's group plan or the government. Other people not required to have health insurance are people in prison or undocumented immigrants. Compliance with the minimum essential coverage requirement is monitored by the IRS. The individual shared responsibility provision of the Affordable Care Act requires taxpayers and family members to have qualifying health coverage, qualify for an exemption from it, or make an individual shared responsibility payment when filing returns.

6 **Explain the costs of premiums and implementation related to the PPACA.**

- People with incomes between 100% and 400% of the Federal Poverty Level can utilize the refundable Advance Premium Tax Credit. It should help low- or moderate-income people purchase insurance. For incomes between 100% and 250% of the FPL, the Cost Sharing Reduction program offers subsidies that can reduce deductibles, co-payments, co-insurance, and total out-of-pocket spending. Purchasing premium subsidies through a marketplace ensures eligibility for tax credit.

- There are four levels: bronze (individual pays 40%, insurance pays 60%), silver (individual 30%, insurance 70%), gold (individual 20%, insurance 80%), and platinum (individual 10%, insurance 90%). "Bronze" premiums are lowest, and the platinum level has the highest premiums. The cost of premiums was 3–4% of income for people at 133–150% of the FPL. Federal subsidies paid remaining premium costs. Average annual premium costs for small businesses have increased by double digits for about half of the United States. The average increase in overall premiums was between 3% and 7%. The cost of the Affordable Care Act should reach $1.207 trillion by 2025.

7 **Compare differences between insurance coverage in states that have or have not expanded Medicaid.**

- By 2015, the Medicaid expansion was utilized by 30 states, with two others and Washington, D.C. considering it. Of the states that declined it, about 10% of citizens could not get government health care due to income guidelines for Medicaid and the health exchanges. In states that did expand Medicaid, the uninsured rate fell from 28% to 17% for people with incomes lower than 100% of the FPL. In states that did not expand Medicaid, the uninsured rate was near 36%.

8 **Which ethnic group is most likely to be uninsured in the United States, and why are some people in this group not eligible for coverage?**

- Latinos are most likely to be uninsured in the United States. About 16% of Latinos are not eligible for coverage because they are not legal immigrants.

9 **Explain the advantages of the PPACA during its first enrollment period.**

- Approximately 15 million individuals were able to obtain health coverage during the first PPACA enrollment period (from October 2013 to March 2015). The percentage of uninsured Americans went from 17% to 10%. It also gave coverage to about 12 million lower-income adults and children enrolled in Medicaid or CHIP.

10 Summarize the disadvantages of the PPACA.

- The PPACA is very complex, and involves many different entities for its implementation. There is a shortage of health care professionals and higher drug costs. The Act has higher costs for certain people, has resulted in millions of insurance policies being canceled, is more expensive for about 39% of Americans than previous coverages, still causes cancelations and denials due to pre-existing conditions if you had a plan existing before 2010 that did not change substantially, resulted in many states opting out of Medicaid expansion, reduced options, does not address long-term care, and penalizes the uninsured.

Summary

Health care reform in the United States has been the subject of much argument over many years. The Patient Protection and Affordable Care Act has attempted to solve many problems related to health insurance, but is still highly controversial. Though millions of Americans have received coverage under the Act, millions more have lost pre-existing coverage because it did not correspond to the regulations set out in the Act. Many Americans were told by President Obama that they could keep their insurance plans, but this turned out not to be true.

Legal battles over various parts of the ACA have reached the Supreme Court. Many individual states opted out of its proposed Medicaid expansion, and its requirement that most Americans have minimum essential coverage or pay a tax penalty remains extremely unpopular. Employers are being forced to downsize their businesses and lay off employees or face paying costs they may not be able to afford. It is hoped that further implementation of new sections of the Act will address all of these concerns, and make health care accessible and affordable for all.

Review questions

1 What is the purpose of health care reform?
2 What is the concept of the Hospital Readmissions Reduction Program?
3 According to the Affordable Care Act, what is the "individual mandate"?
4 What is the Employer Shared Responsibility Payment?
5 What was the impact of the U.S. Supreme Court on Medicaid expansion?
6 What is the meaning of "minimum essential coverage"?
7 What are the four levels of health insurance plan offered through the marketplace?
8 Under the Affordable Care Act, what do "clinical preventive services" include?
9 What was the purpose of Medicaid expansion?
10 What are "Accountable Care Organizations"?

Bibliography

Amadeo, K. 2015. *The Ultimate Obamacare Handbook (2015–2016 Edition): A Definitive Guide to the Benefits, Rights, Responsibilities, and Potential Pitfalls of the Affordable Care Act*. New York: Skyhorse Publishing. Print.

Blumenthal, M. and Cohn, J. 2015. The Surprising Reason So Many People Still Don't Like Obamacare. Available at: www.huffingtonpost.com/2015/06/21/obamacare-approval-polls_n_7632070.html. Chicago: The Huffington Post, Inc.

Brill, S. 2015. *America's Bitter Pill: Money, Politics, Backroom Deals, and the Fight to Fix Our Broken Healthcare System*. New York: Random House Trade Paperbacks. Print.

Cantor, J.C., et al. 2012. Early impact of the Affordable Care Act on health insurance coverage of young adults. *Health Services Research* 47, no. 5: 1773–1790.

Congressional Budget Office (CBO). 2012. *CBO and JCT's Estimates of the Effects of the Affordable Care Act on the Number of People Obtaining Employment-Based Health Insurance*. Washington, D.C.: Congressional Budget Office.

Dorsey, J. 2016. Arizona Health Insurance – AZ Rate Hikes as High as 116% for Some, 1 Carrier Option for Most. Available at: www.healthinsurance.org/arizona/. St. Louis Park: HealthInsurance.org.

Dorsey, J. 2016. Illinois Health Insurance – State's Exchange Participants Fall from Nine Carriers to Five. Available at: www.healthinsurance.org/illinois/. St. Louis Park: Health Insurance.org.

Dorsey, J. 2016. Minnesota Health Insurance – MN Enacts Enrollment Cap as Premiums Rise 50–67%. Available at: www.healthinsurance.org/minnesota/. St. Louis Park: Health-Insurance.org.

Dorsey, J. 2016. Nebraska Health Insurance – Cornhusker State 1 of 10 with Rate Hikes Over 30%. Available at: www.healthinsurance.org/nebraska/. St. Louis Park: Health Insurance.org.

Dorsey, J. 2016. Pennylvania Health Insurance – PA Uninsured Rate Decreases, Questions Increase. Available at: www.healthinsurance.org/pennsylvania/. St. Louis Park: Health Insurance.org.

Dorsey, J. 2016. Tennessee Health Insurance – TN Insurance Commissioner Calls Exchange 'Very Near Collapse'. Available at: www.healthinsurance.org/tennessee/. St. Louis Park: HealthInsurance.org.

Eastman, A.D., and Eastman, K.L. 2013. Person federal tax issues and the Affordable Care Act: Can tax penalties and subsidized premiums provide sufficient incentives for health insurance purchases. *Journal of Business & Economic Research* 11, no. 7: 315–324.

Grant, D. 2013. House Republicans repeal Obamacare again: Why do they keep doing it? *Christian Science Monitor*, May 16.

Harrington, S.E. 2013. Medical loss ratio regulation under the Affordable Care Act. *Inquiry* 50, no. 1: 9–26.

hCentive Healthcare Blog: Pamela Girardin. 2015. States without Medicaid Expansion Face a New Challenge – Huge Unpaid Hospital Bills. Available at: www.hcentive.com/states-without-medicaid-expansion-face-a-new-challenge-huge-unpaid-hospital-bills/. Reston: hCentive.

HHS.gov. 2016. About the Law – Regulations and Guidance. Available at: www.hhs.gov/healthcare/facts/bystate/statebystate.html. Washington, D.C.: U.S. Department of Health and Human Services.

Internal Revenue Service. 2016. Individual Shared Responsibility Provision – Minimum Essential Coverage. Available at: www.irs.gov/affordable-care-act/individuals-and-families/aca-individual-shared-responsibility-provision-minimum-essential-coverage. Washington, D.C.: Internal Revenue Service.

KFF.org. 2012. Family Health Premiums Rise 4 Percent to Average of $15,745 in 2012,

National Benchmark Employer Survey Finds. Available at: http://kff.org/private-insurance/press-release/family-health-premiums-rise-4-percent-to/. Menlo Park: Kaiser Family Foundation.

KFF.org. 2013. Health Reform Implementation Timeline. Available at: http://kff.org/interactive/implementation-timeline. Menlo Park: Kaiser Family Foundation.

KFF.org. 2016. Uncompensated Hospital Care Fell by $6 Billion Nationally in 2014, Primarily in Medicaid Expansion States; However Many Hospitals Worry About Future Changes in Medicaid Supplemental Payments. Available at: http://kff.org/medicaid/press-release/uncompensated-hospital-care-fell-by-6-billion-nationally-in-2014-primarily-in-medicaid-expansion-states-however-many-hospitals-worry-about-future-changes-in-medicaid-supplemental-payments/. Menlo Park: Kaiser Family Foundation.

Kopp, B., et al. 2013. What's new with the Affordable Care Act? *Employee Benefit Plan Review* 68, no. 2: 7–11.

McCaughey, B. 2014. *Beating Obamacare 2014: Avoid the Landmines and Protect Your Health, Income, and Freedom*. Washington, D.C.: Regnery Publishing. Print.

Medicaid.gov. 2016. Affordable Care Act. Available at: www.medicaid.gov/affordablecareact/affordable-care-act.html. Baltimore: Centers for Medicare and Medicaid Services.

New York State. 2012. Federal Health Care Reform in New York State. Available at: www.healthcarereform.ny.gov/summary. New York: New York State.

Norman, G. 2015. *Medicaid Expansion under the Affordable Care Act: Overview and Opportunities (Health Care in Transition)*. Hauppauge: Nova Science Publishing Inc. Print.

Norris, L. 2016. Oklahoma Marketplace History and News – BCBSOK is Sole Exchange Carrier; Average Rate Increase – 76%. Available at: www.healthinsurance.org/oklahoma-state-health-insurance-exchange/. St. Louis Park: HealthInsurance.org.

Obamacare Facts. 2015. Supreme Court ObamaCare – Ruling on ObamaCare. Available at: http://obamacarefacts.com/supreme-court-obamacare. Washington, D.C.: Obamacare Facts.

Obamacare Facts. 2016. What is the Cost of Obamacare?. Available at: http://obamacarefacts.com/cost-of-obamacare. Washington, D.C.: Obamacare Facts.

Pipes, S.C. 2010. *The Truth about Obamacare*. Washington, D.C.: Regnery Publishing. Print.

Quittner, J. 2013. Two New Legal Challenges Seek to Scuttle Obamacare. Available at: www.inc.com/jeremy-quittner/legal-challenges-ACA.html. New York: Mansueto Ventures.

Robertson, L. 2014. Party Lines – 'Skyrocketing' Premiums. Available at: www.factcheck.org/2014/04/skyrocketing-premiums. Philadelphia: FactCheck.org.

Rockwell, L. 2013. Special Report: Health Care Insurance – An Affordable Care Act Case Study. Available at: www.floridatrend.com/article/16058/an-affordable-care-act-case-study. St. Petersburg, Florida: Florida Trend Magazine.

Shi, L., and Singh, D.A. 2015. *Delivering Health Care in America: A Systems Approach, 6th Edition*. Burlington: Jones & Bartlett Learning. Print.

Supplemental Health Care – Workforce Solutions. 2015. The Pros and Cons of the Affordable Care Act. Available at: www.supplementalhealthcare.com/blog/2012/patient-protection-and-affordable-care-act-snapshot-pros-and-cons. Park City: Supplemental Health Care.

Turner, G.-M. 2016. Middle-Income Americans Take the Biggest Hit with Obamacare. Available at: www.forbes.com/sites/gracemarieturner/2016/10/27/middle-income-americans-take-the-biggest-hit-with-obamacare/#293831fb1393. Jersey City: Forbes Media LLC.

Zephyros Press. 2013. *Obamacare Simplified: A Clear Guide to Making Obamacare Work for You*. Berkeley: Zephyros Press. Print.

Chapter 3

Legal and ethical aspects of health care

Objectives

After completing this chapter, the reader should be able to:

1 Explain why knowledge of law and ethics is important to health care practitioners.
2 Discuss the classifications of law.
3 Define the concept of torts and discuss how the tort of negligence affects health care.
4 Explain the four elements necessary to prove negligence (the four Ds).
5 Differentiate between expressed contracts and implied contracts.
6 Discuss the special requirements for disclosing protected health information.
7 Discuss the patient rights defined by HIPAA.
8 Define moral values and explain how they relate to laws and ethics.
9 Define the basic principles of health care ethics.
10 Compare living wills and durable powers of attorney for health care.

Overview

It is important for all health care professionals to understand how laws and ethics affect their jobs. Patients have specific rights, responsibilities, and concerns about medical laws and ethics. The increasingly quick development of medicine requires similar development of these topics in relation to health care. Along with this development, rising costs for health care impact legal and ethical scenarios even further. Therefore, it is essential to be aware of legal and ethical issues that govern health care for all patients.

Law

The rights of all citizens are designed to be protected by *laws*. It is important that all health care professionals understand the relationships that they have with their clients under the law. *Litigation* may occur when a client is unhappy with their health care treatments, resulting in legal proceedings in a court of law. Litigation is commonly referred to as a *lawsuit*. Laws may fall under federal or state jurisdiction.

Federal law

Federal law is derived from the U.S. Constitution, which delegates powers and responsibilities to the three branches of government – executive, legislative, and judicial. The executive branch actually means the president of the United States, who administers laws and can issue *executive orders* without prior approval of Congress. The legislative branch consists of the two houses of Congress, which are the Senate and the House of Representatives. There are two members of the Senate from each state, in total 100. The membership of the House of Representatives is based on population, and totals 435. Congress primarily writes, debates, and passes bills, which are given to the president for approval. The judicial branch includes the U.S. Supreme Court, and has federal judges and courts in every state.

State law

The governments of each state also have executive, legislative, and judicial branches. The numbers of state legislators differ between states, and are also not the same as the number of federal legislators. The governor of each state heads up its executive branch. State constitutions cannot conflict with the U.S. Constitution.

Classifications of law

Laws are created through four areas, which include *constitutional*, *case*, *statutory*, and *administrative* law. Constitutional law is based on the U.S. Constitution; case law is based on previous legal cases; statutory law results from federal or state legislative bodies; and administrative law controls administrative government operations. Laws are then classified into two broad areas: *substantive law* and *procedural law*. Substantive law is statutory or written, and defines and regulates legal rights and obligations. Procedural law defines rules that enforce substantive law. *Criminal law* and *civil law* are the classifications of law that most often relate to health care. The department of the executive branch of the federal government that is responsible for health-related laws is the Department of Health and Human Service (DHHS).

Criminal law

Crimes are offenses against the state that violate public laws. When a state or federal criminal law is violated, criminal charges against the offender are brought by the government. Federal criminal offenses include treason, border-related crimes, and activities such as kidnapping or hijacking, which may cross state lines. State criminal offenses include murder, rape, burglary, robbery, arson, larceny, mayhem, and practicing medicine without a license.

Criminal acts may be classified as felonies or misdemeanors. Felonies are punishable by death or imprisonment for more than one year. Misdemeanors are less serious crimes, and are punishable by imprisonment for one year or less.

Civil law

Civil law involves wrongful acts against individual persons or groups of persons. Civil lawsuits may be brought by the wronged party against another person, a business, or the government. Most commonly, civil lawsuits involve violations of contracts, libel, slander, product liability, trespassing, traffic accidents, or family matters. Civil penalties often require financial settlements to be paid to the wronged party.

Tort liability

A tort is basically a civil wrong that one individual commits against another, or an individual's property, that causes physical injury or property damage, or deprives the individual of freedom and personal liberty. Torts do not include breach of contract, but are designed to preserve peace, recognize wrongdoers, deter individuals from committing future torts, and provide compensation to those who have had torts committed against them. A tort may be intentional or unintentional (see Table 3.1).

Intentional torts

For an intentional tort, the injured party can bring a civil lawsuit and be financially compensated by the person who committed the tort. If the guilty party is determined to have acted maliciously, punitive damages can also be awarded. The person judged guilty of committing a tort is called a *tortfeasor*. Examples of intentional torts include:

- Assault – the threat of bodily harm to another person, or an action that makes the person feel reasonably threatened of bodily harm.
- Battery – an action causing bodily harm to another person, including any contact made without the person's permission.

Table 3.1 Types of torts

Intentional torts	Unintentional torts
Assault	Negligence:
Battery	Criminal
Defamation of character:	Statutory
Libel	Professional (also called malpractice)
Slander	
False imprisonment	
Infliction of mental distress	
Invasion of privacy	

- Defamation of character – the act of causing damage to a person's reputation by making false and malicious public statements about the person. If occurring using spoken words, it is classified as slander. If occurring using printed words, pictures, or signed statements, it is called libel.
- False imprisonment – the unlawful and intentional confinement or restraint of a person by another person.
- Fraud – the use of deceit to deprive, or attempt to deprive, another person of his or her rights, usually for financial gain.
- **Infliction of mental distress** – includes the causing of grief, despair, public humiliation, shame, and the wounding of pride.
- Invasion of privacy – interfering with a person's right to be left alone. This includes breaches of confidentiality concerning medical records. Confidentiality is the most important concept for health care professionals to keep in mind on a daily basis.

Unintentional torts

Most torts that occur in health care are unintentional. These are not intended to cause harm, and are usually committed without disregard for the outcome. They legally constitute negligence, such as when a health care professional causes patient injury because of failing to take ordinary precautions when working with the patient.

Medical negligence does not follow appropriate conduct or may be careless. It often involves *abandonment*, in which care is stopped by a health care professional without providing suitable replacement care, or when treatment is delayed without an adequate reason. Negligence may involve a committed act, or an omission of an act. Medical negligence cases are sometimes classified in the following ways:

- Malfeasance – misconduct, or an unlawful act; the opposite of this, *nonmalfeasance*, is an ethical principle requiring health care practitioners to avoid causing patients harm
- Misfeasance – a lawful act performed incorrectly
- Nonfeasance – an act that was the duty of the health care professional, or that was required by law, was not performed.

The *four Ds of negligence*, as listed by the American Medical Association, include *duty*, *dereliction*, *direct cause*, and *damages*. If a malpractice suit is sought, the patient must be able to prove all four of these claims, which are explained as follows:

- Duty – the provider owed the patient a duty as part of a provider–patient relationship
- Dereliction – the provider did not comply with professional standards, such as when a standard follow-up test is not performed as required
- Direct cause – any damages must be proven to have been directly caused by a breach of duty
- Damages – actual injuries to the patient that are provable.

> ### You should remember
>
> Negligence committed by a professional is malpractice. However, not all malpractice is negligence.

Respondeat superior

The legal doctrine holding employers responsible for the actions of their employees is called *respondeat superior*, which means "let the higher-up answer" or "let the master respond." Also known as *vicarious liability*, it is used in cases wherein a health care facility is liable for negligent acts of employees, even though the organization itself did not actually commit the acts. The wrongful act of an employee must have occurred within the scope of his or her employment. The employer must possess the right, power, and authority to exercise control over the acts of employees.

Contract law

A **contract** consists of a voluntary agreement between two parties. In a contract, certain promises are made in exchange for a consideration. The delivery of health care occurs under various types of contracts. The obligations set out may be changed or eliminated by another contract. Both written and oral contracts bind parties to act in a predetermined manner, and offer legal recourses. Contract law is affected by the *Uniform Commercial Code*, which provides uniformity to sales and transactions within the United States.

Contracts

In order to be legally binding, there are four elements required in a contract, as follows:

- Agreement – an offer is made by one party, which is accepted by the other. It can relate to the present or future, must be communicated, must be made in good faith, cannot be made under duress or as a joke, must be clearly understood by both parties, and must define the obligations of both parties if it is accepted.
- Consideration – in health care, the provider gives medical service, while the patient pays the provider's fee.
- Legal subject matter – the contract must be for legal services or purposes; if either party fails to comply with the contract terms, **breach of contract** may be charged. A contract that is not legally enforceable is called *void*.
- Contractual capacity – both parties must be capable of understanding all terms and conditions set forth in the contract. Mentally incompetent people cannot enter into legal contracts. If either party is incompetent when a contract is made, the contract may be *voidable*. Also, a *minor*, who is any person under the age of 18 in most states, and under 21 in others, cannot enter into a legal contract without the consent of a responsible parent or legal guardian. A *legal guardian* is a person appointed by a judge to act on behalf of a minor or a mentally incompetent adult. Legal guardians can sign consent forms on behalf of the person they are acting for, who is referred to as the *ward*.

Types of contracts

The two primary types of contracts are *expressed contracts* and *implied contracts*. Their terms are derived from the actions of the parties who are involved.

Expressed contracts

An expressed contract is clearly stated, in either written or spoken words. All terms are explicitly stated, according to the Statute of Frauds for the state where the contract is written. In health care, a contract between a physician and patient is usually terminated when treatment is completed and all bills have been paid. However, these contracts may also be terminated because of failure to pay for services, failure to keep scheduled appointments, failure to follow physician instructions, or when the patient seeks another physician's services. Patients can terminate a physician–patient relationship at any time. If the physician wishes to terminate the relationship, he or she must give the patient formal written notice.

Focus on termination of treatment

When terminating treatment of a patient, the termination letter should advise the patient that termination of treatment will occur within 30 days. It should advise the patient to seek additional medical consultation and offer to send the patient's medical record to any new physician.

Implied contracts

An implied contract is one in which the parties' conduct indicates acceptance, creating the contract. This is instead of "expressed words." Most medical office contracts are implied. When a physician makes services available to a patient seeking treatment, an implied offer to treat the patient has been made. The patient's implied acceptance of treatment is made when the patient allows the physician to examine him or her and to prescribe treatment. Additionally, the patient's payment for services shows implied acceptance. Patients have the right to *informed consent*, which means a full explanation of treatment options in order to make an informed decision about their health care. Informed consent is collected from an individual by a provider, following the guidelines of medical and research ethics.

Informed consent

Informed consent is a process that involves getting permission from a mentally competent individual before conducting a health care intervention. The provider may ask the patient for consent to receive therapy before it is provided, or a clinical researcher may ask a research participant for consent before he or she is enrolled into a clinical trial. The individual is considered to have been *informed* when he or she fully understands the possible results, risks, consequences, and outcomes of what will be performed. Anyone who gives informed consent must be able to cognitively reason normally, and must know all related facts about what will be performed.

The health care provider must obtain the individual's *written* informed consent for the majority of medical procedures. These include surgery and other invasive procedures, experimental drug studies, stress tests and other possibly dangerous procedures, and any other procedure that may have significant risks. The individual's informed consent shows that he or she voluntarily agrees to what will be performed.

Health care professionals should never attempt to convince or force patients to sign a consent form if they do not want to. The patient should never feel pressured to sign an informed consent form. A person's written consent should not be asked for in any of the following situations:

- if the patient is not mentally competent
- if the patient is a minor
- if the patient is under the influence of drugs or alcohol
- if the patient does not understand what is being proposed
- if the patient is unable to read the consent form
- if the patient has any unanswered questions about what is being proposed.

Implied consent

When a patient does not sign a written statement, but does give permission for care to be provided, implied consent has been given. Implied consent also covers situations in which the patient is unconscious but assumed to have given permission for care, such as when someone calls 911, but passes out prior to paramedics arriving.

Expressed consent

Expressed consent is a clear, voluntary indication of preference or choice, which is oral or written. It is given freely, when available options and consequences have been made clear, and is actually a part of informed consent. Expressed consent gives formal permission to undergo a procedure or to allow use of personal information for research or for epidemiology, audit, administration, publication, or release to the public. If expressed consent is not given, use of materials related to these areas must be limited to teaching and training.

Professional liability and medical malpractice

Medical negligence is also called **malpractice**. An example of a malpractice claim is when a patient brings a lawsuit against a physician because of an error in treatment or diagnosis. Often, the patient believes that an essential action was not performed by a health care professional, or that something improper was done, resulting in harm. Examples of malpractice include complications following surgery due to an incorrectly cauterized organ, or when a surgical instrument is left inside a surgery patient. This last example is described as a case of res ipsa loquitur, or "the thing speaks for itself," wherein the surgical instrument may be easily discovered on an X-ray of the patient. Malpractice is part of *civil law*, and is classified as a *tort*.

Malpractice lawsuits often lead to court trials, but are sometimes settled through arbitration, in which qualified people with specialized knowledge are chosen, outside of court, to hear the evidence and decide about the dispute. If the case is proven in the patient's favor, the provider must pay a financial award, known as *damages*, to the patient. When a court case is set, the provider will receive a subpoena requiring his or her presence in court at a specific date and time. Other individuals who might have knowledge about the facts in the case may also be subpoenaed.

To prevent malpractice lawsuits, there are "four Cs" that should be followed:

- Caring – offering personalized patient care, with sincerity
- Communication – earning patient respect and trust with professional communication, and asking for confirmation that he or she has understood
- Competence – job skills and continually updating knowledge via continuing education
- Charting – documentation proving competence, having all reports and consultations reviewed by the physician, and charting all patient interactions.

> ### You should remember
>
> One of the most serious areas of medical malpractice concerns general anesthesia. Prior to it being administered, the anesthesiologist must investigate the patient's history for possible complications, and inform the patient of risks related to not following preoperative instructions.

> ### Focus on "failure to diagnose"
>
> "Failure to diagnose" is a malpractice situation in which a condition is not correctly identified, and that often results in worsening of disease. For example, if a physician fails to diagnose breast cancer, which results in the patient requiring chemotherapy and mastectomy, he may be required to pay all of her medical expenses, lost time from work, and monetary penalties to compensate for emotional distress, pain, and suffering.

Liability

To be *liable* means to be legally responsible for one's own actions, whether at work or in private life. Liability insurance protects against injury or harm in many different situations. In the health care profession, for example, general liability by physicians and other professionals may concern medical facilities, vehicles, and safety in the work environment.

Good Samaritan laws

State laws enacted to relieve health care professionals and, sometimes, common citizens from liability in certain emergency situations (such as accidents) are known as *Good Samaritan laws*. These laws, which exist in all 50 states, encourage assistance to be given at the scene of emergencies in order to help an injured person. Consent does not need to be given, since the caregiver is acting to potentially save the life of the injured person. These laws are actually *statutes* that provide a standard of care defining the scope of immunity for eligible persons under the law. They protect emergency caregivers against liability for negligence.

> ### You should remember
>
> In a Good Samaritan situation, for a physician to be protected from liability, the person needing assistance must be in imminent peril or danger. The physician's actions should not be negligent, and should constitute a "reasonable response." They must be in good faith and not involve receiving any compensation or future compensation.

Standard of care and duty of care

Standard of care describes the level of performance that a health care professional must exhibit when carrying out professional work activities. The obligation of health care professionals in relation to patients or non-patients is called *duty of care*. For example, a physician has a duty of care to patients with whom they have a physician–patient relationship, but also to that patient's family members, former patients, and even office staff members. The *reasonable person standard* enforces health care professionals to be responsible for actions as well as failure to act properly.

Physicians must conform to standards of other practitioners in the same field of medicine, in their communities or in similar communities. Specialists have a higher standard of care than physicians in general practice, but their standard of care is similar to other medical specialists. All health care professionals, regardless of their level or field of medicine, must conform to the standards of their peers.

Guidelines for health care practitioners

Health care practitioners should follow the following guidelines in order to remain within their scope of practice and related laws:

● Always maintain confidentiality
● Use the correct legal and ethical guidelines when releasing information
● Practice within your capabilities and the scope of your training
● Always document everything with accuracy
● Use the professional title that is correct for your education and experience
● Prepare and maintain health records correctly
● Follow proper safety and risk management procedures
● Assist in developing and maintaining manuals that concern personnel, policies, and procedures
● Follow established policies of your employer when dealing with health care contracts
● Follow legal guidelines, and keep aware of health care regulations and legislation
● Comply with governmental guidelines when maintaining and disposing of regulated substances
● Meet all requirements for professional credentialing.

The Joint Commission

The *Joint Commission* or *TJC* is an accrediting organization that sets standards concerned with patient safety and medical mistakes. When a mistake occurs, health care providers are required to report it to supervising physicians and other health care professionals, as well as on the patient's medical record. The provider must then inform the patient that he or she has been harmed as a result of a mistake. When a mistake is not reported and then later discovered, the facility at fault may lose accreditation from the Joint Commission. All accredited facilities must implement the following requirements:

● Improve patient identification accuracy
● Improve communication effectiveness between caregivers
● Improve safe uses of high-alert medications
● Eliminate surgeries that are incorrect in relation to site, patient, and procedure
● Improve safe infusion pump use
● Improve clinical alarm system effectiveness
● Reduce risk of nosocomial infections (those acquired from health care).

> ## Focus on the Joint Commission
>
> The Joint Commission accredits hospitals, home care services, nursing care centers, behavioral health care services, ambulatory care services, and laboratories. Organizations must undergo on-site surveys at least every three years, with laboratories being surveyed every two years.

Provider's rights and responsibilities

Providers, as well as patients, both have distinct rights and responsibilities.

The rights and responsibilities of providers include:

- The right to establish a practice that is within the boundaries of his or her license to practice medicine
- The right to establish an office in a location, and with the practice hours of the provider's choice
- The right to specialize
- The right to decide on which services will be provided, and how
- The responsibility to use adequate care, diligence, judgment, and skill for patient treatments that is used by peers in the same medical specialty
- The responsibility to remain informed of the best and most current methods of diagnosis and treatment
- The responsibility to perform with the best possible ability, regardless of receiving or not receiving a fee
- The responsibility to give complete instructions and information to patients about diagnoses, fees, options, and treatment methods.

Also, providers are not expected or required to do any of the following:

- Guarantee successful outcomes of operations or treatments
- Make correct diagnoses every time
- Return patients to their original states of health
- Treat every patient who is seeking care, unless providing care in a hospital emergency room or a free clinic.

Privacy law and HIPAA

Federal privacy laws are based on four basic principles. These include limiting information that is collected and stored about individuals to only what is necessary for the collecting agency. Access to collected personal information must be limited to employees who need the information for the performance of their jobs. The information cannot be released unless authorized by the person to whom it pertains. Authorization is made through the health care contract with the patient, who authorizes release of private and confidential information. The individual in question must be informed that information is being collected, and also must be allowed to verify that the information is accurate.

Most federal privacy laws are concerned with credit or financial information, or electronic information that has been stolen or illegally disclosed. State laws governing medical record confidentiality are varied. The first federal legislation that focused on medical record privacy was the Health Insurance Portability and Accountability Act, or *HIPAA*, passed in 1996. It provided for civil and criminal penalties for violations of its standards.

Many changes to HIPAA were passed as part of the American Recovery and Reinvestment Act or ARRA, in 2009. Specifically, the section most concerning HIPAA changes was called the Health Information Technology for Economic and Clinical Health (HITECH) Act. There were four categories of changes, which included:

- Changes to HIPAA privacy and security standards
- Changes in HIPAA enforcement
- Changes addressing information held by covered entities or business associates not expressly covered by HIPAA
- Changes concerning HIPAA administration, reports, studies, or educational initiatives concerning health care.

The four sets of HIPAA standards are as follows:

- *Transactions and code sets* – *transactions* concern information transmission between two parties in relation to financial or administrative activities; *code sets* are used to encode data elements, including terminology, medical concepts, diagnostic codes, and procedure codes.
- *Privacy Rule* – to protect patient privacy through electronic transmission or storage of medical records, patient permissions must be utilized; this rule gives patients certain rights concerning their own medical records, which include access to and copies of records, amendments to records, accounting of disclosures of protected health information (PHI), and limits on information about patients provided in hospital directories. Patients have a right to receive a *Notice of Privacy Standards*, which provides information on the privacy practices of their health plans and most of their health care providers.
- *Security Rule* – policies and procedures that ensure confidentiality of protected health information.
- *National identifier standards* – provide unique identifiers for electronic transmissions, which are similar to "addresses" on the Internet; the identifiers are unique for employers, providers, and health plans.

Focus on the HIPAA Privacy Rule

The HIPAA Privacy Rule applies to health plans, health care clearing houses, and most health care providers who transmit health information in electronic form. The covered health care providers are determined by the Secretary of Health and Human Services.

Ethics and health care

Ethics is defined as a standard of behavior, as well as concepts of right and wrong, which exceed laws. The basis for ethics consists of moral values derived from societies, cultures, and families. Though laws are based on ethical considerations, health care professionals are expected to act *ethically* and not just *legally*. They must always act in ways reflecting the ideas of right and wrong as put forth by society. In health care, common ethical dilemmas concern the right to refuse treatment or to choose specific treatments, and, in end-of-life situations, when to stop artificial life-sustaining interventions. *Bioethics* concerns topics such as when life realistically begins, proper treatment of incapacitated or highly vulnerable patients, and the determination of a patient's *death*.

Codes of ethics

Most health care disciplines have their own *codes of ethics*, which are designed to ensure high standards of behavior among professionals. These codes concern ethical conduct, and have been developed by various professional organizations to set standards of professional conduct that keep the quality of care high and promote patient welfare. Ethics are essential, continuing components of health care as well as all other professions. Resources on codes of ethics can be obtained by the professional organization that oversees your area of practice. For example, the code of ethics set out by the American Association of Medical Assistants includes the following points:

- Fully respect the humanity and dignity of patients you serve
- Respect all confidential information unless you are legally authorized or required to share it with specific parties
- Accept and uphold the high principles and honor of your profession
- Seek continuing education for the benefit of patients and colleagues
- Be active in service activities that can improve your community's well-being.

Basically, the main principles of a code of ethics concern *beneficence*, *fidelity*, *veracity*, *justice*, and *autonomy*. **Beneficence** means that all actions are aimed at benefiting patients well, and without prejudice. **Fidelity** involves keeping promises to fulfill patient needs and maintain confidentiality. **Veracity** means always telling the truth. **Justice** is focused on fair and equal law-abiding actions. **Autonomy** is based on self-reliance, dependability, initiative, and reliability.

Values

The beliefs and ideals you hold in guiding your behavior and making decisions are known as *values*. These beliefs and ideals are developed over your lifetime. While values among individuals differ, you must strive to support your working environment's practices and values.

> ### You should remember
>
> The five top ethical issues in health care include: balancing care quality and efficiency, improving access to care, building and sustaining the future health care workforce, addressing end-of-life issues, and allocating limited medications and donor organs.
>
> *Source:* www.amnhealthcare.com/latest-healthcare-news/
> five-top-ethical-issues-healthcare/.

Professional ethics

Professional ethics are those that affect the delivery of professional services, such as health care, to clients. The health and safety of all professionals are protected under the Occupational Safety and Health Administration (OSHA). Health care professionals must always act in ways that are ethical in regard to the treatment of patients. The basic principles of professional ethics include the following:

- Preserving life by giving caring attention
- Doing good by showing respect and courtesy
- Respecting autonomy by making sure that patients have consented to all procedures and treatments
- Upholding justice by following all legal guidelines
- Being honest by admitting errors, focusing on accuracy, and avoiding participation in any fraudulent situations
- Being discreet by never discussing or releasing patient information without proper authorization, keeping documentation from being accessed by non-authorized individuals, and protecting the physical privacy of patients
- Keeping promises by verifying that contracts are complete, and by being careful about what you say to patients
- Doing no harm by providing excellent customer service within your scope of practice, following safety precautions and protocols, asking for help when needed, receiving continuing education, keeping certifications current, and staying informed about health care news.

Patient's rights and responsibilities

Evert patient has a variety of rights and responsibilities that he or she should be made aware of. These include the following:

- The right to see a provider of his or her own choosing, though choices may be limited by a managed care plan
- The right to terminate a provider's services
- The right to receive and review a *patient care partnership*, which is a list of standards for health care
- The responsibility to follow the provider's orders for treatment
- The responsibility to follow all instructions given by the provider, and cooperate as much as possible
- The responsibility to give all relevant information to the provider so that a correct diagnosis can be reached – the provider is not liable if an incorrect diagnosis is made based on incomplete patient information
- The responsibility to pay the fees charged for the provided services.

Biomedical concerns

The term biomedical refers to *biomedicine*, which is the application of the natural sciences, especially biological and physiological sciences, to clinical medicine. It is concerned with the effects of the environment on the body. The application of biomedicine has helped create new types of equipment used for diagnosis, treatment, and patient monitoring. Examples of advances made through biomedical engineering include cardiac pacemakers, heart-lung machines, lasers used in surgery, and ultrasonography.

Biomedical concerns regarding health care professionals include specific training on these types of equipment, along with their continued and detailed maintenance. Technicians may be required to install, test, repair, and service a wide variety of machinery. They often specialize in certain types of equipment.

Special considerations

There are certain medical activities that require special consideration. These include stem-cell research, abortion, health care rationing, organ transplantation, and situations that involve death and dying.

Stem-cell research

Stem-cell research, intended to help preserve life, is highly controversial. Stem cells may replace other cells in a patient that have been damaged by diseases or injuries. Scientific information supports that the most effective stem cells include those from human embryos and aborted fetuses. When cells are taken from an embryo, it will die, and many people feel this is murder. Fortunately, certain adult body tissues also contain cells that can function as stem cells. More recently, human skin cells have been used to create stem cells.

You should remember

Stem cells can copy themselves for an unlimited time period. Adult stem cells are called "multipotent," meaning they can turn into several different types of cells within the same basic cell type. Embryonic stem cells are "pluripotent," and can turn into all body cell types except for egg or sperm cells.

Focus on new stem cell technologies

Using somatic cell nuclear transfer and other new technologies, scientists are attempting to manufacture cell lines that are specific to patients as well as diseases.

Abortion

The termination of pregnancy, by either removing or expelling an embryo or fetus from the uterus, is known as abortion. This elective procedure is a highly controversial one, and challenges both ethics and laws. Most arguments concern exactly when "life begins." A woman's choice to have an abortion is extremely personal, since it concerns her own body and health, and laws concerning abortion are in constant debate. Another major area of discussion concerns the rights of an unborn baby, as well as the rights of its father. It should be noted that an abortion may also occur spontaneously during a woman's pregnancy.

The landmark legislation concerning abortion is called *Roe v. Wade* (1973), which gave support to a woman's right to privacy relating to her own body, which includes how a pregnancy may end. The U.S. Supreme Court has repeatedly attempted to define how individual states may regulate or prohibit abortions. During the first trimester of pregnancy, the decision to have an abortion is between a woman and her physician. Under *Roe v. Wade*, in the second trimester, a state may have the power to regulate an abortion in ways reasonably related to the health of the mother. However, by the time of the third trimester of pregnancy, the state may be able to prohibit an abortion unless the health of the mother is in proven jeopardy.

> ## You should remember
>
> Approximately four out of ten unplanned pregnancies in the United States are terminated by abortion. Though overall the abortion rate has declined, poorer women are having these procedures more frequently, suggesting a distinct socioeconomic factor.
>
> *Source:* www.womenscenter.com/abortion_stats.html.

Health care rationing

Because of increasing health care costs, concerns are being raised that rationing of health care may become a serious issue. Already, insurance providers determine certain tests and treatments that they will not cover, meaning that the patient is required to pay in full if these tests and treatments are desired. For making decisions regarding rationing of health care, the likelihood of benefit to the patient is the first concern. Will the treatment improve the patient's quality of life, and how long will the benefits last? How urgent is the patient's condition concerning the needed care? Another consideration is the amount of resources needed for successful treatment.

Organ transplantation

Rationing may also affect which patients are more likely to receive a needed organ transplant, since there are many more people awaiting organs than there are organs available. Fortunately, many people agree to donate their own organs, or those of family members, following death. However, it is illegal to use organs for transplantation that were not donated. Payments cannot be given to organ donors or their family members. The physician who pronounces the death of a patient also cannot participate on the organ transplant surgical team. Anyone wishing to be an organ donor must inform his or her family members. Many states signify the words "organ donor" on driver's licenses, but intentions to donate must be discussed with family members so that following death, transplantation can occur promptly to benefit as many recipients as possible.

Death and dying

According to psychologist Elisabeth Kübler-Ross, five distinct stages of grief occur when an individual learns that he or she is dying. Though each person handles these stages in different ways, the same overall reactions occur. The stages of grief may not occur in the same order for everyone. They are summarized as follows:

- *Denial* – a defense mechanism that may be signified by seeking another opinion, stating that test results must be incorrect, looking for a "miracle cure," or acting as if nothing has changed
- *Anger* – as denial begins to decline, the patient may ask, "Why is this happening to me?," and may be envious of others, irritable, or resentful
- *Bargaining* – as the patient begins to deal with the reality of his or her situation, a last attempt is made to make a "bargain" in order to live; this is often religious in nature
- *Depression* – when bargaining fails, the patient usually shows signs of deep depression and loses hope; he or she may feel guilty for things that were done during life, as well as for leaving loved ones behind
- *Acceptance* – the individual accepts death and the fact that every living thing eventually dies, and that their own death will occur soon; though not resulting in happiness, acceptance is generally free of negative feelings, and the patient usually feels exhausted.

Though every health care provider is obligated to protect life, as a patient nears death, there may be a conflict between this obligation and the patient's own wishes. Patients are allowed to choose whether life-sustaining treatments are used. Life-sustaining measures include ventilators and feeding tubes. When a patient cannot communicate his or her wishes concerning life being sustained, health care professionals must follow any previous instructions given by the patient as part of an *advanced care directive*.

There are several types of advanced care directives. A living will lists any steps requested by the patient that must be taken to save or prolong his or her life. This document takes effect when the patient becomes *incapacitated*, meaning that he or she is unable to make any more medical decisions about care. A living will must be signed and dated by two witnesses who are not blood relatives or beneficiaries of the patient. The living will must be discussed with the patient's physician and a copy placed in the patient's medical record. Another type of advanced care directive is the durable power of attorney *for health care*, which names another person who will make health care decisions on behalf of the patient once he or she becomes incapacitated.

End-of-life issues

The factors that come into question near the end of life concern patient pain and whether it can be relieved, suffering from terminal conditions, being in a coma with little chance of regaining consciousness, lack of brain function, and if a patient actually asks for his or her life to be terminated (euthanasia, or *assisted suicide*). The withdrawal of artificial life-sustaining equipment, also called *passive euthanasia*, has been done many times according to the requests of patients or individuals who were given durable power of attorney for health care (see Figure 3.1). When a patient has not given an advance directive concerning the removal of artificial life-sustaining equipment, it may be legally impossible for health care providers to discontinue its use.

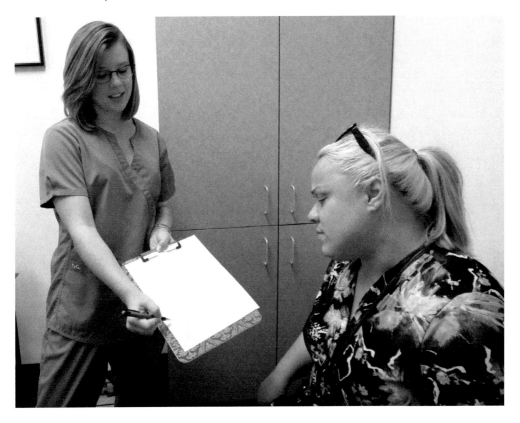

Figure 3.1 A nurse discussing a durable power of attorney with the family member of a patient.

Euthanasia is commonly referred to as *mercy killing*, and is a highly controversial practice that results in the death of a patient, according to the patient's own wishes. The term *active euthanasia* is defined as providing the patient with a lethal dose of medication that results in death. Controversy arises around the idea that if legalized, euthanasia might be ordered by a family member for a sick relative who otherwise would not have made the request. Another factor could be the use of euthanasia upon a patient by health care providers in an effort to manage costs. Health care providers must follow the laws of their states concerning euthanasia. Only Oregon and Washington have passed physician-assisted life termination laws. Though it is clear that *killing* a patient can never be justified, *allowing* a patient to die by removing artificial life-sustaining measures, per the patient or appointed caregiver's request, is a different situation entirely.

In determining what steps to take in these situations, it is also important to understand when a patient is considered to be legally dead. Legally, this is defined as when there is no respiration, heartbeat, or pulse. Today's medical equipment can sustain heartbeat and respiration even when the patient is declared *brain dead*. It is generally accepted that *irreversible cessation of brain function* constitutes death. However, families of patients described as being in a *persistent vegetative state* cannot necessarily order the removal of artificial nutrition. This is a complex area of personal, family, state, and federal government contention that has had many different outcomes, and will continue to be litigated.

One other area of importance is a *do-not-resuscitate order* or *DNR*. These are physician orders instructing that there should be no patient resuscitation in the event of cardiac or respiratory arrest. They are based on scientific evidence that due to diminished quality of life, the patient should not receive any "heroic" rescue methods in these cases because they are not in the patient's best interests. A DNR must be written, signed, and dated by the patient's physician, and consent must be obtained either from the patient or his or her appointed representative. These orders must be statutorily compliant, short in length, and reviewed regularly to determine if the condition of the patient or other circumstances have changed in any significant ways.

You should remember

Treatment can be stopped without a "living will" if everyone involved agrees. Over two-thirds of adults have no living will or other advance directive.

Focus on "legal death"

Though the term "legally dead" has traditionally meant that the heart and lungs have irreversibly ceased to function, there have been cases in which an unconscious patient has remained in this state up to ten years before the heart and lungs finally failed.

CASE STUDY

An elderly patient with severe dementia has been living in a nursing home, with coverage paid for by Medicaid, for five years. She has no family and never issued any directives about her health care prior to losing her cognitive abilities. When the patient develops chest congestion and a fever, and begins having labored breathing, she is taken to the local hospital's intensive care unit. She is intubated and put on a ventilator, but has to be restrained in order to stop her from pulling out her breathing tube. She also has to be given sedatives so that she does not attack the ICU staff. She begins to refuse food and a determination needs to be made about inserting a feeding tube.

1 Do you think it is ethical for a feeding tube to be inserted in this case?
2 If intubation and ventilation were required, was it ethical to restrain this patient since pulling out the breathing tube could cause harm or even the patient's death?
3 If this patient suffered cardiac arrest because of her possible panic at not understanding how she is being treated, what legal outcomes could occur?

Chapter highlights

This section answers the Objectives found at the beginning of the chapter.

1 **Explain why knowledge of law and ethics is important to health care practitioners.**

- Health care professionals are expected to act ethically and not just legally. They must act in ways reflecting the ideas of right and wrong as put forth by society. Health care professionals must respect patient humanity and dignity, and all confidential information unless legally authorized or required to share it; uphold professional principles and honor; seek continuing education; and be active in community service activities.

2 **Discuss the classifications of law.**

- Laws are created through constitutional, case, statutory, and administrative law, and classified into substantive and procedural law. Substantive law is statutory or written, and regulates legal rights and obligations. Procedural law defines rules that enforce substantive law. Criminal law concerns offenses against the state that violate public laws, with criminal acts classified as felonies or misdemeanors. Civil law involves wrongful acts against individuals or groups, and often requires financial settlements.

3 **Define the concept of torts and discuss how the tort of negligence affects health care.**

- A tort is a civil wrong that one individual commits against another, or the individual's property. Torts cause physical injury or property damage, or deprive individuals of freedom and personal liberty. Torts may be intentional or unintentional. Negligence may be defined as criminal, statutory, or professional – malpractice is known as professional negligence. When a health care professional causes patient injury because of not taking ordinary precautions, it is termed negligence. Medical negligence often involves abandonment or delayed treatment without an adequate reason. Medical negligence cases may be classified as malfeasance, misfeasance, or nonfeasance.

4 **Explain the four elements necessary to prove negligence (the four Ds).**

- The four Ds of negligence include duty, dereliction, direct cause, and damages. The provider owes a patient a duty as part of a provider–patient relationship. Dereliction refers to a provider not complying with professional standards. Direct cause involves any damages, which must have been directly caused by a breach of duty. Damages are actual injuries to the patient that are provable.

5 **Differentiate between expressed contracts and implied contracts.**

- An expressed contract is clearly stated, in either written or spoken words, according to the governing state's Statute of Frauds. An implied contract is one in which the parties' conduct indicates acceptance, creating the contract, instead of "expressed words." Most medical office contracts are implied.

6 **Discuss the special requirements for disclosing protected health information.**

- Federal privacy laws limit information that is collected and stored about individuals to only what is necessary for the collecting agency. Access to collected personal information must be limited to employees who need the information for the performance of their jobs. The information cannot be released unless authorized by the person to whom it pertains. The individual in question must be informed that information is being collected, and also must be allowed to verify that it is accurate.

7 Discuss the patient rights defined by HIPAA.

- HIPAA defines patient rights under its Privacy Rule. These include access to and copies of their own medical records, amendments to these records, accounting of disclosures of protected health information (PHI), and limits on patient information that can be provided in hospital directories.

8 Define moral values and explain how they relate to laws and ethics.

- Moral values concern the personal concept of right and wrong of every individual. They are formed through the influence of family, culture, and society. They are the basis for ethics, and laws are based on ethical considerations.

9 Define the basic principles of health care ethics.

- Most health care disciplines have their own codes of ethics, which are designed to ensure high standards of behavior among professionals. These codes help keep quality of care high, and promote patient welfare. Ethics are essential, continuing components of health care. The main principles of a code of ethics concern beneficence, fidelity, veracity, justice, and autonomy.

10 Compare living wills and durable powers of attorney for health care.

- A living will lists any steps requested by a patient that must be taken to save or prolong his or her life. This document takes effect when the patient becomes incapacitated, meaning that he or she is unable to make any more medical decisions about care. The durable power of attorney for health care names another person who will make health care decisions on behalf of the incapacitated patient. Both the living will and the durable power of attorney for health care are examples of "advanced care directives."

Summary

Health care professionals must understand how laws and ethics affect their relationships with their clients. This includes federal and state legislation. Criminal and civil law are the classifications of law most often related to health care. An example of a related criminal violation would be practicing medicine without a license, and an example of a related civil violation would be violating a health care contract with a patient. Torts are civil wrongs that cause physical injury, property damage, or deprive someone of freedom and personal liberty. The intentional tort called invasion of privacy may concern a breach of confidentiality involving medical records, and is a critical component of health care practice. However, most health care-related torts are unintentional, and constitute negligence.

The relationship between a health care provider and a patient is established through an expressed contract. When a health care provider acts negligently toward a patient, a malpractice claim may be filed. Malpractice lawsuits often lead to court trials. Liability insurance protects health care professionals against injury or harm in many different situations. For people who act as good Samaritans in emergency situations, all states in America allow for them to provide care without consent of the patient, since such care may save the patient's life. These laws protect against liability for negligence. The most important concepts of health care practice guidelines include confidentiality under HIPAA, practice within scope of training, accurate documentation, property safety procedures under OSHA, following legal and ethical regulations, and proper professional credentialing.

Special considerations are given to certain medical activities. Stem-cell research is controversial, and designed to help preserve life by replacing cells that have been damaged. Abortion, the termination of pregnancy, challenges ethics and laws because of the determination of when life actually begins. Rationing of health care, whether based on insurance requirements or other factors, must always take patient care into the utmost consideration. Another concern is organ transplantation from donors, and who is able to legally determine the donor's intentions and follow through on them. For people who are terminally ill, advanced care directives are encouraged so that, once the patient becomes incapacitated, his or her wishes concerning measures that may prolong life are respected and acted upon. In a few states, patients may seek euthanasia, which is the assisted termination of their lives – a highly contested legal and ethical issue.

Review questions

1 Why is law and ethics important to health care practitioners?
2 What is tort liability?
3 What is contract law?
4 What is the relationship between laws and ethics?
5 Define professional liability and medical malpractice.
6 What are privacy laws and HIPAA?
7 What are professional ethics?
8 Explain the term "code of ethics."
9 What is the purpose of stem-cell research?
10 Describe the concepts of death and dying.

Bibliography

Amadeo, K. 2015. *The Ultimate Obamacare Handbook (2015–2016 Edition)*. New York: Skyhorse Publishing. Print.

Barua, B. 2013. *Diagnosis: Medically Unreasonable*. Vancouver, British Columbia: The Fraser Institute.

Brzezinski, R. 2014. *HIPAA Privacy and Security Compliance: Simplified (2014 Edition)*. Seattle: CreateSpace. Print.

Darr, K. 1991. *Ethics in Health Services Management, 2nd Edition*. Baltimore: Health Professions Press.

Emanuel, E.J., et al. 2000. What makes clinical research ethical? *Journal of the American Medical Association* 283, no. 20: 2701–7211.

FindLaw. 2016. Health Care Law. Available at: http://healthcare.findlaw.com. Eagan: Thomson Reuters.

HG.org. 2016. Legal Resources – Health Care and Social Law. Available at: www.hg.org/health-law.html. Houston: HG.org – HGExperts.com.

Kavaler, F., and Alexander, R.S. 2012. *Risk Management in Healthcare Institutions: Limiting Liability and Enhancing Care, 3rd Edition*. Burlington: Jones & Bartlett Learning. Print.

Larson, J. 2013. AMN Healthcare – News – Five Top Ethical Issues in Healthcare. Available at: www.amnhealthcare.com/latest-healthcare-news/five-top-ethical-issues-healthcare. Del Mar: AMN Healthcare, Inc.

Markkula Center for Applied Ethics – Better Choices. 2016. End-Of-Life Decision Making. Available at: www.scu.edu/ethics/practicing/focusareas/medical/conserved-patient/case1.html. Santa Clara: Santa Clara University.

McWay, D.C. 2014. *Legal and Ethical Aspects of Health Information Management, 4th Edition*. Boston: Delmar Cengage Learning. Print.

Morrison, E.E., and Furlong, B. 2013. *Health Care Ethics: Critical Issues for the 21st Century, 3rd Edition*. Burlington: Jones & Bartlett Learning. Print.

National Commission on Correctional Health Care. 2016. Ethical and Legal Issues – Ethical Concerns. Available at: www.ncchc.org/cnp-ethical-legal. Chicago: National Commission on Correctional Health Care.

Orlando Women's Center. 2016. Abortion Statistics – Abortion Facts Around the World – Facts About Abortion in the United States. Available at: www.womenscenter.com/abortion_stats.html. Orlando: Orlando Women's Center.

Pozgar, G.D., and Santucci, N. 2015. *Legal Aspects of Health Care Administration, 12th Edition*. Burlington: Jones & Bartlett Learning. Print.

Teitelbaum, J.D., and Wilensky, S.E. 2012. *Essentials of Health Policy and Law (Essential Public Health), 2nd Edition*. Burlington: Jones & Bartlett Learning. Print.

Unit II

Financial management

Contents

4 Health care financing and payment for
services   81

Overview   81
Reimbursement for health care services   82
Government-funded health care   82
Privately funded health care   87
Insurance and managed care   91
Direct payments from patients   93
Comparisons of U.S. health care with other countries   94
Case study   95
Chapter highlights   95
Summary   97
Review questions   98
Bibliography   98

5 Customer service   100

Overview   100
Quality of care   101
Dimensions of quality   101
Quality assurance   103
Quality improvement   106
Quality improvement organizations   107
Customer satisfaction   107
Case study   111
Chapter highlights   111
Summary   113
Review questions   114
Bibliography   114

Chapter 4

Health care financing and payment for services

Objectives

After completing this chapter, the reader should be able to:

1 Describe reimbursements for health care services.
2 Explain how Medicare, Medicaid, and TRICARE originated.
3 Summarize the four parts of Medicare.
4 Explain the three classifications of people who qualify for Medicaid.
5 Describe the four requirements needed to qualify for CHAMPVA.
6 Define the terms "indemnity" and "capitation."
7 Briefly explain when workers' compensation does and does not apply.
8 Discuss what type of person usually uses a medical savings account, and what is covered by withdrawals (distributions) from this type of account.
9 Compare and contrast HMOs and PPOs.
10 Briefly describe the five models of health maintenance organizations.

Overview

Health insurance has changed and grown since World War II, with the United States mostly utilizing private insurance, while other countries of the world use government-provided health care. The U.S. government established Medicare and Medicaid to cover elderly, disabled, and low-income individuals as well as those with certain health conditions.

After many years, with the aging of the population and the complexities of the U.S. health system, costs of health insurance have dramatically increased. Many Americans still cannot afford health insurance. It has become more critical than ever before to find ways to keep health care services at a high standard, while attempting to manage ever-increasing costs. The Affordable Care Act was established in an attempt to manage these costs. Since its passage in 2010, there are still millions of Americans uninsured, and the complexities of the Act must still be addressed.

Reimbursement for health care services

Most health care services are reimbursed using *fee-for-service payments* that occur when the service or services are carried out. Definitions of health care services and what they include are sometimes hard to define. Fees vary widely between practitioners and locations in the country. Public and private health coverage utilize *capitation*, which uses fixed amounts that are paid from insurers to providers for certain services. Fee-for-service pays for particular services that are rendered (itemized) at a specific time. The third means of reimbursing health care services is through salaries, in companies where other incentives are provided to practitioners in order to increase productivity. Hospitals are also reimbursed using similar methods, with one difference, which is reimbursement based on number of days of care. Often, hospitals "average" payments among patients instead of using individualized costs.

Government-funded health care

The federal government of the United States first began to provide health insurance, on a significant basis, because many Americans did not have it due to lack of employment. Medicare was developed to provide health insurance for the elderly, disabled, and patients with end-stage kidney disease. Medicaid was first designed to insure low-income children who did not have parental support, and was later enlarged to cover all low-income people. TRICARE began as CHAMPUS, covering dependents of active-duty military personnel.

As a result of these and other programs, the federal government became the primary insurer for millions of Americans. Huge increases in health care costs related to the government managing coverage for so many people contributed to inflation and harmed employers, resulting in lower wages paid to their employees. Since Medicare and Medicaid, the most significant change in health legislation has been the Patient Protection and Affordable Care Act.

> ### You should remember
>
> In 1965, President Lyndon B. Johnson signed into law the bill that led to the development of Medicare and Medicaid. Originally, Medicare only included Part A, which covered hospital insurance, and Part B, which covered medical insurance.

Medicare plans

Medicare is a federal program that has become the largest single health care program in the United States. It is administered by the Centers for Medicare and Medicaid Services (CMS), which is part of the U.S. Department of Health and Human Services. Medicare was designed to provide patients with the same benefits and health care services that people with private insurance receive. Though set up as a two-part program, Medicare actually includes four separate coverage areas.

- *Part A* or *Medicare Hospital Insurance* reimburses institutional providers for inpatient, hospice, and certain home health services. It pays for critical care access and skilled nursing facility stays. Medicare Part A is funded through a tax paid by working individuals on all of their earned income. Anyone eligible for Medicare Part A may also obtain Part B coverage. However, they must apply and pay a premium to obtain Medicare Part B or to enroll in one of the Medicare Advantage plans. Former federal employees, who received federal employee pensions rather than Social Security and are not covered by Medicare Part A, can purchase Medicare Part B coverage.
- *Part B* or *Medicare Medical Insurance* reimburses institutional providers for outpatient and physicians for inpatient and office services, and also covers durable medical equipment and certain medical services not covered by Part A. Under Part B, after paying an annual deductible, the patient is responsible for 20% of the allowable charge. The amount of the deductible is adjusted yearly.
- *Part C* or *Medicare Advantage* was previously called *Medicare + Choice*; it includes managed care and private fee-for-service plans, which provide contracted care to Medicare patients. It is an alternative plan that is reimbursed under Part A.
- *Part D* or *Medicare Prescription Drug Plans* add prescription drug coverage, certain Medicare Cost Plans, certain Medicare Private Fee-For-Service Plans, and Medicare Medical Savings Account Plans. The medical savings plans set up by the Medicare Modernization Act are similar to private medical savings accounts. They carry high *deductibles* in a fee-for-service plan, as well as a tax-exempt trust that pays for qualified medical expenses.

You should remember

When filing a Medicare claim, the "CMS-1500" form is required. Providers must, according to law, file this form for all eligible Medicare patients.

Beneficiaries can also obtain supplemental Medigap insurance, which help to cover costs not reimbursed by the original Medicare plan. More than one type of Medicare may be available to people, based on the part of the country in which they live.

General Medicare eligibility requires the covered individual or their spouse to have worked for at least ten years in employment covered by Medicare, who are a minimum of 65 years old, and who are citizens or permanent residents of the United States. Individuals under age 65 who have a disability or end-stage renal disease can also qualify for Medicare. A "disability" is defined as something that makes the covered entity unable to do work as before or, if adjustments cannot be made, to do other work due to a medical condition. The disability must last, or be expected to last, one year, or to result in death.

Focus on the various parts of Medicare

For Medicare Part A, most people don't pay a premium for hospital insurance, but for Part B (medical insurance), most people pay a monthly premium. Part C (Medicare Advantage) must be at least equivalent to Parts A and B, and provides much more coverage. Part D covers prescription drugs, for which most people pay a monthly premium.

Medicaid plans

Medicaid is a federally mandated but state-administered medical assistance program. It covers individuals with incomes below the federal poverty level (FPL). Individual states may assign their own variations of the name of this program, such as *MediCal* (in the state of California). States determine eligibility rules and additional benefits. Individual states receive matching funds from the federal government that range between 50% and 76%, based on each state's per-capita income (see Table 4.1). This means that states with higher per-capita income receive lower federal matching funds, and vice versa.

Overall, Medicaid provides medical and health-related services to individuals and families with low incomes and limited resources (known as "medically indigent"), who are U.S. citizens or legal immigrants. It includes the same services as private insurance, including dental and vision care, transportation, and even translation services. Most low-income children have Medicaid coverage, as do about one in three children, regardless of their family income level. It covers more than one-third of all births, and is also the largest source of public funding related to family planning services. The majority of Medicaid spending is for elderly people and for disabled children and adults. Most Medicaid expenditure is for acute care, but it also covers nursing home and long-term care.

Medicaid does not cover all "poor" people, however, and guidelines for eligibility differ between states. The following is a brief overview of eligibility for Medicaid:

- Categorically needy – families who meet Temporary Assistance for Needy Families (TANF) eligibility; caretakers who are relatives or legal guardians of children under age 18, or age 19 if still in high school; individuals and couples living in medical institutions who have a monthly income up to 300% of Supplemental Security Income (SSI); pregnant women and children under age six whose family is at or below 133% of the FPL; SSI recipients (or, in some states, aged, blind, and disabled people meeting more restrictive requirements).
- Medically needy – families that pay monthly premiums equal to the difference between family income and the income eligibility standard; individuals to spend down to Medicaid eligibility by incurring medical/remedial care expenses to offset excess income – this reduces their income to below the maximum allowed by the Medicaid plan of their state.
- Special groups – qualified Medicare beneficiaries, with incomes at or below 100% of the FPL, whose resources are at or below twice the standard allowed under SSI; qualified working disabled individuals, with incomes below 200% of the FPL and resources not more than twice the standard allowed under SSI; qualifying individuals, with incomes between 120% and 175% of the FPL; specified low-income Medicare beneficiaries, with incomes between 100% and 120% of the FPL.

Table 4.1 Medicaid enrollment and payouts (%)

Enrollment	Payouts
Children 48	Disabled 41
Adults 27	Elderly 23
Elderly 21	Children 21
Disabled 15	Adults 15

Source: http://files.kff.org/attachment/issue-brief-medicaid-moving-forward.

> ### You should remember
>
> Nearly all elderly Americans have Medicare, but many people find themselves in financial "gaps" that reduce their coverage. Medicaid assists low-income Medicare beneficiaries with premiums, cost-sharing, and coverage for prescription drugs and long-term care services.

TRICARE and CHAMPVA

TRICARE (formerly *CHAMPUS*) was developed in 1967, to provide military medical care for families of active-duty members. Once reorganized as TRICARE, it became a regionally managed health care program, supplementing the health care resources of the uniformed services with networks of civilian health care professionals. TRICARE supports active-duty uniformed military members, their families, retirees and their families, and survivors who are not eligible for Medicare. It covers members of the Air Force, Army, Coast Guard, Marine Corps, National Oceanic and Atmosphere Administration, Navy, and Public Health Service. TRICARE also covers unmarried children, including stepchildren, or active duty or retired service members.

National Guard and Reserve Component members on active duty for more than 30 days under federal orders are also covered, as are their spouses and unmarried children. Retired National Guard and Reserve Component service members and their families are also covered. Widows or widowers and unmarried children of deceased active-duty or retired service members, Medal of Honor recipients and their family members, and certain eligible former spouses of active-duty or retired service members are additionally covered by TRICARE.

TRICARE options include *Prime*, *Extra*, and *Standard*. TRICARE Prime mostly utilizes military treatment facilities. TRICARE Extra is a preferred provider organization (PPO) option. TRICARE Standard is a fee-for-service option.

CHAMPVA is the abbreviation for the *Civilian Health and Medical Program of the Department of Veterans Affairs*. Under CHAMPVA, this department shares costs of covered health care services and supplies with eligible beneficiaries. It is administered by the Health Administration Center. To be eligible, a beneficiary must be at least one of the following:

- Spouse or child of a veteran rated permanently, totally disabled for a service-connected disability
- Surviving spouse or child of a veteran deceased because of a VA-rated service-connected disability
- Surviving spouse or child of a veteran who died while rated as permanently and totally disabled because of a service-connected disability
- Surviving spouse or child of a military member who died in the line of duty, not due to misconduct; these individuals may be eligible for TRICARE instead of CHAMPVA.

> ### Focus on CHAMPVA
>
> Individuals qualified for CHAMPVA can receive inpatient, outpatient, mental health, prescription medication, and nursing care, but not long-term care.

Indian Health Service

Health services for Native Americans were established in 1921 by the Snyder Act. Today, the Indian Health Service (IHS) is administered by the U.S. Department of Health and Human Services (DHHS). Members of federally recognized tribes and their descendants are eligible for coverage. The current budget for the program is just under $4 billion every year. Out of the 3.4 million American Indians and Alaska Natives in the United States, fewer than two million are serviced by the IHS.

Individual insurance market

Many people in the United States today still sign up and pay for their own health insurance. Approximately 16.3 million people buy their own coverage, or coverage for their family members. When the Affordable Care Act was implemented, individual coverage grew quickly, totaling eight million people initially, which is expected to increase to 24 million by 2024. This is partially due to significant premium subsidies under the Act, as well as the tax penalties imposed on people who meet criteria for buying individual policies. In total, about 15 million people have purchased subsidized private insurance after the Act was implemented.

COBRA

The Consolidated Omnibus Budget Reconciliation Act of 1985 (COBRA) allows employees to continue health care coverage after the termination date of their benefits. This includes coverage under a health maintenance organization (HMO). COBRA amended the Employment Retirement Income Security Act or ERISA to include provisions for health care coverage continuation, applying to group health plans of employers with two or more employees. At their own expense, enrollees maintain health care plan coverage that would have been lost due to termination of employment or other events. The cost of COBRA is comparable to what it would be if the individual were still a member of the employer's health care coverage group.

The COBRA Act required employers with 20 or more employees to allow employees and their dependents to keep their employer-sponsored group health insurance coverage for up to 18 months because of death of the employed spouse, loss of employment or reduction in work hours, or divorce. COBRA allowed former employees, spouses, domestic partners, retirees, and eligible dependent children who lose coverage because of certain events to have temporary continuation of health coverage at group rates. COBRA benefits can actually continue for up to 36 months, based on the qualifying event. When a patient has left a company and has elected to continue coverage in the group health plan under federal COBRA rules, Medicare is considered to be the primary payer.

> **You should remember**
>
> COBRA coverage is often more expensive than the amount employees are required to pay for group health coverage. Normally, employers usually pay part of employee coverage costs. Under COBRA, all of these costs are charged to the employee.

Children's Health Insurance Program

Overseen by the CMS, the Children's Health Insurance Program (CHIP), established in 1997, is overseen by the CMS but managed by the individual states. The plan was expanded when President Obama signed the Children's Health Insurance Program Reauthorization Act in 2009. This program is administered and partially funded on a statewide basis, with children in some states being enrolled in Medicaid. Basically, CHIP provides low-cost health coverage for children whose families earn too much money to qualify for Medicaid. It also covers parents and pregnant women in certain states.

Though CHIP benefits vary widely between the states, comprehensive coverage does include physician visits, dental and vision care, emergency services, immunizations, inpatient and outpatient hospital care, laboratory and X-ray services, prescriptions, and routine check-ups. Many services are free, but some require co-pays, and certain states charge a monthly premium for CHIP coverage. Regardless of your state, you never have to pay more than 5% of your family's income for the year in order to be covered by CHIP.

Focus on "CHIP"

For most families, the Children's Health Insurance Program (CHIP) is free. It covers uninsured children and teenagers for routine physician visits, prescriptions, dental visits, eye care, immunizations, mental health visits, up to 90 days of hospitalization per year, and much more.

The Patient Protection and Affordable Care Act

The *Patient Protection and Affordable Care Act* was passed in 2010, and focused on private health insurance reform. It is the most important piece of health legislation in the United States since Medicare and Medicaid were enacted in 1965. It was discussed in detail in Chapter 2.

Privately funded health care

Privately funded health care in the United States began with BlueCross in 1929. It has grown to become the most popular form of health insurance, and also includes many Medicare beneficiaries who use private insurance to supplement their coverage. After a person retires, privately funded health care may be provided by a previous employer through retirement benefits, or purchased by the individual. Employment-based insurance has declined, as the rate of coverage has increased (up to 2000) and declined since. Privately funded health care has declined slightly since 1994.

There are variances between privately funded health care and employment-based health care. These include comprehensiveness of benefits, premiums, types of available plans, and cost-sharing that may be required. Private health plans offer many different choices of coverage and cost. In general, it is significantly more expensive for an individual to pay for his or her own health insurance than to be part of employment-based health care. In private health insurance, there are many of the same options available in other areas, such as point-of-service, health maintenance organizations, preferred provider organizations, exclusive provider organizations, and indemnity or *fee-for-service plans*. Unfortunately, many private health plans involve high premiums, restricted options, underwriting, lack of guarantees, and recissions.

BlueCross–BlueShield

The popular *BlueCross* and *BlueShield* insurance programs began separately, as two *prepaid health plans* for individuals or groups. They were designed to cover specified medical expenses while premiums were paid up to date. BlueCross began in 1929, guaranteeing up to 21 days of hospitalization per year for subscribers and their dependents, for just a $6 annual premium. BlueShield began in 1938, with physicians' fees for covered medical services paid in full by the plan if the subscriber earned less than $3,000 per year. Once earning more, a small percentage of the physician's fee was required to be paid by the patient. Therefore, originally, BlueCross covered hospital bills while BlueShield covered physician services. In 1977, BlueCross combined with BlueShield, and further consolidation occurred in 1986.

Once joining, BlueCross–BlueShield (BCBS) maintained negotiated contracts with caregivers, making prompt and direct payments of claims, maintaining regional representatives to assist with claims, and providing educational events and materials to keep providers up to date with insurance procedures. BCBS plans are non-profit, receiving tax relief, and cannot cancel coverage for an individual because of poor health, or because payments to providers have exceeded the average of these payments. Policies can only be canceled when premiums are not paid, or if the plan can prove fraud that involves applications for coverage.

BCBS plans must be approved by state insurance commissioners for any increases in rates or changes to benefits that affect that state's members. They must also allow conversion from group to individual coverage, and guarantee transferability of membership from one local plan to another when a covered entity moves to an area served by a different BCBS organization.

Focus on BlueCross–BlueShield

Nationwide, more than 96% of hospitals and 92% of professional health care providers contract directly with BlueCross and BlueShield companies. They cover more than 105 million Americans.

Sources: www.obamacare-health-care.com/Blue-Cross-Blue-Shield-Association; www.bcbs.com/news/press-releases/blue-cross-blue-shield-association-study-reveals-disparities-post-heart-attack.

Kaiser Foundation Health Plan

Henry Kaiser, during World War II, created clinics in California that provided inpatient and outpatient care for shipyard workers. They later were opened to other employers and individuals, becoming called the *Kaiser Permanente Program*. Employers paid fixed amounts per worker over a certain time period, for all required medical care. This payment system is called capitation, and this type of program is also known as a prepaid health plan. Kaiser Permanente became the largest health maintenance organization in the United States, for many years.

The Kaiser Foundation Health Plan was one of three components comprising Kaiser Permanente. It is a non-profit organization that works with employers, employees, and individual members, offering prepaid health plans and insurance. Its funds are reinvested in Kaiser Foundation Hospitals. The Permanente medical groups are owned by physicians, which provide and arrange for the health care of Kaiser Foundation members in respective regions of the country.

> **You should remember**
>
> The Kaiser Permanente plan was the first to establish prepaid health plans, physician group practices, focused preventive medicine, and consolidated, organized health care delivery systems.

Workers' compensation

Both federal and state laws require employers to provide workers' compensation that meets minimum requirements, and covers most employees for work-related illnesses and injuries. Workers' compensation does not apply if a worker was negligent in performing work duties, and was injured or became ill as a result. When a covered injury or illness occurs, the employee receives health care and, if applicable, monetary awards. Dependents of an employee who is killed at work receive benefits.

Workers' compensation laws protect employers and the other workers in the working environment by limiting the amount an injured employee can receive. They also eliminate the liability of coworkers in most accident situations. In federal workers' compensation programs, federal employees or workers employed in significant interstate commerce roles are covered. The workers' compensation laws of individual states apply to most employers there, and establish comprehensive coverage programs. There may be differing limits of liability, a requirement for employees to get workers' compensation coverage for future claims, and the development of a state fund to pay claims when employers have not obtained coverage.

Examples of related federal workers' compensation programs include the Federal Employees' Compensation Act (FECA) Program, the Occupational Safety and Health Administration (OSHA), and the Federal Employment Liability Act (FELA). These programs exist for many different federal employers and industries. For state workers' compensation programs, each state has created a Workers' Board, which may also be called a Workers' Compensation Commission. These boards or commissions administer related laws and handle appeals when claims are denied, or when compensation is insufficient according to an affected employee.

Workers' compensation insurance provides weekly cash payments and reimbursements of health care costs. To qualify, an employee must be injured while working within the scope of his or her job description, while performing a job-related required service, or must have developed a condition that is directly linked to the working environment (see Figure 4.1). An employee injured away from the workplace, such as when driving a company vehicle carrying paperwork or equipment related to work activities, is also covered. Workers' compensation may also cover certain stress-related disorders, which may relate to jobs such as air-traffic control and emergency services.

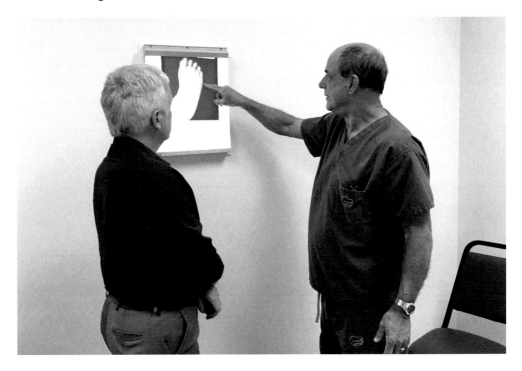

Figure 4.1 An injured employee discusses workers' compensation with an employer.

Focus on federal workers' compensation

Workers' compensation involves four major disability compensation programs for federal workers or their dependents, which include wage replacement benefits, medical treatments, vocational rehabilitation, and other benefits.

Self-insured plans

Self-insured, employer-sponsored group health plans allow larger employers to assume the financial risks of their employees' health care benefits. Employers do not pay fixed premiums to health insurance payers. Instead, a trust fund, of both employer and employee contributions, is established. From this fund, claims are paid.

Medical savings accounts

A *medical savings account* (MSA) is one into which tax-deferred amounts from a person's income can be deposited. These amounts are usually called *contributions*, and may be made by an employee, an employer, or both – based on the appropriate governmental law. The money in a medical savings account is expected to be used for medical expenses.

Withdrawals from the account are usually called *distributions*, which may or may not be subject to income tax. If a withdrawal is made without adequate documentation as to what it is being used for, a penalty may result.

In the United States, MSAs are usually associated with self-employed individuals. Withdrawals are tax-free if used for *qualified medical expenses*. These accounts must be coordinated with a *high-deductible health plan*. Withdrawals from MSAs go toward paying the annual deductible. Funds from MSAs can cover most health care expenses, disability costs, dental care, vision care, and long-term care, regardless of whether expenses were billed through the qualifying insurance or not. Once the annual deductible is met, the high-deductible health plan will pay any remaining covered medical expenses for that year. At the end of the year, if funds remain in the MSA, they can either roll over for the next year, or can be withdrawn as *taxable income*.

Focus on medical savings accounts

Medical savings accounts are similar to the *health savings accounts* that were established in 2003 as part of the Medicare Prescription Drug, Improvement, and Modernization Act.

Insurance and managed care

Managed care health insurance plans are offered by both private insurers and government insurance plans. The term *managed care* refers to various types of *health maintenance organization* and similar types of organization that were established later. The goal of managed care is to control costs while improving preventive care. These plans negotiate reimbursements and limit patients to being treated by providers and facilities with which they have contracts. Managed care plans include five basic concepts:

- The patient chooses one **primary care provider** (PCP), who will provide most of his or her care and also decide what other services are required.
- Care is commonly restricted to providers, hospitals, and laboratories that have accepted the plan's fee schedule or capitation payments.
- The patient may, or may not, have access to providers and services outside the managed care plan. Often, he or she must pay more for services obtained outside the plan. Sometimes the patient must pay the difference between an amount allowed by the plan and the amount actually charged for outside services.
- The plan may require referrals from a PCP for consultations with specialists, physical therapy, speech therapy, certain diagnostic tests, and other services.
- The plan commonly requires prior notification as well as *utilization review* before referral will be authorized to specialists, therapists, surgeons, and for certain procedures or other types of care.

Health maintenance organizations

The first health maintenance organizations (HMOs) were developed as a result of the Health Maintenance Organization Assistance Act of 1973, which authorized federal grants and loans to private organizations in order to develop HMOs. These organizations provide health care services to subscribers in certain areas of the country for fixed fees. Comprehensive health care services are provided to enrolled members on a prepaid basis. Preventive care services are provided to promote good health. This reduces overall costs of medical care. Annual physical examinations are encouraged, and resources such as health risk assessment surveys are available. Primary care providers are responsible for coordinating services and referring enrollees to other health care providers.

A *co-payment* or *co-pay* is usually required, which the enrollee pays to the provider when health care services are rendered. Co-pays range from $1 to $35 per visit. Some services are exempt because co-insurance payments are required instead. Individual state commerce divisions or departments of corporations control the operations of HMOs, depending upon which states they are located in. There are five models of HMOs, as follows:

- Direct contract model – an "open-panel" model, in which contracted health care services are delivered by individual physicians in the community.
- Individual practice association – an "open-panel" model, in which services are delivered by physicians who remain in their independent office settings; also called independent practice associations; physicians are paid on either a fee-for-service or capitation basis.
- Network model – an "open-panel" model, in which services are provided by two or more physician multispecialty group practices.
- Group model – a "closed-panel" model, in which services are delivered by physicians who are members of an independent multispecialty group practice, which can be owned or managed by the HMO, or just contracted with the HMO.
- Staff model – a "closed-panel" model, in which services are provided by physicians employed by the HMO. All ambulatory services are usually provided within HMO corporate buildings.

All BlueCross–BlueShield organizations offer at least one HMO plan, but some HMOs are not easily recognized as BCBS plans because of their names.

A large component of managed forms of health care is called utilization review, which evaluates the appropriateness of provided services. It is designed to ensure that adequate levels of services are given, cost-efficiency is maintained, and subsequent planning of care occurs. Quality of care is a large component of utilization review. Because of the cost of prescription drugs, drug utilization review is a significant practice to prevent patient harm and wasting of drug resources. Prospective utilization review determines appropriateness of health care components prior to care actually being delivered. Concurrent utilization review is a daily determination of length of hospitalization, use of ancillary services, and appropriateness of medical treatments. It is linked to *discharge planning*, focusing on post-discharge continuity of care. Retrospective utilization review examines health care services after they have been delivered, which helps with future health care planning outcomes.

Focus on Health Maintenance Organizations (HMOs)

Coverage provided by HMOs is usually less per month than other types of health insurance. You work with one primary care physician who is responsible for assigning all other caregivers to you, except for emergency room or OB/GYN visits. However, HMOs are not available everywhere and may not cover all the services you need.

Preferred provider organizations

A preferred provider organization (PPO) is also known as a *participating provider organization*. In a PPO, physicians and hospitals join with insurers, employers, and other organizations to provide health care to subscribers for a discounted fee. While contracts for pharmacy or laboratory services are not regularly made, there usually are contracts with specific hospitals that are offered at reduced rates. The majority of PPOs allow patients to use non-PPO providers, but this results in larger out-of-pocket expenses. The co-payments, deductibles, and premiums for a PPO are usually less than those for fee-for-service plans, but more than those for HMOs.

The PPO offered by BlueCross–BlueShield utilizes the word "subscriber" instead of "policyholder." Subscribers must remain within networked PPO providers, and must request referrals to PPO specialists whenever possible. They also must follow the managed care requirements of the policy, such as getting second surgical opinions. If not followed, the subscriber will have claims denied or reduced payments made to providers.

> ### Focus on preferred provider organizations (PPOs)
>
> PPOs are usually more flexible in their health care coverage than HMOs, but are also usually more expensive. With a PPO, you are basically paying for their more flexible coverage.

Organizational cost control

Since health care financing and cost control are closely related, organizational cost control can be said to be reflective of affordable insurance. Insurance is the primary factor that determines the actual amount of demand for medical services. *Demand* is defined here as the quantity of health care purchased. One consideration is when providers have a financial interest in additional treatments, which create an artificial *provider-induced demand*. The quantity of health care consumed is referred to as *utilization of health care services*.

When financing for health insurance is restricted, expenditures for health care are eventually affected. On the other hand, if health insurance is extended to the uninsured, without supply-side rationing, total health care expenditures will increase. Insurance and payments influence availability of health services. When provider reimbursements are reduced, there is a direct influence upon health care expenditures. Reimbursement cuts have previously been made to slow the growth of health care expenditures.

Direct payments from patients

Patients who lack health insurance must pay cash for health services. Those using out-of-network providers also pay cash and then request reimbursement. Increasing numbers of physicians have become out-of-network providers – especially those who are specialists in urban markets with wealthier clients. More insurers are moving to narrow provider networks, and find they can offer lower rates if they focus on doing business with only a small set of providers. More and more individuals and employers are willing to give up access to larger networks of providers in order to reduce costs. Hospitals and other providers have begun setting high rates for patients who pay out of pocket, and often do not itemize the costs prior to collecting payments. As a result, people are requesting more transparency from health care providers regarding the costs of services.

Comparisons of U.S. health care with other countries

While the United States has traditionally relied on private, employer-based health insurance, the majority of other developed countries have not. Great Britain, France, Canada, and other countries spend much of their gross domestic product (GDP) on the financing of health care. Examples of various government-funded health care services are as follows:

- *Great Britain* – The National Health Service (NHS) is primarily funded through taxation. It provides a comprehensive range of health services, which are mostly free for legal residents. Approximately two-thirds of general practitioners and dentists are reimbursed primarily through capitation, with the remainder mostly from fee-for-service payments based on performance. Clinical commissioning groups control most of the health system budget, and purchase hospital and specialty care for patients. A newer *Payment by Results* system is now in place, based on average costs of procedures or treatments across the entire health system. Great Britain has 2.8 practicing physicians per 1,000 population. The NHS is one of the largest public service organizations in Europe, having more than one million employees and more than 2,500 hospitals. Though the British have made significant efforts to reduce inefficiencies in their system, they have been partially blocked by opposition from medical professionals, and the separation that exists between general practitioners, hospitals, and community health organizations.
- *Canada* – National health care is also primarily funded through taxation. It is mostly free at the point of use and has most services provided by private entities. The Canadian health system is unique in that prescription drugs are not covered. Primary care physicians are paid on a fee-for-service basis, using a relative value scale for reimbursable procedures or codes. Fee schedules vary widely between the various provinces of Canada. A newer method of blended capitation, relying on payments adjusted for age and gender, is being used in some areas of the country. Financial incentives are used to encourage evidence-based guidelines. Canada has 2.4 practicing physicians per 1,000 population. Hospitals are mostly private and non-profit, but almost totally funded by the public, meaning they have extremely tight budgets. Since most physicians must refer patients to hospitals for diagnoses and tests, there are often extended waiting times.
- *France* – The French health system is partially funded by taxation, as well as by government funding, and users who must pay small amounts of costs for the health care they receive. Physicians in private hospitals and ambulatory facilities are reimbursed via a fee schedule decided upon by their associations, health system funds, and the government. Between 15% and 25% of physicians extra-bill beyond negotiated fees, but these are primarily specialists. Physicians in public hospitals receive salaries. France has 3.3 practicing physicians per 1,000 population. The country also has more hospital beds than the United States, Great Britain, or Canada. Problems exist in coordination between hospitals and community-based physicians.

Comparatively, the United States pays much higher prices for medical care. This is primarily because our health care system does not operate within a budget, and does not aggressively negotiate prices with providers. The United States has 2.5 practicing physicians per 1,000 population.

> ## CASE STUDY
>
> Lack of ability to pay for health care often means that an individual waits too long to seek treatment for a condition, then goes to an emergency department when it intensifies. Unfortunately, it may be too late. An example of this scenario is a woman who failed to get treatment for lupus due to a lack of insurance. One night, her condition worsened so much that she had a seizure. The woman was rushed to the emergency department by her mother, and the hospital did everything they could to treat her. Regardless of their help, the woman died within a few months.
>
> 1 List some reasons why this woman may not have been able to get insurance coverage that she could afford.
> 2 Research how an emergency department bill can be paid off if the patient does not qualify as indigent.
> 3 Use the Internet to find out how many Americans die every year who lack health insurance.

Chapter highlights

This section answers the Objectives found at the beginning of the chapter.

1 Describe reimbursements for health care services.

- Most health care services are reimbursed using fee-for-service payments, when the service or services occur. Fees vary widely between practitioners and locations. Public and private health coverage utilize capitation, which uses fixed amounts paid from insurers to providers for certain services. Fee-for-service pays for particular services rendered (itemized) at a specific time. The third means of reimbursing health care services is through salaries, in companies where other incentives are provided to practitioners in order to increase productivity.

2 Explain how Medicare, Medicaid, and TRICARE originated.

- Medicare originated to provide health insurance for the elderly, disabled, and patients with end-stage kidney disease.
- Medicaid originated to insure low-income children who did not have parental support, and was later enlarged to cover all low-income people.
- TRICARE began as CHAMPUS, covering the dependents of active-duty military personnel.

3 Summarize the four parts of Medicare.

- Part A – Hospital Insurance – reimburses institutional providers, pays for critical care access and skilled nursing facility stays
- Part B – Medical Insurance – reimburses institutional providers and physicians; covers durable medical equipment and services not covered by Part A
- Part C – Advantage – includes managed care, private fee-for-service plans that provide contracted care; it is reimbursed under Part A
- Part D – Prescription Drug Plans – add prescription drug coverage, certain cost plans, certain fee-for-service plans, and medical savings account plans

4 **Explain the three classifications of people who qualify for Medicaid.**

- Categorically needy – either meet the Temporary Assistance for Needy Families eligibility, are caretakers, live in medical institutions and have monthly income up to 300% of SSI, are pregnant women or children under age six at or below 133% of the FPL, or are SSI recipients
- Medically needy – pay monthly premiums equal to the difference between family income and the income eligibility standard; individuals spending down to eligibility by incurring expenses to offset excess income
- Special groups – beneficiaries with income at or below 100% of the FPL, at or below twice the SSI-allowed standard; working disabled individuals with incomes below 200% of the FPL and resources not more than twice the same standard; those with incomes between 120% and 175% of the FPL; and those with incomes between 100% and 120% of the FPL.

5 **Describe the four requirements needed to qualify for CHAMPVA.**

- Spouse or child of a veteran who is permanently, totally disabled because of a service-connected disability
- Surviving spouse or child of a veteran deceased because of a VA-rated service-connected disability
- Surviving spouse or child of a veteran who died as permanently and totally disabled because of a service-connected disability
- Surviving spouse or child of a military member who died in the line of duty, not due to misconduct.

6 **Define the terms "indemnity" and "capitation."**

- Indemnity is a type of health insurance plan also called "fee-for-service," in which patients can direct their own health care and visit nearly any physician or hospital; the insurer pays a set portion of total charges
- Capitation is a payment arrangement for providers that pays them a certain amount for each enrolled person assigned to them, for a certain period, regardless of whether that person seeks care.

7 **Briefly explain when workers' compensation does and does not apply.**

- Workers' compensation covers most employees for work-related illnesses and injuries. Injury must occur while working within the scope of the job description, performing a job-related required service, or be due to a condition directly linked to the working environment. An employee injured away from the workplace, such as when driving a company vehicle, is also covered. Stress-related disorders, which may relate to jobs such as air-traffic control and emergency services, may be covered.
- It does not apply if a worker was negligent in performing work, and was injured or became ill as a result. It limits the liability of coworkers in most accident situations.

8 **What type of person usually uses a medical savings account, and what is covered by withdrawals (distributions) from this type of account?**

- Medical savings accounts are usually associated with self-employed individuals. Withdrawals (distributions) should be used for qualified medical expenses. They go toward paying the annual deductible associated with a high-deductible health plan.

Funds can cover most health care expenses, disability, dental care, vision care, and long-term care, regardless of whether expenses were billed through the qualifying insurance or not.

9 **Compare and contrast HMOs and PPOs.**

- Health maintenance organizations (HMOs) provide services in certain areas, for fixed fees. Comprehensive services are provided to members on a prepaid basis. Preventive services are provided to promote good health. Primary care providers coordinate services and refer enrollees to other providers. A co-payment is usually required when services are rendered. An HMO may be: a direct contract model, individual practice association, network model, group model, or staff model. Utilization reviews are important components of HMOs.
- Preferred provider organizations (PPOs), or participating provider organizations, consist of physicians and hospitals that join with insurers, employers, and others to provide care to subscribers for a discounted fee. There are usually contracts with specific hospitals, offered at reduced rates. Most PPOs allow patients to use non-PPO providers, resulting in larger out-of-pocket expenses. Co-payments, deductibles, and premiums are usually less than those for fee-for-service plans, but more than those for HMOs.

10 **Briefly describe the five models of health maintenance organizations.**

- Direct contract model – services by individual physicians in the community
- Individual practice association – services by physicians in independent offices; also called independent practice associations; physicians paid by fee-for-service or capitation
- Network model – services by two or more multispecialty group practices
- Group model – services by physicians in an independent multispecialty group practice, owned or managed by the HMO, or contracted with it
- Staff model – services by physicians employed by the HMO; ambulatory services usually provided within HMO corporate buildings.

Summary

In regard to health care financing in the United States, the federal government has developed health insurance programs for the unemployed, elderly, disabled, low-income, and military personnel and their dependents, plus those with certain chronic conditions. Therefore, the government became the primary insurer for millions of Americans. Prior to the Affordable Care Act, these programs included Medicare, Medicaid, TRICARE, CHAMPVA, COBRA, and CHIP. Privately funded health care began with BlueCross, and also includes BlueShield, the Kaiser Foundation Health Plan, and workers' compensation. Self-insured plans, medical savings accounts, health maintenance organizations, preferred provider organizations, and various organizational cost controls were developed to help offer more alternatives to Americans to manage their health care needs.

> ### Review questions
>
> 1 What are various methods of reimbursement for health care services?
> 2 Compare the various plans offered by Medicare and Medicaid.
> 3 What is the difference between TRICARE and COBRA?
> 4 What is Medicare Part C?
> 5 What is the Kaiser Foundation Health Plan?
> 6 What is the Children's Health Insurance Program?
> 7 Compare self-insured plans and medical savings accounts.
> 8 What is a health maintenance organization?
> 9 What is workers' compensation?
> 10 What is a primary care provider?

Bibliography

Austin, D.R., et al. 2013. Small increases to employer premiums could shift millions of people to the exchanges and add billions to federal outlays. *Health Affairs* 32, no. 9: 1531–1537.

Barr, D.A. 2011. *Introduction to U.S. Health Policy: The Organization, Financing, and Delivery of Health Care in America, 3rd Edition*. Baltimore: Johns Hopkins University Press. Print.

Berarducci, J., et al. 2012. New partnership opportunities for payers and providers. *Healthcare Financial Management* 66, no. 10: 58–61.

Blanchfield, B.B., et al. 2010. Saving billions of dollars and physicians' time by streamlining billing practices. *Health Affairs* 29, no. 6: 1248–1254.

BlueCross BlueShield. 2016. Blue Cross Blue Shield Association Study Reveals Disparities in Post-Heart Attack Treatment between Women and Men. Available at: www.bcbs.com/news/press-releases/blue-cross-blue-shield-association-study-reveals-disparities-post-heart-attack. Chicago: Blue Cross Blue Shield Association.

Bronstein, M. 2012. *U.S. Investment in Health Research: 2011*. Alexandria: Research America.

Claxton, G., et al. 2010. *Employer Health Benefits: 2010 Annual Survey*. Menlo Park: The Kaiser Family Foundation.

CMS.gov. 2015. Health Care Financing Review. Available at: www.cms.gov/Research-Statistics-Data-and-Systems/Research/HealthCareFinancingReview/index.html. Baltimore: U.S. Centers for Medicare and Medicaid Services.

Cohen, A.B., Colby, D.C., Wailoo, K.A., and Zelizer, J.E. 2015. *Medicare and Medicaid at 50: America's Entitlement Programs in the Age of Affordable Care*. New York: Oxford University Press. Print.

Conn, J. 2013. Tipping point. *Modern Healthcare* 43, no. 25: 14–15.

Employee Benefit Research Institute (EBRI). 2013. *Fast Facts: Why Uninsured? Most Workers Cite Cost*. No. 243. Washington, D.C.: Employee Benefit Research Institute.

Fronstin, P. 2012. *Sources of Health Insurance and Characteristics of the Uninsured: Analysis of the March 2012 Current Population Survey*. Issue Brief No. 376. Washington, D.C.: Employee Benefit Research Institute.

Green, M.A. 2014. *Understanding Health Insurance: A Guide to Billing and Reimbursement, 12th Edition*. Boston: Delmar Cengage Learning. Print.

Hartman, M., et al. 2011. Health spending growth at a historic low in 2008. *Health Affairs* 29, no. 1: 147–155.

Ho, V., et al. 2013. State deregulation and Medicare costs for acute cardiac care. *Medical Care Research & Review* 70, no. 2: 185–205.

Holahan, J. 2011. The 2007–09 recession and health insurance coverage. *Health Affairs* 30, no. 1: 145–152.

Hussey, P.S., et al. 2012. *Bundled Payment: Effects on Health Care Spending and Quality*. Rockville: Agency for Healthcare Research and Quality.

Hwang, W., et al. 2013. Effects of integrated delivery system on cost and quality. *American Journal of Managed Care* 19, no. 5: e175–e184.

Krugman, P. 2008. Health Care Horror Stories. Available at: www.nytimes.com/2008/04/11/opinion/11krugman.html?_r=0. New York: The New York Times.

McQueen, M.P., and Meyer, H. 2013. A different kind of Medicaid expansion. *Modern Healthcare* 43, no. 30: 6–16.

Medicaid.gov. 2016. Keeping America Healthy – Home Page. Available at: http://medicaid.gov. Baltimore: U.S. Centers for Medicare and Medicaid Services.

Medicare.gov. 2016. MyMedicare.gov – Home Page. Available at: www.medicare.gov. Baltimore: U.S. Centers for Medicare and Medicaid Services.

Mulvaney, C. 2013. Insurance market reform: The grand experiment. *Healthcare Financial Management* 67, no. 4: 82–86, 88.

National Prevention Council. 2011. *Nation Prevention Strategy: America's Plan for Better Health and Wellness*. Washington, D.C.: U.S. Department of Health and Human Services.

Obamacare Health Care. 2016. About the BCBSA (Blue Cross and Blue Shield Companies). Available at: www.obamacare-health-care.com/Blue-Cross-Blue-Shield-Association. New York: Obamacare Health Care.

Paradise, J. 2015. The Kaiser Commission on Medicaid and the Uninsured – Medicaid Moving Forward. Available at: http://files.kff.org/attachment/issue-brief-medicaid-moving-forward. Menlo Park: Kaiser Family Foundation.

Robinson, J. 2011. Hospitals respond to Medicare payment shortfalls by both shifting costs and cutting them, based on market concentration. *Health Affairs* 30, no. 7: 1265–1271.

Sorenson, C., et al. 2013. Medical technology as a key driver of rising health expenditures: Disentangling the relationship. *ClinicoEconomics and Outcomes Research* 5: 223–234.

TRICARE. 2016. TRICARE – Home Page. Available at: www.tricare.mil. Falls Church: Defense Health Agency / Military Health System.

U.S. Department of Veterans Affairs. 2016. VHA Office of Community Care – CHAMPVA. Available at: www.va.gov/hac/forbeneficiaries/champva/handbook/chandbook.pdf. Washington, D.C.: U.S. Department of Veterans Affairs.

Wall Street Journal. 2010. Republicans and ObamaCare. *Wall Street Journal – Eastern Edition*, March 23: A20.

WorkersCompensation.com. 2016. Workers Compensation – Home Page. Available at: www.workerscompensation.com. Sarasota: WorkersCompensation.com, LLC.

Yee, T., et al. 2012. Small employers and self-insured health benefits: Too small to succeed? *Issue Brief No. 138*. Washington, D.C.: Center for Studying Health System Change.

Chapter 5

Customer service

Objectives

After completing this chapter, the reader should be able to:

1 Define the term "quality of care."
2 Differentiate between the terms "quality assessment," "quality assurance," and "quality control."
3 Explain what the terms "macro quality" and "micro quality" mean.
4 Briefly explain the four factors required to maintain quality of health care.
5 Suggest how health insurance reviewers may compromise a physician's ability to determine the best health care for each patient.
6 Identify how quality assessment and performance improvement (QAPI) programs affect quality improvement.
7 Briefly explain "continuous quality improvement."
8 List two examples of methods used to improve quality of care while reducing costs.
9 Give examples of methods that provide better customer satisfaction.
10 Define "constructive criticism."

Overview

In the health care professions, the term *customer* refers to both internal and external individuals. *Internal customers* are people who work in the health care industry, including physicians, nurses, dietitians, social workers, physical therapists, administrators, and many others. *External customers* include patients, customers, clients, or consumers. All external customers expect to receive care that is of high quality and is delivered professionally.

Determining a patient's quality of care includes many factors, such as courtesy, timeliness, proper scheduling, adequate instructions and education, obtaining of consent for procedures, compassion of caregivers, comfortable patient environments, and personal treatment.

More than any other factor, quality of care is based on the patient's perception of mutual trust and respect with caregivers. Health care professionals must always attempt to build constructive, positive relationships with all patients. Quality of care involves methods such as quality assurance and quality control, which use continued monitoring of care to provide quality improvement. Other measures such as **utilization review** are also implemented. Collectively, these various methods combine to provide customer satisfaction, which results in high levels of excellent customer service.

Quality of care

The **quality of care** that a patient receives is of the utmost concern in every health care profession. It must be documented so that there is a record of care that was provided to patients by health care professionals. When a deficiency in the quality of care is discovered, the individuals involved can receive specific training to improve all future quality of care.

In health care, **quality** may be evaluated by communities, individuals, or populations. It is not always easy to measure. Desired health **outcomes** are emphasized, based on their scientifically identified improvements by the provided services. When it is scientifically impossible to compare quality measures, it is not certain whether the medical system is at fault. Higher health care payments do not mean better health. High-quality care must be cost-effective. For **quality assessment** of health care, there is an increasing need to incorporate its cost. Quality assessment of health care means how quality is measured against established standards. The process of improving quality of care and taking into account all of these factors is ongoing.

Dimensions of quality

Quality can be evaluated in both "micro" and "macro" approaches. **Micro quality** concerns the point at which health care services are delivered, the effects of these services, and the performance of individuals and organizations. **Macro quality** is concerned with populations, and the performance of the entire health care system. It evaluates how often certain health conditions occur, and how life expectancy and mortality rates are affected by various conditions.

The micro approach to evaluating quality includes clinical and interpersonal factors, as well as quality of life. It focuses on technical quality of health care facilities and caregivers, treatments that are used, cost-efficiency, and health outcomes. *Medical errors*, which are preventable adverse effects of health care, are linked to a lack of clinical quality. They may or may not be evident or harmful to patients, and include the following:

- Behavioral outcomes caused by errors
- Diagnoses that are inaccurate or incomplete
- Infections caused by errors
- Injury to the patient
- Syndromes that develop because of errors
- Treatments that are inaccurate or incomplete.

> ## Focus on medical errors
>
> In 2014, the first case of Ebola occurred in the United States, in Dallas, Texas. A man who had traveled from West Africa, where there was an Ebola outbreak, went to the local hospital with flu-like symptoms. One of the nurses there who took the patient's history did not ask about any traveling the man might have done. He was, therefore, treated for the flu and released. Within 48 hours, he returned with signs and symptoms of Ebola. The CDC recommended testing for the disease, which was confirmed. As a result of this medical error, this patient died, and other people contracted Ebola.

Types of medical error include **medication errors** (adverse drug events), **surgical errors**, **diagnostic errors**, and **systemic factors**, which include organization of health care and how resources are distributed. Interpersonal factors involve how patients perceive their caregivers. It is a proven fact that positive patient–caregiver interactions greatly contribute to better patient health outcomes. The way a patient is treated, from the first person that greets them at the front desk to the specialist who performs a difficult procedure upon them, influences patient perceptions – and, therefore, health outcomes. Patient satisfaction surveys play an important role in gauging interpersonal factors between caregivers and patients.

> ## You should remember
>
> Approximately 98,000 Americans die each year as a result of medical errors, with nearly 7,000 of these attributable to actual medication errors.
> *Sources:* www.nationalacademies.org/hmd/~/media/Files/Report%20 Files/1999/To-Err-is-Human/To%20Err%20is%20Human%201999%20%20 report%20brief.pdf; www.ahrq.gov/sites/default/files/wysiwyg/ professionals/quality-patient-safety/patient-safety-resources/resources/ advances-in-patient-safety/vol4/nosek.pdf.

There is a variety of methods that are used to reduce the numbers of deaths and adverse outcomes caused by medical errors. These methods include:

- *Root cause analysis* – this identifies the primary causes of medical errors, which involves understanding of the actual error, when it happened, where it happened, and its outcome
- *Failure mode and effects analysis* – this looks at vulnerable areas or processes in health care, to identify potential areas where errors are more likely to occur in the future
- *Better information sharing* – the use of computerized information sharing systems helps to make sure that all health care professionals involved in any patient's treatment are able to share up-to-date information and cross-check for inaccuracies
- *Appropriate patient education* – informing patients in terms they can understand about all of the information related to their health care condition, and then having them explain what they were told back to the health care provider, is an excellent way to increase their knowledge and to help avoid possible errors, primarily in relation to medication usage
- *Better error reporting* – ongoing improvements in electronic health record systems allow for automatic data reporting, which eliminates many steps formerly handled by health

care professionals; mobile technologies are offering more widespread sharing of information concerning medical errors; new technologies for data and pattern analysis are allowing for error reporting to be analyzed more deeply.

Each patient's *health-related quality of life* involves perceptions of health quality, ability to function, limitations caused by physical or emotional problems, and personal happiness. There are also *disease-specific* perceptions related to impairments, treatments, and adverse effects of treatments. Another area of perception with regard to quality of life is related to institutions such as hospitals. This focuses on patient perceptions concerning their comfort within an institution, if they are able to have self-governance, and basic human factors. Comfort factors include cleanliness, noise, odors, safety, air quality, lighting, temperature, and furnishings within a modern health institution (see Figure 5.1). A patient's self-governance concerns his or her own freedom to make decisions or complaints, and the staff's accommodation of things the patient does and does not like. Human factors include how caregivers treat and show compassion for patients, privacy levels, respect of confidentiality, patient dignity, and freedom from all forms of abusive situations.

Quality assurance

Quality assurance is defined as a method of ensuring high-quality performance in all business activities. It is designed to provide quality improvement, and is based on total quality management. Quality control is a program that monitors all phases of business activities to ensure high quality.

Unfortunately, recent studies have shown that the United States currently ranks *in last place* when the quality of its health care is compared to the following ten nations:

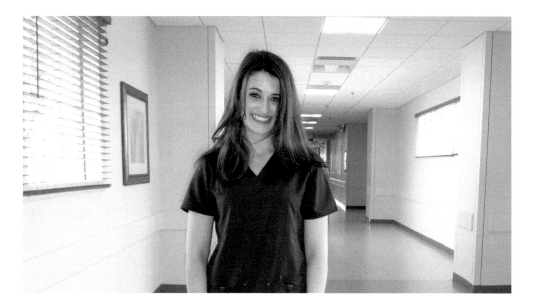

Figure 5.1 A modern health institution (showing a neat, clean, and well-lit area of a hospital).

Australia, Canada, France, Germany, the Netherlands, New Zealand, Norway, Sweden, Switzerland, and the United Kingdom. While the United States spends more of its gross domestic product on health care than any other country, it only ranks as the 37th best in patient outcomes.

Quality in health care is the degree to which services increase the likelihood of desired health outcomes. This definition covers individuals and groups of patients, including people who seek care and those that do not. There are six "dimensions" of quality: safety, effectiveness, patient-centered focus, timeliness, efficiency, and equitability.

Today, health care providers find it difficult to balance high-quality care with cost control. Just because care costs more in certain places than in others, it does not guarantee the highest level of care. Regarding their quality of care, patients are concerned that services are delivered well, that outcomes are good, and that there is easy access to services. Patients expect their care to be delivered quickly and safely, and that continued care is well coordinated.

Factors to consider when considering quality of care include patient education, length of hospitalizations, management of complications, pre-existing conditions, and the availability of family members and friends who may need to assist patients. Quality of care may differ because of location of medical facilities, percentages of elderly patients in comparison to other age groups, socioeconomic factors, and many other complicated issues. The goal is, obviously, to provide 100% correct care without errors, but this is extremely difficult realistically. However, all health care professionals must attempt to provide care that is always appropriate, competent, and conscientious.

Focus on health care quality assurance

Health care quality assurance consists of activities and programs designed to assure or improve the quality of care in either a defined medical setting or a program. It addresses medical errors, cross infections, evidence-based medicine, and patient satisfaction.

To maintain quality of health care, the following are required:

- *Clinical practice guidelines* – descriptions that accurately represent preferred clinical processes for specific conditions
- *Cost-efficiency* – also called cost-effectiveness; services are cost-efficient when received benefits are greater than costs incurred to provide services. Overuse or *overutilization* occurs when additional care is delivered, but costs or risks of treatment outweigh benefits. Underuse or *underutilization* occurs when benefits or interventions outweigh risks or costs, but the benefits or interventions are still not used.
- *Critical pathways* – methods of case management that are based on outcomes and are centered on patients. They work between many medical disciplines and help care to be coordinated between many caregivers and clinical departments. Timelines identify planned medical interventions as well as expected patient outcomes for certain classes of cases or specific diagnoses.
- *Risk management* – proactive efforts designed to prevent adverse events in clinical care and facilities operations. It focuses on preventing medical malpractice, while encouraging cost-efficiency.

Insurance company reviewers are another area of concern. They make many patient care decisions, determining whether procedures are medically "necessary" and if lower-cost alternative procedures are available. Some procedures must be *preauthorized* before they can be performed, such as certain surgeries and hospital admissions for non-emergencies (see Figure 5.2). However, these reviewers may not have a lot of medical training, and base their decisions on statistics about average patients with similar diseases or conditions.

Reviewers have the ability to approve or deny procedures that are recommended by physicians. They may approve cheaper procedures instead of those that were recommended, or only a limited number of treatments. They may only approve a surgery if it is done on an outpatient basis. This compromises the physician's ability to determine the best health care for each patient. Patients may worry that they are not receiving needed care. However, the number of unnecessary surgeries and procedures has actually decreased.

Focus on health insurer denials for diagnostic tests

There is usually a good reason behind a health insurer's denial of coverage for diagnostic tests. The tests may not be necessary, may not reveal any new information because of similar tests already performed, or a less expensive test is available that will reveal the same information.

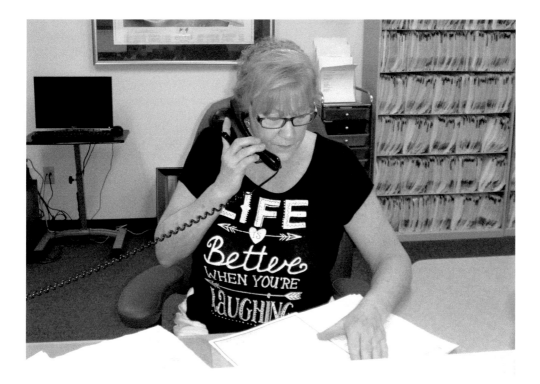

Figure 5.2 A medical assistant calling an insurance company for preauthorization.

Quality improvement

Quality improvement is described as improving or preserving quality of care while decreasing costs. Agencies such as the Centers for Medicare and Medicaid Services (CMS) have developed monitoring systems within the various health care organizations it oversees. This monitoring identifies ways to decrease costs while still keeping quality of care at proper levels.

To improve quality, health care facilities should establish a *quality assessment and performance improvement* (QAPI) program. The basic elements of these programs affect quality improvement in the following ways:

- They are evaluated regularly.
- They evaluate continuity and coordination of patient care.
- They include consumer satisfaction measures.
- They evaluate and monitor high-risk and high-volume services as well as care of acute and chronic conditions.
- They provide access to collected information when this is necessary to monitor and ensure quality of care.
- They establish written protocols for utilization review, which are based on current medical practice standards.
- They allow for health care professionals to review all processes.
- They allow for data collection, analysis, and reporting – this means that quality care indicators are presented.
- They create or change ways of medical practice, based on identified areas needing improvement.
- They are able to detect underutilization and overutilization of services.
- They can evaluate services, informing providers and enrollees of results.
- They can base utilization review protocols on medical practice standards.
- They can publish information that helps provide more coverage options.
- They can offer systematic follow-up to assess effectiveness of programs.

You should understand that the term *quality*, in relation to patient care, means the degree that delivered services meet both professional standards and good outcomes of care. Good quality health care involves procedures that are correct and timely, properly performed on the correct patient, and achieve the best possible outcome. Basically, the "Golden Rule" applies to patient care – correctly choosing the best treatments and procedures for a patient that you would, as a health care professional, choose for yourself. The best interests of the patient should always be of utmost importance.

Continuous quality improvement involves follow-through in gathering and assessing data. This data can then provide future improvements in health care efficiency. Programs have different names, one of which is total quality management, but they all focus on meeting internal needs of health care facilities. This takes time, but offers higher degrees of care than ever before.

You should remember

Continuous quality improvement encourages all health care professionals to ask the questions, "How are we doing?" and "Can we do it better, more efficiently, or more quickly?"

Utilization review or *utilization management* is the evaluation of health care services, facilities, and procedures. It focuses on their appropriateness, efficiency, and necessity. Utilization review can be performed by public agencies or peer review groups. It usually involves comparing specific cases to an aggregate (collected) set of cases, according to certain benchmarks, data, or protocols. Mostly, utilization review focuses on patient records and bills, and is one of the main ways that health insurers control costs and overutilization, while managing care. Utilization review was discussed in greater detail in Chapter 4.

Focus on utilization review

Utilization review is utilized by health insurers and providers to determine if diagnoses and treatments are medically necessary. It is usually done after services are delivered and varies between different states. A utilization review usually involves three stages: case review by a licensed practitioner that is reviewed by a physician, an appeal for a second review, and a review by a specialist.

Quality improvement organizations

Quality improvement organizations are private and usually not-for-profit. They are run by physicians and other health care professionals, and focus on Medicaid and Medicare. These organizations assess whether care is provided, and if it is necessary and reasonable. Examples of methods used to improve quality of care while reducing costs include:

- Avoiding the prescribing of broad-spectrum antibiotics, in favor of using cultures followed by more specific antibiotics
- Using disposable bibs to prevent hospitalized patient gowns from becoming soiled and requiring laundering
- Addressing individual complaints, appeals, and violations to avoid related problems in the future
- Offering education and outreach to better inform patients, families, and providers about quality improvement methods.

Examples of quality improvement organizations are listed in Table 5.1.

Customer satisfaction

Patient satisfaction is an essential component of quality of care. Health care facilities often mail out questionnaires to their customers to determine levels of provided care and patient satisfaction. They may also call their customers and ask for responses about care (see Figure 5.3). It is important in the competitive market of health care that the providers' organizations and characteristics are focused on customer satisfaction.

To ensure good customer satisfaction, health care professionals must attempt to understand their thoughts, avoid interrupting, and not make an attempt to defend themselves or their facilities. Every health care professional in his or her facility is responsible for patient

Table 5.1 Quality improvement organizations

Organization	Description
Community quality collaboratives	Regional organizations that are active in encouraging community engagement, facilitating quality improvement, and public reporting
Employers and employer organizations	Individually and as a group, they seek to incentivize higher quality and value; they are very large, and are concerned with both employee health and health care costs; examples include the *National Business Group on Health* and the *National Business Coalition on Health*
Institute for Healthcare Improvement (IHI)	A non-profit organization that seeks to organize and mobilize quality improvement and transformation; it does this with learning networks and collaboration
National Committee for Quality Assurance (NCQA)	Accredits and certifies health care programs, focusing on health plans, disease management organizations, primary care medical homes, and accountable care organizations; also maintains Healthcare Effectiveness Data and Information Set (HEDIS) measures of health plans
National Quality Forum (NQF)	A non-profit, membership-based organization that focuses on quality measurement, endorses standards for performance measurement, and promotes measures for use in public reporting and payment
Quality improvement organizations (QIOs)	Health quality experts, clinicians, and consumers who work with the CMS to improve care for Medicare beneficiaries and also review quality concerns; the QIOs that do quality improvement are separate from those doing reviews
The Joint Commission	A non-profit organization that accredits and certifies health care organizations and programs, critical to hospitals and other organizations since the CMS requires accreditation in order to participate in the Medicare program
University research programs	At major universities, these are funded by the National Institutes of Health, AHRQ, and private foundations; they develop quality and safety measures along with evidence on how quality and safety can be improved on all levels

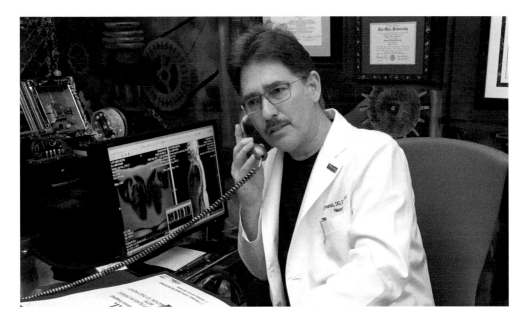

Figure 5.3 A physician giving a follow-up call to a patient.

satisfaction. Every unhappy patient is likely to tell many other people about his or her perceived inadequate health care. Health care professionals must understand that patient satisfaction is subjective, and determine all patient concerns. Small events such as long waiting
times often result in patients telling others about poor treatment (see Figure 5.4). Methods
that help to provide better customer satisfaction, for both internal and external customers,
are listed in Table 5.2.

Figure 5.4 Patients sitting for a long time in a waiting room.

Table 5.2 Methods to provide better customer satisfaction

Method	Steps you should take
Identify problems	Be open-minded to complaints Attempt to understand the complainant's feelings Do not interrupt, but ask clarifying questions Avoid showing verbal or non-verbal defensiveness Thank the complainant for the information, which will help establish their satisfaction
Find a resolution	If the complainant has a personal issue with you, it is appropriate to apologize, thank them for feedback, and assure them that you will try your best not to repeat the error If you need more information before being able to resolve the problem, let the complainant know when you will be able to respond Provide the complainant with any information he or she may be missing, determining if he or she is open-minded about it Use wording that is non-defensive and does not place blame on the complainant If you are not authorized to deal with the complaint, refer the complainant to the correct person, or ask the correct person to contact the complainant
Confirm customer satisfaction	Find out if the complainant feels that the problem has been satisfactorily resolved

For internal customers, make sure to praise them as well as constructively criticize them whenever required. Helping coworkers to feel proud of their contributions is just as important as pointing out areas in which they need to improve. Constructive criticism is optimistic in nature. It should be used to encourage coworkers or subordinates that occurrences resulting in negative outcomes can be learned from and improved upon. Constructive criticism offers basic steps that individuals can follow to improve their work. Remember that employees who are satisfied with their jobs and self-effectiveness will be able to better satisfy their customers.

You should remember

Patient satisfaction surveys can show that a medical practice is interested in quality of care. These surveys work best when they are short, clear, and consistent. They can help a practice identify ways of improving, which results in better care and happier patients.

```
CASE STUDY
```

Derek went to see a specialist for a gastrointestinal condition. When he arrived early for his appointment at the facility, the front desk administrator asked him if he was a new patient or a returning patient. When he said "new patient," she told him rather rudely to "sit over there and I'll bring you paperwork to fill out in a while." Derek waited for 15 minutes before she did so. She then told him he had to fill out the paperwork as fast as he could because the doctor was "backed up" and she needed to get his information into the computer system before he could be seen. When Derek finished, he asked where the bathroom was, and the administrator said, "You walked right by it after you entered the building – you must not have been paying attention." Derek waited another 20 minutes to see the doctor, who finally saw him a half-hour after his scheduled appointment. He felt rushed by the doctor, who didn't seem to care about all the details of his condition.

1 How could the woman behind the front desk have made Derek feel more welcome?
2 If the doctor and the administrator knew they could not see Derek on time, what should they have done?
3 What do you think the results of a patient satisfaction survey would be if Derek filled it out for this specialist's office?

Chapter highlights

This section answers the Objectives found at the beginning of the chapter.

1 Define the term "quality of care."

- Quality of care is the level of a patient's treatment in relationship to the best possible outcome, lowest possible costs, and overall satisfaction; it involves quality assurance, quality control, and continued quality improvement. The quality of care is of the utmost concern in every health care profession.

2 Differentiate between the terms "quality assessment," "quality assurance," and "quality control."

- Quality assessment = how quality is measured against established standards.
- Quality assurance = a method of ensuring high-quality performance in all business activities, designed to provide quality improvement, based on total quality management. It addresses medical errors, cross infections, evidence-based medicine, and patient satisfaction.
- Quality control = monitoring business activities to ensure high quality.

3 Explain what the terms "macro quality" and "micro quality" mean.

- Macro quality is concerned with populations, and performance of the entire health care system. It evaluates when certain health conditions occur, and how life expectancy and mortality rates are affected by various conditions.

- Micro quality evaluates clinical and interpersonal factors, and quality of life. It focuses on technical quality of health care facilities and caregivers, treatments that are used, cost-efficiency, and health outcomes.

4 **Briefly explain the four factors required to maintain quality of health care.**

- Clinical practice guidelines – descriptions that accurately represent preferred clinical processes for specific conditions
- Cost-efficiency (cost-effectiveness) – received benefits are greater than costs incurred to provide services
- Critical pathways – methods of case management based on outcomes and centered on patients
- Risk management – proactive efforts designed to prevent adverse events in clinical care and facilities operations.

5 **Suggest how health insurance reviewers may compromise a physician's ability to determine the best health care for each patient.**

- Health insurance reviewers may approve or deny procedures that are recommended by physicians, cheaper procedures instead of those that were recommended, or only a limited number of treatments. They may only approve a surgery if it is done on an outpatient basis. This compromises the physician's ability to determine the best health care for each patient.

6 **Identify how quality assessment and performance improvement (QAPI) programs affect quality improvement.**

- Regular evaluation
- Evaluate continuity and coordination of patient care
- Include consumer satisfaction measures
- Monitor high-risk, high-volume services; acute and chronic conditions
- Provide access to collected information when this is necessary
- Establish written protocols for utilization review
- Allow for health care professionals to review all processes
- Allow for data collection, analysis, and reporting
- Create or change ways of practice, based on areas needing improvement
- Able to detect underutilization and overutilization of services
- Can evaluate services, informing providers and enrollees of results
- Can base utilization reviews on medical practice standards
- Can publish information to help provide more coverage options
- Can offer systematic follow-up to assess program effectiveness.

7 **Briefly explain "continuous quality improvement."**

- Continuous quality improvement involves follow-through in gathering and assessing data so that health care efficiency can be improved
- Programs may be called total quality management or other names
- All programs focus on meeting internal needs of facilities
- This takes time, but offers higher degrees of care than previously
- Ask "How are we doing?," "How can we improve?"

8 List two examples of methods used to improve quality of care while reducing costs.

- Avoid prescribing broad-spectrum antibiotics, in favor of using cultures followed by more specific antibiotics
- Use disposable bibs to prevent hospitalized patient gowns from becoming soiled and requiring laundering.

9 Give examples of methods that provide better customer satisfaction.

- Mailing out questionnaires to customers
- Calling customers and asking for responses about care
- Documenting complaints, attempts to resolve them, and customer satisfaction
- Showing empathy
- Being courteous and asking clarifying questions
- Avoiding defense statements
- Reducing long waiting times
- Thanking customers who complain for the information
- Assuring complainants that you will try not to repeat errors
- Providing needed information
- Making sure the correct person handles each complaint.

10 Define "constructive criticism."

- Constructive criticism is the process of offering valid, well-reasoned opinions about others' work, involving positive and negative comments; it is optimistic, and should be used to encourage coworkers or subordinates that occurrences resulting in negative outcomes can be learned from
- Constructive criticism offers basic steps that individuals can follow to improve their work.

Summary

Every health care provider must be concerned with the quality of care provided to patients. Quality is determined through assessment, which measures care against established standards. It is difficult to balance high-quality care with cost control. The determination of quality of care involves clinical practice guidelines, cost-efficiency, critical pathways of case management, and management of risks. Quality improvement focuses on improving or preserving quality of care while lowering costs. Ideally, this should be performed on a continuous basis to improve the effectiveness of every health care facility. Utilization reviews evaluate all health care facilities, facilities, and procedures. Since most patients voice their opinions when they are dissatisfied with care, rather than when they are satisfied, it is important to communicate with patients to determine their perceptions about treatment. Patient satisfaction surveys identify areas needing improvement.

Review questions

1 How may quality health care be evaluated?
2 Why does the quality of health care in the United States currently rank in last place in Western countries?
3 How is quality assurance different from quality control?
4 What factors may influence quality of care?
5 What is risk management?
6 What is the role of the Centers for Medicare and Medicaid Services regarding quality improvement?
7 What is total quality management?
8 What is utilization review?
9 Why is customer satisfaction regarding health care important?
10 What are the characteristics of patient satisfaction surveys?

Bibliography

Agency for Health Care Administration. 2016. Utilization Review – Quality Assurance/ Quality Improvement – Prior Authorization and Quality Improvement. Available at: www.fdhc.state.fl.us/Medicaid/Utilization_Review/index.shtml. Tallahassee: Agency for Health Care Administration.

Agency for Healthcare Research and Quality. 2016. Standardizing Medication Error Event Reporting. Available at: www.ahrq.gov/sites/default/files/wysiwyg/professionals/quality-patient-safety/patient-safety-resources/resources/advances-in-patient-safety/vol4/Nosek. pdf. Rockville: Agency for Healthcare Research and Quality.

Brumley, S. 2016. Key Concepts of Total Quality Management Within a Health Care Organization. Available at: http://smallbusiness.chron.com/key-concepts-total-quality-management-within-health-care-organization-77731.html. Houston: Houston Chronicle/ Hearst Newspapers, LLC.

DeLaet, R. 2011. *Introduction to Health Care & Careers*. New York: Lippincott, Williams, & Wilkins. Print.

Fleurence, R., et al. 2013. How the Patient-Centered Outcomes Research Institute is engaging patients and others in shaping its research agenda. *Health Affairs* 32, no. 2: 393–400.

Health Resources and Services Administration. 2016. Quality Improvement Methodology. Available at: www.hrsa.gov/quality/toolbox/methodology/qualityimprovement/index. html. Rockville: Health Resources and Services Administration.

Inozu, B., Chauncey, D., Kamataris, V., and Mount, C. 2011. *Performance Improvement for Healthcare: Leading Change with Lean, Six Sigma, and Constraints Management*. New York: McGraw-Hill Education. Print.

Institute of Medicine – Shaping the Future for Health. 1999. To Err Is Human: Building a Safer Health System. Available at: nationalacademies.org/hmd/~/media/Files/Report%20 Files/1999/To-Err-is-Human/To%20Err%20is%20Human%201999%20%20 report%20brief.pdf. Washington, D.C.: Committee on Quality of Health Care in America/National Academy of Sciences.

Joint Commission. 2012. *Fundamentals of Health Care Improvement: A Guide to Improving Your Patients' Care, 2nd Edition*. Oak Brook: Joint Commission Resources. Print.

Kelly, D.L. 2011. *Applying Quality Management in Healthcare, 3rd Edition*. Chicago: Health Administration Press. Print.

Knickman, J.R., and Kovner, A.R. 2015. *Jonas and Kovner's Health Care Delivery in the United States, 11th Edition.* New York: Springer Publishing Company. Print.

Leebov, W. 2012. *Customer Service for Professional in Health Care: Key Behaviors That Enhance the Patient and Family Experience.* Seattle: CreateSpace. Print.

Leebov, W., Scott, G., and Olson, L. 2012. *Achieving Impressive Customer Service: 7 Strategies for the Health Care Manager.* Seattle: CreateSpace. Print.

Mclaughlin, A. 2012. Medical Practice Customer Service from the H.E.A.R.T. Available at: www.physicianspractice.com/blog/medical-practice-customer-service-heart. New York: UBM Media, LLC.

Medicare.gov. 2016. Find Contact Information. Available at: www.medicare.gov/contacts. Baltimore: U.S. Centers for Medicare and Medicaid Services.

Mitchell, D., and Haroun, L. 2011. *Introduction to Health Care, 3rd Edition.* Boston: Delmar Cengage Learning. Print.

National Association for Healthcare Quality. 2016. NAHQ – Home Page. Available at: www.nahq.org. Chicago: National Association for Healthcare Quality.

NCQA. 2016. NCQA – Home Page. Available at: www.ncqa.org. Princeton: National Committee for Quality Assurance.

Office of Disease Prevention and Health Promotion – HealthyPeople.gov. 2016. Access to Health Services – Overview and Impact – Life Stages and Determinants. Available at: www.healthypeople.gov/2020/topics-objectives/topic/Access-to-Health-Services. Washington, D.C.: U.S. Department of Health and Human Services.

Payne, R.K. 2014. *Bridges to Health and Healthcare: New Solutions for Improving Access and Services.* Houston: Aha! Process. Print.

Reinhard, S.C., et al. 2011. How the Affordable Care Act can help move states towards a high-performing system of long-term services and supports. *Health Affairs* 30, no. 3: 447–453.

Ross, J.S., et al. 2010. State-sponsored public reporting of hospital quality: Results are hard to find and lack uniformity. *Health Affairs* 29, no. 12: 2317–2322.

Ross, T.K. 2014. *Health Care Quality Management: Tools and Applications.* San Francisco: Jossey-Bass. Print.

Shapiro, L. 2013. *Quality Care, Affordable Care: How Physicians Can Reduce Variation and Lower Healthcare Costs.* Williamsport: Greenbranch Publishing. Print.

Sollecito, W.A., and Johnson, J.K. 2011. *McLaughlin and Kaluzny's Continuous Quality Improvement in Health Care, 4th Edition.* Burlington: Jones & Bartlett Learning. Print.

Sox, H. 2012. The Patient-Centered Outcomes Research Institute should focus on high-impact problems that can be solved quickly. *Health Affairs* 31, no. 10: 2176–2182.

Timbie, J.W., et al. 2012. Five reasons that many comparative effectiveness studies fail to change patient care and clinical practice. *Health Affairs* 31, no. 10: 2168–2175.

U.S. Department of Health and Human Services. 2016. Topic: Outcomes. Available at: www.ahrq.gov/health-care-information/topics/topic-outcomes.html. Rockville: Agency for Healthcare Research and Quality.

World Health Organization. 2016. Management of Quality Assurance and Quality of Care. Available at: www.who.int/management/quality/assurance/QualityCare_B.Def.pdf. Washington, D.C.: Pan American Health Organization.

Professionals and professional practice

Contents

6 Careers in the health care profession 119

Overview 119
Therapeutic divisions of the health care system 120
Diagnostic divisions of the health care system 150
Health care management 157
Health care education 157
Case study 158
Chapter highlights 158
Summary 160
Review questions 160
Bibliography 162

7 Professionalism in health care 164

Overview 164
Professionalism 165
Professional behavior 166
Stress management 174
Personal health 177
Personal hygiene 179
Case study 180
Chapter highlights 180
Summary 182
Review questions 182
Bibliography 183

Chapter 6

Careers in the health care profession

Objectives

After study of the chapter, readers should be able to:

1 Describe the roles of physician assistants.
2 List the top five jobs in this chapter that have the highest projected growth.
3 Differentiate between the job descriptions of dental hygienists and dental assistants.
4 Describe the job duties of emergency medical technicians and paramedics.
5 Explain the differences between chiropractors and physical therapists.
6 Outline the education required to become a psychologist.
7 Describe the duties of health care administrators and health information technicians.
8 Explain the roles of dietitians in the health care profession.
9 Describe the roles of clinical laboratory technologists.
10 Explain the activities of various health educators.

Overview

The many different types of career in health care are subdivided into therapeutic, diagnostic, management, and education divisions. The primary therapeutic professionals include physicians, nurse practitioners, physician assistants, dentists, and pharmacists. The primary diagnostic professionals include radiologists, cardiovascular technologists, and various types of clinical laboratory technologists. Health care administrators handle the management of many different health care facilities, and health care educators work in a variety of settings,

119

teaching many different types of people about health and wellness. There are many career opportunities in the ever-growing health care field, and students should have an optimistic outlook about the potential of these various jobs.

Therapeutic divisions of the health care system

This chapter focuses on therapeutic and other divisions of the health care system. The therapeutic divisions discussed include physicians, nurses, physician assistants, medical assistants, surgical technologists, dentists, dental hygienists, dental assistants, occupational therapists, respiratory therapists and technicians, emergency medical technicians and paramedics, optometrists, ophthalmologists, audiologists, pharmacists, pharmacy technicians, dietitians, chiropractors, physical therapists and therapist assistants, massage therapists, psychologists, medical social workers, and rehabilitation counselors.

Physicians

Physicians are medical professionals who diagnose illnesses, prescribe and administer medications and treatments, examine patients, obtain medical histories, counsel patients on lifestyle choices and behaviors, and interpret diagnostic tests. The two types of physician are the *medical doctor (MD)* and the *doctor of osteopathic medicine (DO)*. The DO focuses on the musculoskeletal system, preventive medicine, and holistic care. Various physician specialties are listed in Table 6.1.

Many physicians work in private offices or clinics and are assisted by nurses and other health care professionals. However, more physicians today work in groups or health care organizations. Work hours are often long, more than 50 hours per week. There are more than 661,000 physicians in the United States, with most working in private offices. About 55% work in specialty areas while the remainder are in primary care. A vast majority (up to 80%) of physicians are located in metropolitan areas, while the rest are in rural areas.

A physician usually needs about eight years of education after high school, plus 3–8 years of internship and residency. They must be licensed to practice in all of the United States and its territories. The average student studying to be a physician will go through four years of undergraduate school, four years of medical school, and then the 3–8 years of internship and residency, the length of which is based on the specialty selected. Some medical schools offer combined undergraduate and medical studies that last only 6–7 years. Studies include biology, physics, mathematics, English, chemistry, humanities, and social sciences. Most applicants to medical school have at least a Bachelor's degree.

There are at least 129 medical schools accredited for the MD degree by the Liaison Committee on Medical Education (LCME), while there are 25 schools accredited for the DO degree by the American Osteopathic Association. Competition is very intense, and acceptance is based on fantastic school transcripts, high scores on the Medical College Admission Test, letters of recommendation, personality of the candidate, participation in extracurricular activities, and school interviews.

Instruction involves classrooms and laboratories, with courses in anatomy, physiology, biochemistry, pharmacology, microbiology, psychology, medical ethics, pathology, and medical law. During the final two years of schooling, students work with patients while supervised by licensed physicians, to learn acute, chronic, preventive, and rehabilitative health care. Experience is gained as the student experiences rotation through family practice, internal medicine, gynecology and obstetrics, pediatrics, psychiatry, and surgical

Table 6.1 Types of physician specialties

Specialty	Description
Anesthesiologist	Evaluates and treats surgical patients, focusing on pain relief; works to maintain heart rate, temperature, blood pressure, and breathing during surgery
Family physician	Assesses and treats most conditions for regular, long-term patients
General internist	Diagnoses and provides non-surgical treatments; are usually primary care specialists
General pediatrician	Provides a variety of treatments for infants, children, teenagers, and young adults
Gynecologist/ obstetrician	Specializes in women's health, pregnancy, childbirth, and postpartum care
Psychiatrist	Primary caregiver that utilizes psychoanalysis, psychotherapy, and medications
Surgeon	Performs surgeries to treat and correct all types of conditions
Miscellaneous specialty areas	These include allergists, cardiologists, dermatologists, emergency physicians, endocrinologists, gastroenterologists, neurologists, ophthalmologists, pathologists, and radiologists

environments. Most MDs enter a residency once they leave medical school. This usually takes place in a hospital. For DOs, most go through a 12-month rotating internship after graduation but before residency, which can last 2–6 years.

More than 85% of new physicians are in significant debt for their educational expenses as they began actual practice. Licensure is through the United States Medical Licensing Examination (USMLE). Reciprocity throughout various states is usually not limited, but may be limited between certain states. Physicians of both major types who want to become certified in a specialty can spend up to seven years in residency training. For certification by the American Board of Medical Specialists or the American Osteopathic Association, a different examination is required after residency or after 1–2 years of practice.

Job opportunities for physicians are excellent, with 22% growth expected up to the year 2022. Many colleges are increasing their enrollments for new physicians. Salaries for physicians are higher than many other occupations, with primary care physicians averaging $200,000 per year, and specialists averaging $400,000 per year.

> ### Focus on primary care physicians
>
> Today, fewer students than ever choose to become primary care physicians (PCPs). As older PCPs retire early and others move into hospital work environments, only about 30% of all physicians practice primary care. Fifty years ago, this percentage was 70%.
>
> *Sources:* www.primarycareprogress.org/blogs/16/394; www.kevinmd.com/ blog/2014/02/shortage-primary-care-physicians.html.

Nurses

Nurses fall into two major categories: registered nurses (RNs) and licensed practical nurses (LPNs). The job of a nurse is to treat and educate patients, give advice and emotional support to family members of patients, record information, assist with diagnoses, analyze test results, operate medical equipment, administer medications, and assist with follow-up visits and rehabilitation. RNs establish treatment plans and direct LPNs and nursing aides. RNs may specialize in certain settings or treatments, certain health conditions, certain organs or body systems, or certain populations. For example, *critical care nurses* focus on patients who have acute, complex illnesses or injuries and need extremely close monitoring as well as medications and other therapies.

RNs are employed in nearly every type of health care setting. Some RNs become advanced practice nurses (APNs), working independently of or alongside physicians, often focusing on primary care. A nurse practitioner may be both a primary and specialty care provider, and most often specialize in family practices, adult practices, pediatrics, geriatrics, women's health, or acute care. RNs may work many different types of schedule based on the facilities in which they are employed. Since most nurses come into close contact with patients, they must always observe strict guidelines for protective clothing and equipment.

Nursing is the largest health care occupation, with at least 2.6 million nurses being employed in the United States. Most nurses work in hospitals, but also may work in physician offices, home health care, nursing care facilities, employment services, government agencies, educational institutions, and social assistance agencies. Nursing programs usually give Bachelor's degrees, Associate's degrees, or a diploma. A national licensing examination is then taken in order to earn a nursing license. Nurses who must earn a Master's degree include clinical nurse specialists, nurse anesthetists, nurse midwives, and nurse practitioners.

Bachelor's degree nursing programs usually take four years to complete, and result in a Bachelor of Science degree in nursing (BSN). Associate's degree nursing programs usually take 2–3 years to complete, and result in an Associate of Science degree in nursing (ASN). Diploma programs, which are administered by hospitals, take about three years to complete, but are less common than the other two types of programs. There are also *RN-to-BSN* programs, in which students are employed as nurses after earning an ASN, and then work toward their BSN. There is also an Accelerated Master's degree in nursing (MSN) that takes 3–4 years to complete with full-time study, with students being awarded both BSN and MSN degrees.

Students who have Bachelor's degrees in other fields may also enroll in accelerated BSN programs, which last 12–18 months. Similarly, there are MSN programs for individuals with Bachelor's degrees – these usually last two years. Nursing programs always combine classroom instruction with supervised clinical experience in a variety of health care facilities.

Courses studied include anatomy, physiology, chemistry, microbiology, nutrition, psychology, behavioral sciences, and actual nursing subjects.

The national nursing licensure examination is called the National Council Licensure Examination or NCLEX-RN. Certain states have other eligibility requirements for licensure – these are listed at each state board of nursing. Job opportunities for RNs are excellent, with 22% growth expected up to the year 2022. Employment is expected to grow more slowly in hospitals than in other work areas, with more jobs in physician offices being anticipated than any other area. RNs average between $43,410 and $92,240 in annual salaries.

Licensed practical nurses are also known as *licensed vocational nurses*. They may work under the direction of physicians or registered nurses. Most LPNs work standard 40-hour weeks, though they may also be on-call and be required to work different shifts as needed. There are just under 754,000 LPN jobs in the United States, with the majority being in nursing care facilities and hospitals. Most training programs for LPNs require about one year of study, and are available from vocational or technical schools as well as community or junior colleges. Like RNs, study involves both classroom instruction and supervised clinical practice.

Licensure of LPNs is also through the National Council Licensure Examination, but with an *NCLEX-PN* designation, featuring different questions. The exam covers safe and effective care environments, health promotion and maintenance, psychosocial integrity, and physiological integrity. LPNs may go on to receive credentials in specialty areas such as gerontology, IV therapy, long-term care, or pharmacology. They may also become RNs by attending LPN-to-RN training programs. Job opportunities for LPNs are projected to grow 21% by the year 2022. Annual salaries for LPNs range from $28,260 to $53,580.

Focus on nurses

Nurses are injured on the job more than construction workers, and assaulted more than prison guards. One out of every five nurses meets the criteria for post-traumatic stress disorder.

Sources: www.nursingworld.org/especiallyforyou/staff-nurses/staff-nurse-news/npr-series-on-nurse-injuries.html; www.evergreennursing.ca/images/policy-pdf/workplace-violence-prevention-policy.pdf; www.uchealth.org/today/news/cu-researchers-take-aim-at-ptsd-burnout-in-the-icu.

Physician assistants

In the 1960s, because of a lack of primary care physicians, the new job title of *physician assistant* (PA) was developed. PAs assist physicians in providing personal health services. They are specially trained to assist doctors of medicine or osteopathy, and are directly responsible for their own actions while working. They are considered *middle-level health workers*, with skills that lie between licensed physicians and registered nurses.

Following 2–4 years of college and some health care work experience, PAs must complete an accredited postgraduate program of at least two years, pass a national examination, and then obtain a license to practice. Most PA programs are in allied health schools, four-year colleges, academic health centers, or medical schools. Others are found in community colleges, hospitals, and the military. There are more than 170 education programs for PAs, including certificate programs or Associate's, Bachelor's, and Master's degrees. The job outlook is extremely good, since facilities are hiring more PAs in order to control costs. Employment of PAs is expected to grow 38%, from 86,700 to 120,000, by the year 2022.

This includes traditional medical practices and even telemedicine. The pay range for PAs is currently from $64,100 to $134,720.

Focus on shortages of physicians and physician assistants

Because of the increase in people who have access to health care under the Affordable Care Act, there is a shortage of physicians. Therefore, there is also a need for more physician assistants.

Training as a physician assistant includes coursework in biochemistry, human anatomy and physiology, microbiology, pathology, clinical medicine, clinical pharmacology, disease prevention, geriatric care, home health care, and medical ethics. Clinical training includes family medicine, internal medicine, prenatal care, gynecology, surgery, emergency medicine, geriatrics, pediatrics, and psychiatry.

The Physician Assistant National Certifying Exam (PANCE) is given by the National Commission on Certification of Physician Assistants (NCCPA). It can be taken only by graduates of accredited PA programs. Once successfully completing the exam, an individual may use the credential "Physician Assistant – Certified." Every two years, a PA must complete 100 hours of continuing medical education in order to remain certified. Every ten years, a re-certification examination must be completed, or an alternative program may be completed that includes continuing education and an at-home examination. Many PAs go on to specialize in a specific area by seeking additional postgraduate education.

A PA can provide, under the supervision of a physician and according to state law, routine diagnostic, preventive, and therapeutic health care services. Job duties include examining patients, taking medical histories, coordinating X-rays and laboratory tests, making preliminary diagnoses, applying casts or splints, suturing wounds, recording progress notes, managing the practice, ordering supplies, supervising other health care professionals, and counseling patients. In all states except Florida, Hawaii, Kentucky, and Oklahoma, PAs can even prescribe most types of medications without seeking medical board approval.

Physician assistants often work on their own without direct supervision of a physician, though the physician eventually reviews all of the activities performed by the PA. They often handle visits to nursing facilities, clinics, hospitals, and even patient households. PAs most commonly work in emergency medicine, family practices, general or orthopedic surgery, geriatric facilities, internal medicine, pediatric facilities, and thoracic surgery. More than 58% of physician assistant jobs are in the offices of various types of physician.

Medical assistants

Medical assistants perform administrative and clinical tasks in many different types of health care office. Though their duties differ between health care settings, they generally coordinate medical records and insurance forms; answer telephones (see Figure 6.1); greet patients; schedule appointments; handle all forms of correspondence; assist with billing, accepting payments (see Figure 6.2), and bookkeeping; and arrange for laboratory tests and hospital admissions. Generally, medical assistants work regular 40-hour weeks, but may be required to work evenings, weekends, or on a part-time basis.

There were about 560,800 medical assistant jobs in the United States in 2012, with the majority being in physician offices. Medical assisting programs are offered by community

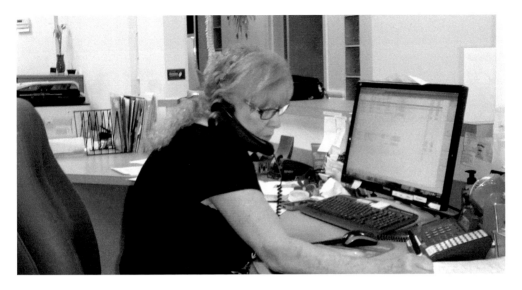

Figure 6.1 A medical assistant answering the phone.

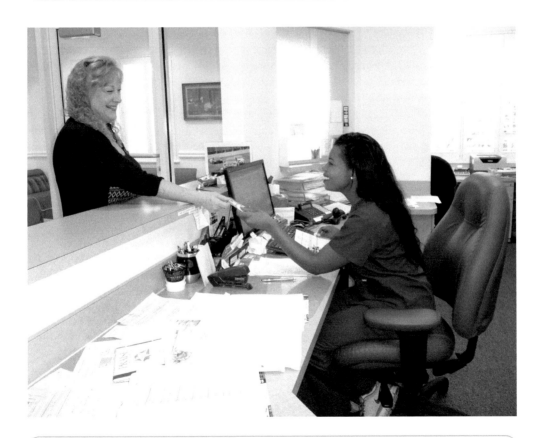

Figure 6.2 A medical assistant accepting payment from a patient.

and junior colleges, postsecondary vocational schools, and even vocational-technical high schools. Programs usually last 1–2 years, and result in a certificate, diploma, or Associate's degree. Students receive instruction in both administrative and clinical areas. Though formal training is usually preferred, it is not always required, and on-the-job training of medical assistants still occurs.

Certification of medical assistants may be obtained through one of three organizations. The *Certified Medical Assistant* credential is given through the American Association of Medical Assistants (AAMA). The *Registered Medical Assistant* credential is given through the American Medical Technologists (AMT). The *Certified Clinical Medical Assistant* credential is given through the National Healthcareer Association (NHA). Medical assisting is one of the fastest-growing areas in health care. Job opportunities are expected to grow 34% up to the year 2022. Average annual earnings range between $20,600 and $39,570.

Surgical technologists

Surgical technologists are also called *surgical technicians*, *operating room technicians*, or, more commonly, *scrubs*. They assist in surgeries by preparing operating rooms, setting up equipment and supplies, preparing and transporting patients, positioning patients, monitoring vital signs, assisting the surgical team with putting on surgical clothing, and verifying information on patient charts. During actual surgical procedures, surgical technologists pass instruments and supplies, and basically account for everything used as part of the surgery. They assist in the operation of equipment, handle specimens, apply surgical dressings, restock supplies, maintain hemostasis, assist with anesthesia, and document procedures.

Surgical technologists usually work a 40-hour week, but may work on a rotating basis during evenings, weekends, and holidays. There were about 98,500 surgical technology jobs in 2012, mostly in hospitals. Community and junior colleges, vocational schools, hospitals, and the military offer surgical technology programs. The *Commission on Accreditation of Allied Health Education Programs* (CAA-HEP) recognizes more than 450 accredited training programs that last from nine to 24 months. They lead to a certificate, diploma, or Associate's degree. A high school diploma is usually required for applicants to these programs. Training combines classroom instruction and supervised clinical experience.

Certified surgical technologists are preferred by employers, and voluntary certification can be obtained after graduation from an accredited program by passing the national certification exam administered by the *Liaison Council on Certification for the Surgical Technologist (LCCST)*. Those who pass can use the *Certified Surgical Technologist (CST)* credential. Certification must be renewed every four years, which requires continuing education or re-examination. The *National Center for Competency Testing (NCCT)* also approves certification, with passing individuals receiving the *Tech in Surgery-Certified (TS-C)* credential. This certification is renewed every five years via continuing education or re-examination. Job opportunities for surgical technologists are expected to grow 25% up to the year 2022. Average annual earnings range between $27,510 and $54,300.

> **You should remember**
>
> The term "surgical technologist" is relatively new, being developed in 1973. Previously, this role was often described as an "instrument nurse" or "instrument tech."

Dentists

Dentists specialize in the teeth and tissues of the mouth, and may be general practitioners or a specialist in one of the nine areas listed in Table 6.2.

General dentists counsel patients in order to help prevent future problems from developing, including instruction on brushing, flossing, diet, fluoride use, and other areas. They may fill cavities, remove tooth decay, examine X-rays, seal children's teeth with plastic substances, repair tooth fractures, or straighten teeth (see Figure 6.3). They may also extract teeth, create models of dentition in order to replace missing teeth, take measurements, administer anesthetics, and write medical prescriptions.

A dentist must be familiar with the use of a large variety of equipment, including drills, mouth mirrors, probes, forceps, brushes, scalpels, lasers, digital scanners, computers, and X-ray machines. During procedures, dentists wear gloves, masks, and safety glasses to protect against transmission of infections (see Figure 6.4). In private practice, dentists often handle administration, inventory, and the supervision of other staff members, such as dental hygienists, laboratory technicians, assistants, and receptionists.

Focus on OSHA and bloodborne pathogens

The Occupational Safety and Health Administration (OSHA) requires that dentists, dental hygienists, and dental assistants protect themselves from bloodborne pathogens by wearing gloves, gowns, goggles, and masks as needed. Bloodborne pathogens may be transferred through body fluids, including blood.

Table 6.2 Types of dental specialties

Specialty	Description
Dental public health specialist	Focuses on community dental health promotion and disease prevention
Endodontist	Focuses on root-canal therapies
Oral/maxillofacial radiologist	Diagnoses head and neck diseases using various imaging techniques
Oral/maxillofacial surgeon	Performs surgeries involving the teeth, gums, mouth, jaws, head, and neck
Oral pathologist	Focuses on diagnosis of oral diseases
Orthodontist	Uses braces and other appliances to straighten teeth
Pediatric dentist	Focuses on children and "special needs" patients
Periodontist	Focuses on the gums and bones that support the teeth
Prosthodontist	Replaces teeth with bridges, crowns, dentures, or other fixtures

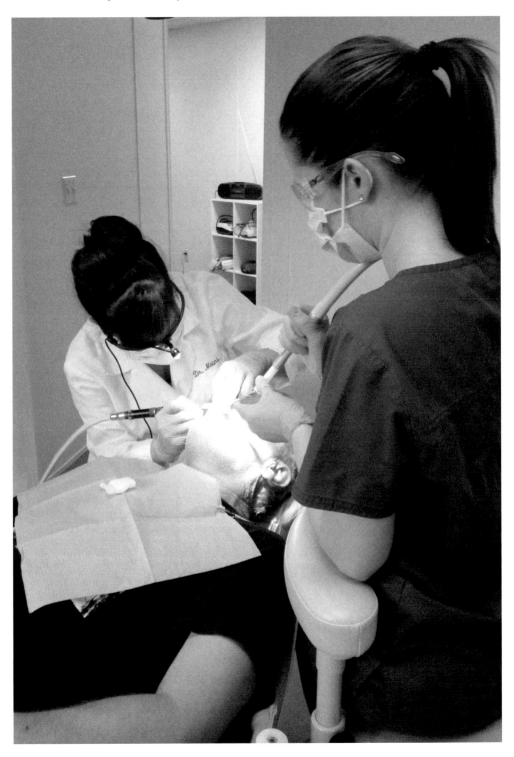

Figure 6.3 A dentist performing a procedure on a patient.

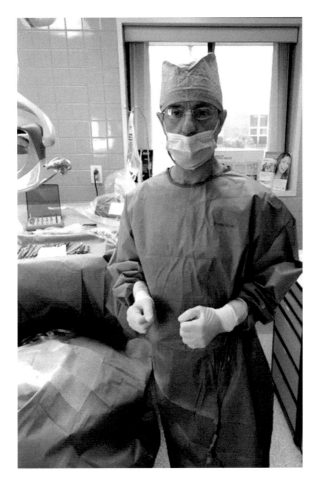

Figure 6.4 A dentist wearing protective garb.

The majority of dentists own "solo" practices, while some have partners or associates. There are more than 147,000 dentists of all types in the United States, with general practitioners making up nearly 126,000 of these. About 15% of all dentists are specialists, and about one in four dentists are self-employed in private practice, and not part of a corporation. Dentists must be licensed in order to practice, which requires them to graduate from an accredited dental school as well as pass written and practical examinations.

The American Dental Association accredits 65 dental schools in the United States, which require a Bachelor's degree in Science prior to entering dental school. Before dental school, important areas of study include biology, chemistry, health, mathematics, physics, and many different science courses. A Dental Admissions Test (DAT) is required by all dental schools upon application, and competition for admission is extremely high.

Dental school usually involves four years of study, including anatomy, physiology, biochemistry, laboratory techniques, and microbiology. In the final two years of study, dental students treat patients (usually in clinics) while licensed dentists supervise. Most dental schools award a Doctor of Dental Surgery (DDS) surgery, but some award a Doctor of Dental Medicine (DMD) degree. For licensing following dental school, the written requirements may be fulfilled by passing the National Board Dental Examination administered by the state government or a regional testing agency.

To become a specialist, most requirements involve two years of postgraduate education in the specialty area (while some require three or four years), plus completion of a special state examination. There may also be a required postgraduate residency term of up to two years. In most states, a license to practice allows a dentist to be a general practitioner or a specialist. For those who want to teach or become a researcher, there is usually 2–5 years of additional dental training, in either a dental school or a hospital. Job prospects for all types of dentist are excellent, with the field projected to grow by 16% up to 2022. Also, since routine services can be handled by hygienists and assistants, opportunities for those positions are also expected to grow.

General dentists' salaries average just under $143,000 per year – based on location, years in practice, and hours of practice. Specialists may earn more, and self-employed private practice dentists generally earn more than salaried dentists.

> ### You should remember
>
> Salaried dentists usually receive better insurance coverage, including malpractice insurance, than self-employed private practice dentists.

Dental hygienists

The role of the dental hygienist is to educate patients about good oral hygiene, while also providing oral examinations, recording all findings, cleaning the teeth of bacterial build-up and stains, providing other types of preventive dental care, taking and developing X-rays, applying fluorides and other agents, and sealing pits and fissures in the teeth (see Figure 6.5). Certain states allow dental hygienists to administer local anesthetics and gases, complete fillings and periodontal dressings, remove sutures, and complete metal restorations. Hygienists often teach patients about diet, tooth brushing, flossing, and other good dental practices. They may also seek additional education in order to teach or conduct research.

Equipment used by dental hygienists includes lasers, ultrasonic devices, hand and rotary instruments, X-ray equipment, syringes, needles, tooth models, gloves, surgical masks, and safety glasses. The Consumer-Patient Radiation Health and Safety Act set standards for dental hygienists. These standards include:

- Techniques, procedures, and methods that minimize unnecessary radiation exposure
- Eliminating the need for retakes of diagnostic radiologic procedures
- Eliminating unproductive screening programs
- Providing optimum diagnostic information with minimum radiologic exposure
- Therapeutic application of radiation to individuals in the treatment of disease.

The jobs of dental hygienists often involve flexible scheduling on an as-needed basis. More than half of all dental hygienists work part time. The amount of jobs held by dental hygienists, therefore, is just under 192,800 in the United States, as of 2012. Nearly all dental hygienists work in dentist offices.

To practice as a dental hygienist, you must become licensed in your state. This requires a degree from an accredited dental hygiene school, and a licensure examination. A dental hygiene program requires a high school diploma and completion of a college entrance test

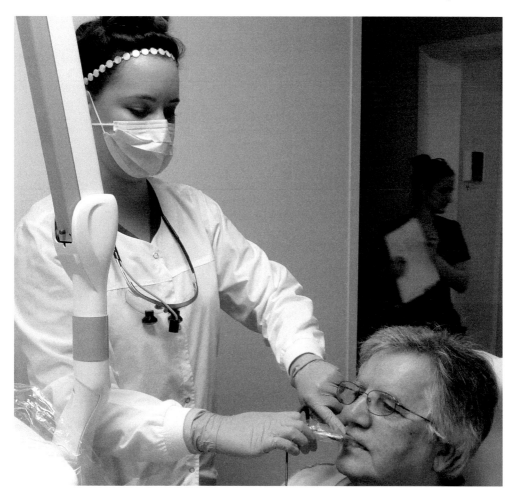

Figure 6.5 A dental hygienist taking an X-ray.

with an adequate score. Prior to the program, coursework should include biology, chemistry, and mathematics. Dental hygiene programs require at least one to two years of college prior to admittance. There are approximately 330 programs accredited by the Commission on Dental Accreditation. The student will study anatomy, physiology, chemistry, microbiology, nutrition, pharmacology, histology, radiography, pathology, periodontology, clinical dental hygiene, dental materials, and even behavioral and social sciences.

Most dental hygiene programs award an Associate's degree. To work in a private dental office, an Associate's degree or certificate is usually all that is required, while Bachelor's or Master's degrees in dental hygiene lead to research, teaching in colleges, or clinical practice in programs for the general public.

State licenses for dental hygiene usually require graduation from an accredited dental hygiene school, and passing both written and clinical examinations. The written examinations are given by the American Dental Association's Joint Commission on National Dental Examinations. The clinical examinations are given by state or regional testing agencies. Most states also require an examination about legal topics involved in dental hygiene.

One state, Alabama, allows students to take its licensure examinations if they have trained in an approved on-the-job program in a dentist's office.

The outlook for dental hygienist jobs is excellent, with 36% growth expected through the year 2018. It is one of the fastest-growing occupations in all of health care. Dental hygienists earn between $49,190 and $97,390 a year based on location, type of employer, and amount of experience. Benefits for this position also vary widely, based on the practice setting and whether employment is part- or full-time.

Dental assistants

A dental assistant is involved in a large variety of dental care for patients, as well as in office and laboratory support work. They assist dentists during examinations and treatments, help patients to feel comfortable during procedures, prepare patients for treatment, access dental records, use suction and other treatment-related devices, disinfect and sterilize equipment, prepare dental equipment trays, and educate patients about oral health care (see Figure 6.6). A dental assistant may also be required to assist with X-ray and other imaging, and if approved by state laws, assist in suture removal, apply anesthetics and other agents, place dental devices, and remove excess filling cements and other materials. In some states, they may be allowed to complete dental polishing and other restorative functions. They often wear gloves and masks while working to protect against infection transmission.

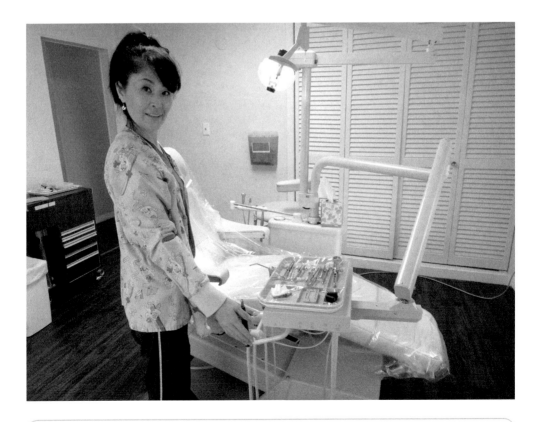

Figure 6.6 A dental assistant preparing a tray.

In the laboratory setting, dental assistants may make tooth and mouth casts from impressions, make temporary crowns, and clean and polish dentures and other removable appliances. In the dental office, they may handle appointments and patient reception, organize records, handle billings and payments, and order supplies. Dental assistants are support personnel to dentists and dental hygienists. Their schedules are often flexible and may be part- or full-time.

More than 303,200 dental assisting jobs exist in the United States, with nearly all of them being in dentist offices. Often, skills are learned through on-the-job training, though increased amounts of training programs are available through colleges, trade schools, the military, or technical institutes. These programs usually take only one year to complete. Dental assistants do not require licensure or certification unless they are required to perform more advanced activities or to be involved with radiological procedures. To become a dental assistant, an individual should study biology, chemistry, health, and office practices.

If additional education is desired, there are more than 250 dental assisting certificate or diploma programs in the United States that are approved by the Commission on Dental Accreditation. Community and junior colleges offer two-year Associate's degree programs. For admittance to a dental assistant program, a high school diploma or equivalent is required, and additional requirements may include computer-related or science courses. There are also non-accredited four- to six-month vocational programs in dental assisting. Some states require dental assistants to complete state-approved continuing education, which takes four to twelve hours. For a dental assistant to work with radiological procedures, more than 30 states require completion of the Radiation Health and Safety examination given by the Dental Assisting National Board.

The job outlook for dental assistants is excellent, and is expected to grow 25% up to 2022, one of the fastest-growing occupations in all of health care. The pay range for dental assistants is from $24,580 to $49,540 annually. Benefits vary widely; more than half of all dental assistants receive health and other benefits.

You should remember

In most states, dental assistants do not perform the same tasks as dental hygienists. In most dental offices, they are in charge of infection control procedures, which are closely regulated by OSHA.

Occupational therapists

Occupational therapists (OTs) assist people with a variety of disabilities in coping with daily living, the effects of their disabilities, and how these may affect their ability to work. These therapists often work alongside physicians, nurses, psychologists, and other health care professionals. They use a variety of different activities, some of which may resemble games, to provide needed skills that are targeted to each individual. Examples of activities utilized by occupational therapists include techniques for getting dressed, driving a vehicle, walking, using a bathroom, working with computers, and others.

OTs often focus on specific age groups or people with certain types of disability. Just over half of them work with physically disabled individuals, with the remainder working with developmental, emotional, or psychological problems. In schools, therapists assist children in learning ways to participate and learn more effectively. For mental health therapists, the focus is on mental or emotional disorders, including depression, stress disorders, eating disorders, and alcohol or drug abuse.

Most OTs work a regular 40-hour week, but some have to work evenings and weekends as needed. There were about 113,200 OT jobs in the United States in 2012, most of which were in ambulatory health care facilities. To become an OT, a Master's degree is usually required, but a doctoral degree is another option. In order to take the national certifying exam, the applicant must complete a program accredited by the *Accreditation Council for Occupational Therapy Education (ACOTE)*. There are approximately 150 accredited Master's or combined Master and Bachelor's programs, and four doctoral degree programs in the United States.

All states regulate occupational therapists. To become licensed, they must complete an accredited program and pass the national exam, after which they are awarded the *Occupational Therapist Registered (OTR)* credential. Certain states have other requirements that are based on specialty areas. Certification may also be obtained, on a voluntary basis. Job opportunities for OTs are expected to grow 26% up to the year 2022. Average annual salaries range between $42,820 and $81,290.

Respiratory therapists and technicians

Respiratory therapists are also known as *respiratory care practitioners*. They evaluate and treat patients who have breathing or cardiopulmonary disorders. They have primary responsibility for all related treatments, and also supervise respiratory technicians. Respiratory therapists also focus on life support in intensive-care units. They work with all ages of patients, and must be knowledgeable about a large variety of respiratory conditions, including asthma, emphysema, and related conditions such as heart attack or stroke.

A respiratory therapist interviews patients, performs simple physical examinations, and conducts diagnostic tests of breathing capacity, blood gases, and pH. They may utilize aerosol medications, chest physiotherapy, and oxygen or oxygen mixtures in their work. They often teach patients how to take medications and improve their breathing. Therapists may be required to place patients onto mechanical ventilators. They regularly assess patients as well as equipment. Today, respiratory therapists are working more than ever with areas such as disease prevention, pulmonary rehabilitation, smoking cessation, case management, and polysomnography, which diagnoses breathing disorders during sleep.

Respiratory therapists usually work less than 40 hours per week, and may be required to work evenings and weekends. There are about 119,300 respiratory therapist jobs in 2012, the vast majority of which are in hospitals. A Bachelor's degree is the minimum requirement to be a respiratory therapist, and is obtainable from many colleges, universities, medical schools, vocational or technical schools, or the military. The Committee on Accreditation for Respiratory Care (CoARC) accredits more than 500 respiratory therapy programs in the United States.

All states except Alaska and Hawaii require respiratory therapists to be licensed, and most employers require them to maintain their CPR certification. The *National Board for Respiratory Care* gives the *Certified Respiratory Therapist (CRT)* credential to students graduating from accredited programs. For a CRT who graduates from an advanced program and passes two separate examinations, a *Registered Respiratory Therapist* certification is awarded. Job opportunities for respiratory therapists are expected to grow 21% up to the year 2022, with most work being in hospitals. Respiratory therapists average annual salaries of $55,870.

Respiratory therapy technicians usually need an Associate's degree, but entry-level students may have an accredited postsecondary certificate. There is limited demand for technicians due to the majority of work in respiratory care being handled by respiratory therapists. There were approximately 10,610 respiratory therapy technicians employed in the United States in 2012. Average annual wages for respiratory therapy technicians are approximately $47,810.

Focus on respiratory therapy

Respiratory therapy is a relatively new field of medicine that began in the 1920s with oxygen therapy. This was followed by use of the iron lung for polio patients, then intermittent positive pressure breathing therapy, then nebulizers, and today's latest methods of therapy.

Emergency medical technicians and paramedics

Emergency medical technicians (EMTs) and paramedics provide fast and potentially life-saving care as they treat and transport patients to hospitals and other medical facilities. They are usually dispatched by 911 operators to emergency scenes, and regularly work alongside firefighters and the police. They assess each patient's immediate condition and determine any pre-existing conditions. Specialized equipment is used by EMTs, including devices to measure vital signs and backboards that immobilize patients before transport. EMTs and paramedics may travel in ambulances, other motor vehicles, and even helicopters.

There are five levels of qualification and training for EMTs and paramedics, as follows: first responder, EMT-basic, EMT-intermediate (1985), EMT-intermediate (1999), and paramedic. Each state has its own certification program and may use different names and titles for these levels. Paramedics are trained to provide the most extensive patient care, and may also give oral and intravenous drugs, perform endotracheal intubations, interpret electrocardiograms, use more complex equipment, and perform other high-level services. However, all states have specific guidelines as to what EMTs and paramedics can legally do.

Most professional EMTs and paramedics work in excess of 40 hours per week, on an as-needed basis. There were more than 235,760 of these jobs in 2012, with most paid positions being located closer to metropolitan areas, and most volunteer positions being located in more rural areas. Nearly half of all EMTs and paramedics work in private ambulance services.

To enter EMT or paramedic training, a high school diploma is usually required, but a formal training and certification process must also be completed. Coursework increases in difficulty depending on whether the applicant wants to be trained at the basic, intermediate, or paramedic levels. Applicants will be trained in respiratory, trauma, and cardiac emergencies; patient assessment, bleeding, fractures, airway obstruction, cardiac arrest, emergency childbirth, and equipment use. Those who graduate from an approved EMT-basic program must pass a written and practical examination given by a state agency or the *National Registry of Emergency Medical Technicians (NREMT)*. Intermediate-level students need between 30 and 350 training hours and also learn about advanced airway devices, intravenous fluids, and certain medications.

The *advanced paramedic* training level includes instruction in anatomy, physiology, and advanced medical skills. This usually occurs in community colleges or technical schools, and takes 1–2 years, resulting in an Associate's degree. Much clinical and field experience is also required, and continuing education is available as needed. All states require every level of EMT to be certified, and most require registration with the NREMT. Re-certification must occur (usually) every two years.

Job opportunities for EMTs and paramedics are expected to grow by 19% up to the year 2022. Annual wages range between $20,690 and $54,690, based on geographic location and level of training.

You should remember

According to the Registry of Emergency Medical Technicians, EMTs and paramedics treat between 25 and 30 million patients per year in the United States, at a cost of about $5 billion. Most of these professionals are males, and only 45% have a college degree or higher.

Source: www.nremt.org/rwd/public/data/maps.

Optometrists

Optometrists are the main providers of vision care, and also are referred to as *doctors of optometry*. They examine the eyes of patients, diagnose vision problems, test visual perception, test for glaucoma and other eye diseases, prescribe contact lenses and eyeglasses, and may provide vision therapy or low-vision rehabilitation as well as other treatments (see Figure 6.7). Optometrists may also refer patients to other physicians, prescribe medication, provide pre- or post-operative care, promote nutrition, and educate patients about hygiene that can minimize risks for eye disease.

Most optometrists work in general practice, but some specialize in pediatrics, geriatrics, vision therapy or rehabilitation, contact lenses, and other areas. Other specialty areas include sports vision, occupational vision, vision problems related to head trauma, and more. Some optometrists act as consultants, perform research, or become instructors. The majority of optometrists are private practitioners. Optometrists are not the same as ophthalmologists or *dispensing opticians*. The term "dispensing optician" describes an individual who may fit and adjust contact lenses or eyeglasses.

About 33,100 optometrist jobs were filled in the year 2012. Most salaried positions were located in optometrist offices, physician offices (including those of ophthalmologists), health-related stores, and personal care stores such as those selling optical goods. Optometrist jobs are also found in hospitals, outpatient care centers, and the federal government. To become an optometrist, three years of general study (with science courses emphasized) at an accredited school is required, followed by a four-year *Doctor of Optometry* degree at an accredited school of optometry.

There are only 20 accredited colleges of optometry in the United States, and competition for acceptance into their programs is highly competitive. Due to this limited amount of colleges, graduates from optometry programs number fewer than 2,000 per year. Changes in this field of health care must be made, since as many as one in four optometrists who are currently practicing are approaching the age of retirement. Accreditation of optometry programs is given by the Accreditation Council on Optometric Education of the American Optometric Association.

For acceptance into an optometry program, an applicant must take the Optometry Admissions Test, which measures academic abilities and understanding of scientific princi-

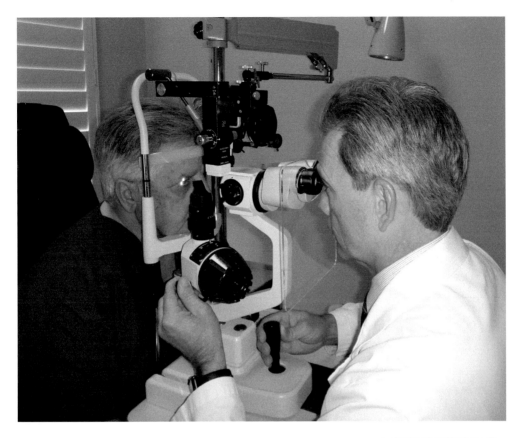

Figure 6.7 An optometrist examining a patient.

ples. It includes areas on biology, general and organic chemistry, physics, quantitative reasoning, and reading comprehension. The test is often taken several times by individuals in order to raise scores. You should note that every school has its own specific prerequisites for undergraduates, and find out what these are for the optometry school of your choice.

All programs include classroom as well as laboratory study, followed by clinical training. One-year postgraduate clinical residencies are available for any optometrist who wants to earn advanced competence in a specialty area, such as family practice optometry, geriatric or pediatric optometry, low-vision rehabilitation, contact lenses, vision therapy, ocular disease, primary eye care optometry, or refractive and ocular surgery. Optometrists intending to do research or teach may continue to study for a Master's degree or PhD in a variety of related areas.

Every state requires optometrists to become licensed in order to practice. After completing the Doctor of Optometry degree, various examinations must be passed. Usually, the student will take written and clinical examinations given by the National Board of Examiners in Optometry while still in college. Many states also require examinations on state laws pertaining to optometry. Optometrists must renew their licenses every 1–3 years, according to the laws of their states, which requires continuing education credits. Employment of optometrists is projected to grow 24% up to the year 2022. Optometrist wages range between $78,000 and $169,115.

> ### Focus on optometry
>
> Of the approximately 78 million primary eye examinations performed every year in the United States, optometrists performed 70% of them. The aging of the U.S. population is increasing demand for eye exams and glasses, as well as opportunities for new optometrists.
>
> *Sources:* www.confluencehealth.org/specialties/optometry/; www.firstresearch.com/industry-research/optometrists.html.

Ophthalmologists

Ophthalmologists are physicians who diagnose and treat eye diseases and injuries, as well as performing eye surgeries of various types. They also can prescribe contact lenses and eyeglasses. Ophthalmologists are specially trained to diagnose and treat more complex eye conditions than optometrists. Since ophthalmologists are medical doctors, they are allowed to prescribe a wider range of prescription drugs than optometrists.

Ophthalmologists receive four or more years of premedical undergraduate training, four years of medical school, and then an additional year of internship in order to earn their doctoral degree. Residency requires three years.

> ### You should remember
>
> Ophthalmologists are trained to perform eye surgery, while optometrists are not. Ophthalmologists may be involved with Lasik® vision correction, cataract removal, or surgery related to burns, eye trauma, or retinal detachment. Some ophthalmologists prefer not to be involved with vision correction via eyeglasses or contact lenses.

There are at least 24,000 ophthalmology jobs in the United States. The examination required to practice as an ophthalmologist is given by the American Board of Ophthalmology, and is known as the Written Qualifying Examination. Job opportunities for ophthalmologists are expected to grow 18% up to the year 2022. Ophthalmologists earn between $215,000 and $354,500 annually.

Audiologists

Audiologists work with people of all ages who have hearing, balance, or related ear problems. They utilize a variety of equipment, such as audiometers, computers, and testing devices to measure hearing ability as well as ability to distinguish specific sounds. They also diagnose balance disorders. Audiologists may counsel patients about adjusting to hearing loss, train them how to use hearing aids, teach communication and listening strategies, and fit hearing aids and equipment. Some audiologists specialize to work with children, the elderly, or the hearing impaired. They may conduct hearing protection programs in factories, schools, and communities.

Most audiologists work standard 40-hour weeks, though weekend and evenings may be required on an as-needed basis. There were about 13,000 audiologists employed in the United States in 2012, most of which were located in physician or other health care practitioner offices. Audiologists require licensure, and requirements vary by state. A Master's degree in audiology is required, but many states are now requiring a doctoral degree. A doctoral degree usually lasts four years, with the student earning an *AuD* designation. Audiology programs are accredited by the *Council on Academic Accreditation*, which is part of the *American Speech-Language-Hearing Association (ASHA)*. There are 70 accredited doctoral programs in audiology.

Some states do not allow audiologists to dispense hearing aids unless they have a separate *Hearing Aid Dispenser* license – check with your state's board of health or medicine for details. A *Certificate of Clinical Competence in Audiology (CCC-A)* may be earned from the ASHA, which satisfies most or all of the requirements for state licensure. Job opportunities for audiologists are expected to grow 25% up to the year 2022. Average annual salaries range between $40,360 and $98,880.

Pharmacists

Pharmacists are medical professionals who dispense medications following the guidelines of prescribers, which include licensed physicians, dentists, and other health professionals. Today, pharmacists play a much smaller role in compounding medications than in the past, since most medications are prepared by manufacturers in the correct dosage and form required.

Pharmacists in community or retail pharmacies often counsel patients about prescription medications, over-the-counter medications, supplements, and other products. Pharmacists routinely use computers to manage drug information for many different customers. In hospital pharmacies, pharmacists advise medical staff members about drug selections and adverse effects. They may also prepare sterile solutions, order supplies, conduct administrative procedures, and educate students and patients. The monitoring of drug regimens and drug use evaluation is a common part of the hospital pharmacist's duties. They may visit patients along with physicians to aid in monitoring medication use – in this case, they are referred to as pharmacotherapists.

In home health care, pharmacists may prepare infusions and monitor drug therapy. Some focus on cancer or psychiatric medications, while *nutrition support pharmacists* help to select drugs needed to improve nutrition. Pharmacists who work with radiopharmaceuticals are also called nuclear pharmacists or *radio-pharmacists*. Pharmacist activities are regulated by both state and federal boards.

Pharmacists are employed in many capacities, some of which require them to wear safety equipment and clothing. Though many pharmacists have regular schedules, some work in 24-hour facilities, requiring flexible scheduling. There are more than 286,400 pharmacist jobs in the United States, with most (61%) in retail pharmacies and about 23% in hospitals. Smaller numbers of jobs exist in the federal government, physician offices, wholesalers, mail order pharmacies, and Internet pharmacies.

Every state requires pharmacists to be licensed, meaning that they must first earn a Doctor of Pharmacy (PharmD) degree from an accredited college, as well as pass several examinations. The Accreditation Council for Pharmacy Education lists 124 fully accredited PharmD programs in the United States. Admittance to a PharmD program requires at least two years of specific professional study, which usually means courses in mathematics, biology, chemistry, physics, humanities, and social studies. Most programs require students to take the Pharmacy College Admissions Test before admittance. Each PharmD program usually takes four years to complete. Students are in classroom settings for about three-quarters of their training, and the remainder is spent in various pharmacy settings, supervised by licensed pharmacists.

Some colleges of pharmacy award the Master of Science or PhD degree after completion of a PharmD, for students who wish to have additional experience in clinical, laboratory, or research settings. Graduate studies include *pharmaceutical chemistry*, *pharmacology*, pharmaceutics, and *pharmacy administration*. Often, a student who attains a Master's degree or a PhD becomes a researcher for a drug manufacturer or a professor at a university. Pharmacy graduates may also enter one- to two-year residency fellowships or other programs. A residency in pharmacy usually requires a research project to be completed, which is often a mandatory requirement for a pharmacist intending to work in a hospital. Pharmacists who own their own pharmacies often seek an MBA degree (Master's in Business Administration). Others may go on to public administration or public health degrees.

All states require pharmacists who wish to practice to be licensed. A license can only be acquired after graduation from an accredited college of pharmacy and the completion of several examinations, including the North American Pharmacist Licensure Exam (NAPLEX). The majority of states also require the Multistate Pharmacy Jurisprudence Exam (MPJE) on pharmacy law. The remainder of states require their own pharmacy law exams. These exams are administered by the National Association of Boards of Pharmacy (NABP). Certain states and U.S. territories require their own unique exams in addition to these. Pharmacists may also specialize in specific areas, which include critical care, diabetes, nutrition, oncology, and pediatrics.

Except for California, all U.S. jurisdictions grant license transfers to qualified pharmacists who are already licensed by other jurisdictions. Pharmacists are often licensed to practice in multiple jurisdictions, and most of these require continuing education for licenses to be renewed. Foreign pharmacy school graduates may qualify for licensure in certain U.S. jurisdictions. A variety of exams must be passed by these individuals, including the NAPLEX and MPJE.

Job prospects for pharmacists are slightly better than average (14%) for health care jobs through the year 2022. Aside from community and hospital pharmacies, demand for pharmacists is also increasing in managed care organizations, in the field of *pharmacoeconomics* – which studies cost–benefit analyses of various drug therapies – in disease management, in pharmacy sales and marketing, and in *pharmacy informatics*, which is the use of information technology to improve patient care through medication use. Pharmacists generally earn between $89,320 and $150,550 per year.

You should remember

It is predicted that by the year 2020, 62% of active pharmacists will be women. This reflects the trend of females enrolling in pharmacy programs at higher rates than males.

Source: www.pharmacist.com/sites/default/files/files/ new_pharmacist_supply_Knapp.pdf.

Pharmacy technicians

The role of the *pharmacy technician* is to help the licensed pharmacist in the preparation and compounding of prescription medications, pharmacy administrative duties, labeling, and customer service. A pharmacy technician usually receives prescription requests, counts tablets or capsules, and labels bottles. *Pharmacy technicians* usually answer phones, operate cash registers, and stock shelves.

The practice of pharmacy technicians is regulated by state regulations. All pharmacy technicians are responsible for verifying the accuracy and completeness of information. Their work is supervised and verified by licensed pharmacists. Technicians often manage patient profiles, handle insurance claims, and make sure to refer all customer questions to the pharmacist. Pharmacy technicians may work in all types of pharmacies along with pharmacists, as well as assisted-living facilities and nursing homes. Schedules for pharmacy technicians are often flexible, and may be full-time or part-time.

The majority of pharmacy technicians (75%) work in retail pharmacies, and approximately 17% work in hospitals. There were approximately 355,300 pharmacy technician jobs in 2012. Though no national training standard currently exists, employers prefer individuals who have received formal training or certification, or those who have previous experience. For on-the-job training, a period of between three and 12 months is usually required. Regarding formal education, pharmacy technicians may be trained at a variety of colleges, hospitals, vocational schools, and the military. Programs range between six months and two years, involving work in classrooms and laboratories. There is training in terminology, calculations, record-keeping, pharmaceutical techniques, law and ethics, medication names, drug actions, indications of drugs, and medication dosages. Training often includes *internships* that provide hands-on experience in pharmacies. Graduating pharmacy technician students may receive a certificate, a diploma, or an Associate's degree.

Most states require pharmacy technicians to become registered with their state board of pharmacy. While most states do not require pharmacy technician certification, voluntary certification is available from the Pharmacy Technician Certification Board (PTCB) via their Pharmacy Technician Certification Exam (PTCE), and the National Healthcareer Association's (NHA) Exam for the Certification of Pharmacy Technicians (ExCPT). To take the national certification examinations offered by these organizations, a high school diploma is required, along with no felony convictions. For the PTCE, the applicant cannot have had any drug- or pharmacy-related convictions, even if these are misdemeanors.

Re-certification is required every two years, involving 20 hours of continuing education. These credits can be earned from colleges, training programs, and pharmacy associations. Job-provided continuing education can also be earned, if the technician is under a pharmacist's direct supervision and instruction. Job opportunities for pharmacy technicians are expected to increase 20% up to 2022, while opportunities for pharmacy aides are expected to decrease by 6%, because the job descriptions for pharmacy technicians are enlarging to encompass many areas only previously handled by pharmacy aides.

Average wages for pharmacy technicians are between $29,320 and $42,400, while average wages for pharmacy aides are between $17,451 and $37,918. For pharmacy technicians, those with certification often earn more than those who are not certified.

Dietitians

Dietitians and *nutritionists* assist with selection and preparation of meals, promote healthy eating habits, evaluate patient diets, and suggest changes (see Figure 6.8). They also research the best diets for individual patients and groups. Major types of dietitian are listed in Table 6.3.

Most dietitians work regular 40-hour weeks, though about one in five work only part time. There are about 60,300 dietitian and nutritionist jobs in the United States, with more than half in hospitals, nursing care facilities, outpatient care centers, or other health facilities.

A Bachelor's degree or higher in dietetics, foods and nutrition, food service systems management, or a related area is required to become a dietitian or nutritionist. Each state has its own licensure, certification, or registration requirements. There are at least 275 Bachelor's

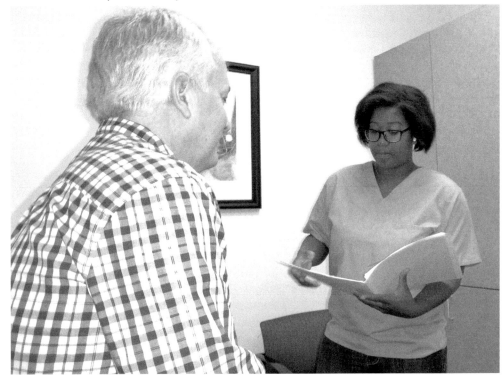

Figure 6.8 A dietitian consulting with a patient.

degree programs and 18 Master's degree programs that are approved by the American Dietetic Association. Today, 35 states require licensure, 12 require certification, and one requires registration – check with your state board of health.

There is a non-required credential called *Registered Dietitian* that is awarded by the *Commission on Dietetic Registration of the American Dietetic Association*. It requires 75 credit hours in approved continuing education every five years. Supervised internships are required for certification and last 4–5 years, or may be replaced by 900 hours of supervised practice in one of 243 accredited internships that last six months to two years based on part-time or full-time practice. Growth in the dietitian or nutritionist area of health care is about 9%, projected up to the year 2022. Annual wages range between \$31,460 and \$73,410.

You should remember

Some dietitians specialize in areas such as renal, diabetic, cardiovascular, or pediatric dietetics. The area of pediatric dietetics is expected to grow much faster (21% up to the year 2022) than the general percentage of growth in dietetics.

Sources: www.studentscholarships.org/salary/594/dietitians_and_ nutritionists.php?p=2; www.publichealthonline.org/nutrition/ #context/api/listings/prefilter.

Table 6.3 Types of dietitian specialties

Specialty	Description
Business dietitian	Develops products, designs menus, and acts as a food stylist, sales/purchasing agent, and marketing expert
Clinical dietitian	Provides services in hospitals, clinics, physician offices, or nursing homes
Community dietitian	Educates people in HMOs, home health agencies, and meal delivery companies
Consultant dietitian	Conducts nutrition screenings; works with health facilities and private practices
Educator dietitian	Teaches in schools, hospitals; performs research; writes articles and books
Management dietitian	Handles food services in cafeterias, hospitals, prisons, and schools
Research dietitian	Conduct studies in medical centers, schools, and community health programs

Chiropractors

A chiropractor treats health problems of the neuromusculoskeletal system, which includes nerves, muscles, ligaments, tendons, and bones. They utilize spinal adjustments, manipulation, and other techniques to improve health and reduce back and neck pain. There are approximately 44,400 chiropractors in the United States. In order to become a chiropractor, students must earn a Doctor of Chiropractic (DC) degree, which takes at least three years of undergraduate college education and four years of chiropractic study.

The chiropractic qualification examination is given through the National Board of Chiropractic Examiners. Job opportunities for chiropractors are expected to grow 15% up to the year 2022. The average annual wage for chiropractors is approximately $67,000.

Physical therapists and therapist assistants

Physical therapists help to identify and correct dysfunctions of normal body movement. They help to restore and maintain overall health and fitness. Physical therapists often work with patients who have or have had arthritis, stroke, heart disease, lower-back pain, cerebral palsy, fractures, and head injuries. They may utilize therapeutic exercise, a variety of assistive devices (see Figure 6.9), electrical therapies, physical agents, joint or soft tissue mobilization, bronchopulmonary therapies, and training or retraining involving neuromuscular movement and ambulation. Therapists often test and measure muscular strength and endurance, joint motion, reflexes, perceptions and sensations, nerve integrity, and how activities of daily living will be impacted by a movement disorder.

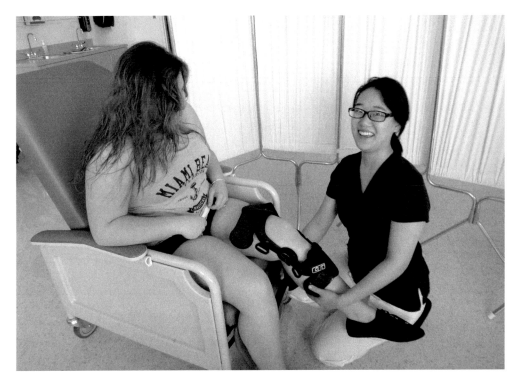

Figure 6.9 A physical therapist putting a knee brace on a patient.

Other treatments involved in physical therapy may include hot packs, cold compresses, ultrasound, deep-tissue massage, traction, and at-home exercise programs. Physical therapists often interact with many different health care professionals. Some therapists specialize in working with children, the elderly, athletes, or those with orthopedic, neurologic, or cardiopulmonary impairments. The majority of physical therapists work a normal 40-hour week, but some work evenings and weekends as needed. About one in four physical therapists work part time.

There were about 204,200 physical therapy jobs in 2012, with most occurring in hospitals or physical therapy offices. The *American Physical Therapy Association (APTA)* accredits entry-level programs in physical therapy, of which there are approximately 215. Most of these award doctoral degrees over three years, but a few award Master's degrees over two to 2.5 years.

Though eligibility requirements vary, all states regulate the practice of physical therapy. Licensure is based on graduation from an accredited program, passing the National Physical Therapy Examination, and meeting state requirements such as *jurisprudence examinations*. Continuing education is often required to maintain licensure. Job opportunities for physical therapists are expected to grow 30% up to the year 2022. Average annual wages are between $50,350 and $104,350.

Physical therapist assistants assist physical therapists in providing treatment to patients. They may demonstrate the use of equipment to patients, assist with exercises, give massages or electrical stimulation, apply traction or hot/cold packs, perform ultrasound techniques, or document patient information. Therapist assistants are directly supervised by therapists or other physical therapist assistants. Though usually working full time, about one in four physical therapist assistants work only part time.

There were about 121,400 physical therapist assistant jobs in the United States in 2012, mostly in physical therapy offices or hospitals. They usually must have a high school diploma, and can receive on-the-job training. However, most states require them to have an Associate's degree. According to the APTA, there are 237 accredited programs, which usually last for two years. Assistants must be certified in CPR and other first aid, and receive instruction in anatomy, physiology, algebra, biology, chemistry, and psychology.

Some states require licensing or registration for physical therapist assistants. Licensure may involve certain educational or examination criteria. A minimum number of hours of clinical experience is often required. State licensing boards can provide detailed information. Job opportunities for physical therapist assistants are expected to grow 35% up to the year 2022. Average annual wages range from $28,580 to $63,830.

> ## You should remember
>
> The jobs of physical therapists and therapist assistants are mentally and physically demanding. They often have to collect medical information needed for diagnosis and treatment, explain proposed therapies, assist and move patients, demonstrate exercises, and help with physical conditioning to motivate patients.

Massage therapists

Massage therapists manipulate muscles, connective tissue, tendons, and other soft body tissues, to improve joint mobility and range of motion. They do not work with the skeleton, since this type of body manipulation falls under the scope of *chiropractic*. Massage therapy is used to relieve pain and stress, improve circulation, promote relaxation, aid in general wellness, and improve quality of life for patients with many different conditions (see Figure 6.10). Massage therapists take thorough medical histories from patients in order to identify areas of manipulation that will release muscle tightness. There are many different forms of specialized massage, including deep-tissue, sports, and Swedish massage.

Massage involves manipulation via the therapist's fingers, hands, forearms, elbows, and even feet. Massage lotions or oils are often used, and therapy sessions may last from five minutes to more than one hour. Massage therapists often instruct patients about techniques they can use at home such as muscle strengthening, stretching, posture improvement, and relaxation. Massage therapists may be mobile, or work in private offices, hospitals, pain clinics, drug treatment centers, fitness centers, spas, nursing homes, hotels, and even airports.

The area of massage therapy gained popularity in the United States in the 1970s, as part of the *complementary and alternative medicine* movement. However, demand for massage therapists is extremely high. In 2014, 87,670 massage therapists were employed in the United States, mostly as part of massage therapy franchises. The field is expected to grow at a rate of 23% up to the year 2022. Regulation for massage therapy began around 1988, and licensure began as late as 1992 with the *National Certification Board for Therapeutic Massage & Bodywork (NCBTMB)*. The same year, the *Federation of State Massage Therapy Boards (FSMTB)* created its *Massage and Bodywork Licensing Examination*

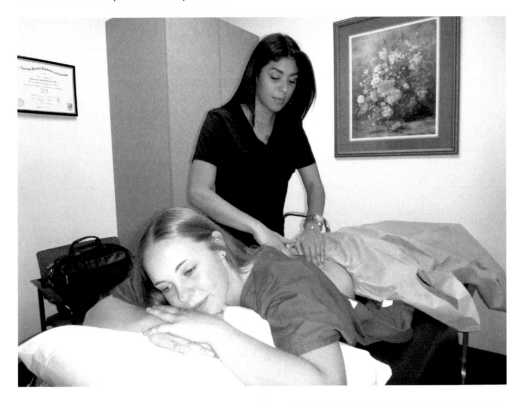

Figure 6.10 A massage therapist working with a patient.

(MBLEx). In 2014, the FSMTB became the only association that administered the MBLEx, while the NCBTMB became responsible for certification of licensed massage therapists. States that do not require licensure include Kansas, Minnesota, Oklahoma, Vermont, and Wyoming.

Most states require massage therapists to be licensed or certified, which usually follows postsecondary education involving 500–1,000 hours of study and clinical experience. Massage therapy programs are found in many private or public institutions or community colleges. Classroom study, which may be part-time or full-time, is combined with laboratory "hands-on" practice. Study areas include anatomy, physiology, kinesiology, diseases and pathology, business management, and ethics. Some programs focus on specialty areas. Programs may assist with job placement and continuing education.

At the end of 2016, all nationally certified massage therapists will be transferred to "Board Certification" because "National Certification" will no longer be valid. This new certification is considered more advanced, requiring passage of the Board Certification Exam for Therapeutic Massage and Bodywork, continuing education, professional hands-on experience, a national background check, and a complete *cardiopulmonary resuscitation certification (CPR)*. Board Certification must be renewed every two years.

Most massage therapists currently work only on a part-time basis, since building up a sufficient client base takes time. Massage therapists are advised to join a professional association in order to find additional clients. The average annual salary for a massage therapist is $41,790, though this may vary widely based on location and types of client.

> ## Focus on massage therapy
>
> Most massage therapists (88%) are female, with an average age of 45 years. They typically work as sole practitioners, but usually belong to a professional organization. The average hourly rate is about $68, though most massage therapists only work 18 hours a week actually providing massage. Other business activities dominate their workweek.
>
> *Source:* www.amtamassage.org/infocenter/
> economic_industry-fact-sheet.html.

Psychologists

Psychologists study the human mind as well as normal and abnormal human behaviors. The term *psychology* refers to the scientific collecting, quantifying, analyzing, and interpretation of human behaviors and their related mental and physical processes. The goal of a psychologist is to identify causes of behaviors, prevent undesirable behaviors, and solve problems related to behavior. Psychology helps to diagnose, treat, and prevent mental illness. It works closely with psychiatry, social work, and psychiatric nursing. Psychology, unlike psychiatry, is not actually considered a "medical" field, but is instead considered a "scientific" field.

The beginning of psychological treatment is focused on the patient's reaction to his or her life and relationships, on all levels. This differs from psychiatric social work, which initially focuses on the circumstances and relationships that surround the patient. Psychologists study both individual and group behaviors, often by utilizing in-depth interviews and tests. People who practice psychology may be employed in private practice, hospitals, mental health centers, or rehabilitation centers. Research in psychology aids in improved diagnoses as well as treatment and prevention of a large variety of mental and emotional disorders. Psychologists may also work with the disabled to diagnose and treat behavioral problems. They often resolve problems in workplaces, educational institutions, and home settings.

Many psychologists teach or work in research. Today, it is becoming more common for psychologists to work as administrators in clinics, community health facilities, and hospitals. They are also found in governmental agencies, business organizations, and the armed forces. Specialty areas of psychology are listed in Table 6.4.

There are more than 160,000 psychologist jobs in the United States, with most employed in educational institutions, followed by health care facilities of different types. When a psychologist has several years of experience and with a doctoral degree, he or she often goes into private practice, research, or consulting.

To be a psychologist, a Master's or doctoral degree, as well as a license, are required. Doctoral degrees include PhDs and Doctor of Psychology (PsyD) degrees. Doctoral degrees usually require five years of graduate study followed by a dissertation that utilizes original research.

Graduate psychology programs in college are highly competitive to enter, and may require an undergraduate major in psychology. Students who obtain a Bachelor's degree in psychology can assist psychologists and others in a variety of mental health, correctional, and rehabilitation facilities, as well as work as research or administrative assistants. The federal government employs psychologists who do not have advanced degrees, but have completed at least 24 semester hours in psychology, plus one course in statistics. Doctoral training programs are accredited by the American Psychological Association (APA), and advanced degree programs in school psychology are provided by the National Association of School Psychologists.

Table 6.4 Types of psychologist specialties

Specialty	Description
Clinical psychologist	Works with smoking cessation, weight loss, stroke and head injuries, and with the elderly
Counseling psychologist	Helps slightly maladjusted people to deal with their problems, preventing or slowing onset of mental illness
Developmental psychologist	Determines origins of behavior; studies the entire lifespan
Educational psychologist	Works in educational, training programs in the public and military areas
Engineering psychologist	Works with systems and environments used by people in daily life
Experimental/research psychologist	Works with human and animal behavior; includes comparative, learning, and physiological psychologist areas
Industrial psychologist	Uses science to improve workplace quality, productivity, and satisfaction
Personnel psychologist	Focuses on employee productivity and job satisfaction
Psychometric psychologist	Measures behavior, conducts studies to assess psychological variables
Rehabilitation psychologist	Focuses on physical, emotional, social, economic needs of the disabled
School psychologist	Develops programs for school children and adult education students
Social psychologist	Studies effects of groups and individuals in public and private areas

Licensing for psychologists varies from state to state, and between the various disciplines in the field. Licensed or certified psychologists must limit their practice to areas in which they have been professionally trained and in which they have enough experience. Most clinical and counseling psychologists require a doctoral degree, an approved internship, and 1–2 years of professional experience. Every state requires applicants to pass an examination, which is often supplemented with additional oral or written essay questions. Continuing education is often but not always required for license renewals.

At the national level, professional competency is recognized via the Nationally Certified School Psychologist (NCSP) designation, which is awarded by the National Association of School Psychologists. This is recognized by 31 states, which allow certified psychologists to transfer their credentials between states without taking another certification exam. To get the NCSP designation, 60 graduate semester hours in school psychology must be completed, as well as a 1,200-hour internship, and each applicant must also pass the National School Psychology Examination.

Certification awarded by the American Board of Professional Psychology includes 13 areas, such as psychoanalysis, forensic psychology, group psychology, rehabilitation, clinical health, school psychology, couple psychology, and family psychology. Candidates must have a doctorate in psychology and a state licensure, postdoctoral training in a chosen specialty, several years of experience, and professional endorsements. The specialty board examination must then be passed.

Industrial and organizational psychologist job opportunities are expected to increase by 53% through 2022. For other areas of psychology, the job growth is expected to be 12%. In general, salaries for psychologists range between $42,230 and $120,670.

Focus on psychology

Many people ask about the basic differences between psychologists and psychiatrists. Psychologists are not physicians and cannot generally prescribe drugs. Training is usually shorter, by several years, for a psychologist. Psychologists focus on changing thinking and behaviors, while psychiatrists focus on curing mental disorders resulting from physical abnormalities.

Medical social workers

Medical social workers help people with their personal and family problems and relationships. Their work may involve diseases, disabilities, housing, substance abuse, unemployment, domestic conflicts, research, advocacy, policy planning, and other areas. When a state requires social workers to be licensed, they may be called *licensed clinical social workers*. Areas of specialization in social work include schools, conflict resolution, child welfare, child protective services, and family services.

Medical and public health social workers give psychological and social support to people coping with all types of illnesses, including AIDS, Alzheimer's disease, and cancer. They often advise patients as well as their families about care options, including nutritional needs. Most medical social workers have 40-hour workweeks, but weekends and evenings may also require their services. There were approximately 133,510 medical social workers in the United States in 2012. The majority of their jobs were located in the health care and social assistance industries.

Social work requires the minimum of a Bachelor's degree, though more advanced degrees are often desired by employers. A Bachelor's degree in social work (BSW) is the most common minimum requirement. The *Council on Social Work Education* accredits 468 Bachelor's degree and 196 Master's degree programs. The *Group for the Advancement of Doctoral Education* lists 74 doctoral programs (DSW or PhD) in the United States. Accredited programs require at least 400 hours of supervised experience working in the field.

Licensure, certification, and registration requirements vary between the various states. The majority of states require two years, or 3,000 hours, of supervised clinical experience. You should check the requirements of your state. Job opportunities for medical social workers is expected to increase 22% up to the year 2022. Annual salaries for medical social workers ranges between $38,370 and $51,470.

Rehabilitation counselors

A rehabilitation counselor assesses clients' abilities, needs, and eligibility for a variety of services. Counselors arrange for evaluations of mental, physical, academic, vocational, and other abilities in order to determine the proper rehabilitation plan for each individual. They often work with clients' families to make sure the plan is followed, and also interact with physicians, psychologists, occupational therapists, and other professionals in order to develop and implement the correct type of plan.

There are more than 117,500 rehabilitation counselors in the United States. This type of job usually requires a Master's degree in rehabilitation counseling. A certificate or license may be required in certain jurisdictions. The National Counselor Examination is a popular choice in order to become licensed as a professional counselor, though there are other examinations more directly focused on rehabilitation counseling. Job opportunities for rehabilitation counselors are expected to grow 20% up to the year 2022. The average annual salary for this job is $33,880.

Diagnostic divisions of the health care system

The diagnostic divisions of the health care that are discussed in this chapter include radiologists, radiologic technologists, cardiovascular technologists and technicians, clinical laboratory technologists and technicians, phlebotomists, pathologists, and pathology assistants.

Radiologists

A *radiologist* is a physician who specializes in interpreting radiographs, which show the various tissues in the body. They are MDs or DOs who have completed a four-year residency focusing on various types of imaging techniques. Radiologists play an essential role in the diagnosis of various conditions and disorders.

Radiologic technologists

Radiologic technologists, along with radiologic technicians, perform diagnostic imaging examinations of patients. The difference is that radiologic technologists work with more complicated equipment, including **computed tomography (CT)**, fluoroscopy equipment, **mammography** equipment, and **magnetic resonance imaging (MRI)**. Radiologic technicians are also called *radiographers*, and work with X-ray films (radiographs). They may specialize in certain types of imaging technology.

There were about 229,300 radiologic technologist jobs in the United States in 2012, most of which were located in hospitals. A large variety of programs are available from hospitals as well as colleges and universities. Graduates receive a certificate (21–24 months of study), an Associate's degree, or a Bachelor's degree. The *Joint Review Committee on Education in Radiologic Technology* accredits 213 certificate programs, 397 Associate's degree programs, and 35 Bachelor's degree programs. Students study in both classroom and clinical scenarios, including instruction in anatomy, physiology, patient care, radiation physics and protection, imaging principles, medical terminology, patient positioning, medical ethics, pathology, and radiobiology.

Though state requirements vary, most states require radiologic technologists to be licensed. You should check with your state board of health for details. Voluntary certification is available through the *American Registry of Radiologic Technologists*, which is given after examinations are passed. Most employers prefer radiologic technologists to be certified. Continuing education involves 24 hours every two years. Job opportunities for radiologic technologists are expected to increase by 21% through the year 2022. Annual salaries range between $35,100 and $74,970.

Radiologic technicians are specially trained to provide diagnostic imaging examinations of patients. They are required to place imaging equipment over appropriate parts of patients' bodies and to program the equipment to the appropriate settings. Radiologic technicians also prepare patients for various diagnostic procedures, educate patients, and position patients. They are skilled at minimizing radiation exposure for patients, other health care professionals, and themselves.

Radiologic technicians earn Associate's degrees through universities, community colleges, technical schools, hospitals, and online universities. Programs are accredited by the Joint Review Committee on Education in Radiologic Technology (JRCERT). Licensing requirements for radiologic technicians vary widely between different states. Many require technicians to pass the *American Registry of Radiologic Technologists (ARRT)* examination in order to be licensed, or specific state licensure examinations. A few states require technicians to be certified, but you should check your state board of medicine's guidelines to determine the specifics.

You should remember

Most radiologists are primarily diagnosticians. They work with radiologic technologists to create and interpret diagnostic images, in collaboration with other physicians. Radiologic technologists specialize in working with radiologic equipment, and ensure patient safety during procedures.

Cardiovascular technologists and technicians

Cardiovascular technologists and technicians work with physicians, assisting in the diagnosis and treatment of cardiovascular conditions. Their work involves appointment scheduling, file reviews, monitoring patients, equipment maintenance, explaining procedures, and identifying abnormal test results. Cardiovascular technologists may specialize in echocardiography, invasive cardiology, or vascular technology. The cardiovascular technologists that specialize in invasive procedures are known as *cardiology technologists*. In general, they assist with cardiac catheterizations. Those who work in echocardiography or vascular technology perform non-invasive tests. Cardiovascular technicians work on basic or general monitoring tests, while technologists work on more complex testing and may even assist in surgical procedures. Technicians designated as *EKG technicians* focus primarily on electrocardiogram monitoring. They test patient heart rates and blood pressure as required. With additional training technicians may also perform more advanced tests and procedures, including exercise stress tests and Holter monitoring. They are usually responsible for maintaining and checking equipment on a regular basis.

Cardiovascular technologists and technicians usually work standard 40-hour weeks, but weekends may sometimes be required. There were about 51,080 cardiovascular technologist or technician jobs in the United States in 2012, mostly in the cardiology departments of hospitals. The separate totals of these jobs are not broken down into individual figures.

Though some are trained on the job, the majority of technologists complete two-year junior or community college programs. Four-year programs are also available and becoming more popular. Cardiovascular technicians usually complete Associate's degrees, though Bachelor's degree and certificate programs are also available. Accreditation is through the *Commission on Accreditation of Allied Health Education Programs (CAAHEP)*, and 34 programs are currently accredited in the United States.

Licensure is usually not required for these jobs, but you should contact your state's medical board for details. There is certification available, either through the *Cardiovascular Credentialing International (CCI)* administration or the *American Registry for Diagnostic Medical Sonographers*. Many employers prefer certification for their employees. Job opportunities for cardiovascular technologists and technicians are expected to grow 24% up to the year 2022. Average annual earnings for cardiovascular technologists average $48,984, while cardiovascular technicians earn $29,270.

Clinical laboratory technologists and technicians

Clinical laboratory technologists assist pathologists in performing the tests needed to determine the presence of disease and to evaluate effective treatments. Clinical laboratory testing is an extremely important component of modern health care. The majority of clinical laboratory technologists are employed in hospitals, but other work settings also exist.

In the laboratory, technologists analyze body fluids, cells, and other media for microorganisms, chemicals, blood typing, drug levels, and additional contents. Technologists are also involved in counting cells, preparing specimens, and searching for abnormalities in the blood and body fluids. They regularly utilize laboratory equipment such as microscopes, cell counters, and testing equipment that may be computerized or automated. Clinical lab technologists analyze results and send them to physicians as well as adding them into the electronic medical records of patients. With advanced technology, the work of technologists in the laboratory has become more analytical, with fewer manual procedures being required. In general, technologists have more complex job duties than technicians in the laboratory.

Lab technologists are regularly involved with complicated biological, chemical, bacteriological, hematological, immunologic, and microscopic testing. Along with lab technicians, technologists are concerned with procedures and programs that help to verify test results in an accurate manner. Technologists supervise technicians in the laboratory. In larger laboratory settings, technologists usually specialize in areas such as blood banking or cytology, clinical chemistry, immunology, and microbiology. Laboratory technologist specialty areas are quite diverse, and are summarized in Table 6.5.

You should remember

Technologists as well as technicians must wear protective clothing and equipment in order to limit potential transfer of pathogens.

Clinical laboratory technologists may have varied work schedules since many laboratories operate on a continuous, 24-hour basis. All types of work shifts are available, and many individuals work on rotating shifts instead of having regular schedules. Laboratory personnel may be "on call" for part of each workweek, or in emergencies.

Table 6.5 Types of laboratory technologist specialties

Specialty	Description
Blood bank technologist	Collects, types, and prepares blood and its components for transfusions
Clinical chemistry technologist	Analyzes body fluid chemicals, hormones; prepares specimens
Cytotechnologist	Prepares body cells on slides and examines them for abnormalities
Immunology technologist	Examines antigens, antibodies, and other immune system components
Microbiology technologist	Examines and identifies microorganisms
Molecular biology technologist	Tests cell samples as part of genetic testing for diseases

As of 2012, there were 325,800 clinical and medical laboratory technologists and technicians in the workforce, with the majority of these jobs being in hospitals, followed by physician offices and both medical and diagnostic laboratories. There is no individual breakdown of clinical or medical laboratory technologist and technician jobs. A very small number of these jobs were in educational facilities and various ambulatory facilities.

A clinical laboratory technologist requires a Bachelor's degree in medical technology or a life science. However, some individuals have attained this position via combined education and specialized training. Medical technology programs are offered by universities as well as hospitals. For individuals who do not live near larger cities, training may be accessed via online and distance learning programs. All students must receive classroom instruction as well as clinical laboratory training, usually in a hospital, that is closely supervised by laboratory staff members. Competition among students to receive clinical rotations in hospitals is high due to a lack of technology training programs to meet demand. Coursework includes study in biological sciences, chemistry, mathematics, microbiology, statistics, and clinical laboratory applications. Business, computer, and management courses are often included in the program.

Clinical laboratory technologists who perform complex testing are required by the *Clinical Laboratory Improvement Act (CLIA)* to obtain at least an Associate's degree. There are about 527 programs for medical and clinical technologists and those who choose to specify in their work. These programs are accredited by the *National Accrediting Agency for Clinical Laboratory Sciences (NAACLS)*. This agency also approves approximately 70 phlebotomy and clinical assisting programs. There are additional accrediting agencies for clinical laboratory workers, including the *Accrediting Bureau of Health Education Schools* and the *Commission on Accreditation of Allied Health Education Programs*.

Various states require lab technologists to be licensed or registered. Further information is available from state health departments or occupational licensing boards. Regarding employment, it is often preferred that applicants be certified by a recognized professional association such as the *Board of Registry of the American Society for Clinical Pathology*

(ASCP), the *American Medical Technologists*, the *Board of Registry of the American Association of Bioanalysts*, or the *National Credentialing Agency for Laboratory Personnel*.

The ASCP's Board of Certification offers a national exam for graduates of a Bachelor's program in medical technology. Once certified under the ASCP, clinical laboratory technologists can add the initials "CLS" after their names. Technologists may become lab supervisors as well as lab managers or chief scientists with continued experience and education. Advancement is faster with a graduate degree in medical technology, a biological science, chemistry, education, or management. To become a lab director, a doctoral degree is usually required. According to federal laws, directors of moderate or high-level complex laboratories must have a Bachelor's or Master's degree along with proper training and experience.

Job opportunities for clinical laboratory technologists are excellent, mostly in hospitals, with growth expected at 14% up to the year 2022. Salaries average $60,560. The highest hourly wages are for cytotechnologists at approximately $33 per hour.

Clinical laboratory technicians are involved in less complicated activities in the laboratory, in comparison with clinical laboratory technologists. However, they also are involved with microscopic examination of blood and other body fluids and tissues for the presence of specific microorganisms. Technicians are basically involved in less complicated testing and laboratory procedures than technologists. They prepare specimens, conduct manual testing, and may operate **automated analyzers**. Their work is usually supervised by a technologist, the lab manager, a research scientist, or a pathologist. Technicians may also work in various specialties or focus on just one area. Examples include *histotechnicians*, who prepare specimens of tissues so that pathologists can examine them microscopically, and *phlebotomists*, who collect samples.

Clinical laboratory technicians usually must have either an Associate's degree from a community or junior college, or a certificate from a hospital, vocational or technical school, or the military. However, some technicians learn their skills through on-the-job training. Along with technologists, lab technicians are trained to work with potentially infectious specimens and utilize proper infection control and sterilization methods.

Regarding licensure, for those who have met postsecondary training requirements and have passed their examination, a Medical Laboratory Technician Certification can be obtained through the American Association of Bioanalysts. Lab technicians can advance through education and experience to become lab technologists.

Job opportunities for clinical laboratory technicians are even better than for technologists, with 30% growth expected up to the year 2022. The Affordable Care Act is anticipated to increase demand for technicians, as well as technologists, since more people have access to health insurance via the health exchanges. Salaries average $40,750 for clinical laboratory technicians. Pay is higher for those who acquire additional education, training, and certification in various subspecialties.

Phlebotomists

Phlebotomists are actually considered a specialty area of *clinical laboratory technicians*. Their job involves drawing blood, transporting it to the lab for processing and analysis, and basic blood testing. They may use centrifuges and other equipment related to blood testing. Phlebotomists may also assist in drawing blood for blood drives, and often are required to explain what they do to patients prior to drawing blood. They also assist when an adverse reaction occurs following a phlebotomy procedure. Phlebotomy involves both venipuncture and skin puncture, based on the type of blood testing that is required (see Figure 6.11). The

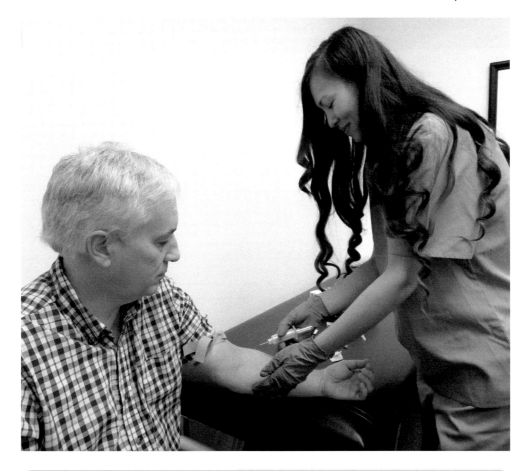

Figure 6.11 A phlebotomist performing venipuncture.

job requires strong interpersonal skills, since phlebotomists must often deal with patients who are apprehensive about blood being drawn.

Phlebotomists work in a variety of facilities, including hospitals, blood donation facilities, diagnostic laboratories, outpatient clinics, and may even work as mobile blood-collection personnel. Because of high, continual demand for their services, phlebotomists have a great number of future job opportunities. Their positions are continually evolving to become part of other job titles, but their skills will always be needed.

Most phlebotomists attain a postsecondary non-degree award from a phlebotomy program in a community college, or a vocational or technical school. Some phlebotomists, however, proceed from a high school diploma into direct on-the-job training. Those who prefer formal education usually receive a certificate or a diploma, and phlebotomy programs usually take less than one year to complete. Instruction involves classroom study and laboratory "hands-on" practice. A phlebotomist will receive instruction in anatomy, physiology, and medical terminology. Except for California, Florida, Louisiana, Nevada, and Washington, phlebotomists are not required to be licensed. However, it is suggested that you check with your state health department or occupational licensing board for updated information.

However, most employers prefer phlebotomists who are certified. This usually involves completion, after education, of an examination that requires demonstration of venipuncture and skin puncture. Laboratory experience is taken into account only if it is within a CLIA-regulated laboratory. Phlebotomy certification can be obtained from the ASCP, the *American Certification for Healthcare Professionals (ACA)*, the *American Medical Technologists (AMT)*, or the *National Center for Competency Testing (NCCT)*. Some phlebotomists seek additional training to become medical assistants or other types of health care professional.

Job opportunities for phlebotomists are projected to grow 27% up to the year 2022. The average salary for a phlebotomist is approximately $32,000 per year.

> ### Focus on phlebotomists
>
> Certified phlebotomists can expect to work with multiple medical professionals, including physicians, nurses, EMTs, paramedics, dialysis technicians, laboratory scientists, and surgeons.

Pathologists

Pathologists are physicians specializing in the diagnosis and study of disease, using laboratory methods. Many pathology jobs require completion of medical school and postgraduate training through residencies. Board certification is available for pathologists. Pathologists are usually clinical or anatomical in their job focus. Clinical pathologists primarily examine body fluids, conduct toxicology tests, work in blood banks, or test immune functions of patients. Anatomical pathologists analyze cell and tissue samples to determine the causes of disease.

There are more than 18,000 pathologist jobs in the United States. The American Society of Clinical Pathologists administers the National Registry Examination. After earning their medical degree, pathologists complete specialized study and then usually become certified through the American Board of Pathology. Job opportunities for pathologists are expected to grow 18% up to the year 2022. The average annual salary for pathologists is $174,544.

Pathology assistants

Pathology assistants work under the supervision of pathologists in preparing and dissecting surgical specimens, as well as in the preparation and selection of tissue samples for analysis. Pathology assistants often are required to document findings and sterilize equipment. They may work as assistants to surgical departments, coroners, medical examiners, and in many administrative capacities. There are more than 51,000 pathology assistant jobs in the United States. Voluntary certification is provided through the ASCP. Pathology assistants need a Bachelor's or Master's degree from an accredited program, plus up to two years of additional experience prior to practice. They may need certification as a pathology assistant. Job opportunities for pathology assistants are expected to grow 30% up to the year 2022. The average annual salary for a pathology assistant is $58,640.

Health care management

The positions involved in health care management that are discussed in this chapter include health care administrators and health information technicians.

Health care administrators

Health care administrators manage health care businesses and coordinate services performed by clinics, physician offices, hospitals, and nursing care facilities. There are more than 250,000 jobs for health care administrators in the United States. Many colleges and universities offer Bachelor's, Master's, and doctoral degrees in health care administration. More than 70 schools have accredited Master's degree programs. Also, certificate or diploma programs exist that often are less than one year in length. For upper-level health care management positions, most employers seek candidates who have at least a Bachelor's degree. Job opportunities for health care administrators are expected to grow 22% up to the year 2022. Average annual wages range between $85,860 and $102,000.

Health information technicians

Health information technicians, or *medical records technicians*, manage health information provided by patients, physicians, and other health professionals. They receive patient forms, medical histories, and test results, which they then analyze for accuracy and completeness. Their primary responsibility is to maintain confidentiality of all health information. There are more than 186,300 health information technician jobs in the United States. Health information technicians usually need an Associate's degree in order to be employed. Job opportunities for health information technicians are expected to grow 22% by the year 2022. Health information technicians usually receive annual wages of $34,160.

Health care education

Health care educators are responsible for teaching health and wellness to people of all ages. The two job areas focused on this chapter are health educators and school health educators.

Health educators

Health educators teach people about behaviors that promote wellness for individuals and communities. They are generally full-time employees that may work in many different settings, including colleges, non-profit organizations, and hospitals. There are more than 99,400 health educators in the United States. Health educators must earn at least a Bachelor's degree, and many employers require them to have the Certified Health Education Specialist credential. Job opportunities for health educators are expected to grow 21% by the year 2022. Average annual wages for health educators are $48,790.

School health educators

School health educators assist children and younger people to develop healthy living skills, working alongside school physicians and nurses, teachers, and other administrative personnel. They most often participate in community health programs. School health educators need at least four years of college education, a Bachelor's degree or Master's degree, and a background in health education as well as the behavioral, biological, and social sciences. They must meet the regular certification standards for teachers in their states. Job opportunities are expected to grow 18% by the year 2022. Average annual wages for school health educators are $41,830.

CASE STUDY

To determine which area of health care you may be best suited for, many colleges offer "aptitude tests" that help to determine your areas of interest, and then match them to health careers. Areas of questioning include demonstrating respect, interpersonal communication, quality orientation, service orientation, and patient centricity. These tests have the potential to help students focus on careers that they really have the most chance of being successful in. Unfortunately, many students base their decisions on lack of information or bad reasoning.

1 Many students choose a specialty based on its earning potential. Can you name the specialties with the highest earning potentials?
2 Often, students choose a specialty based on a false perception that the work hours are "easier" than other specialties. Why do you think being an emergency medical technician, a radiologist, or an anesthesiologist might actually require more unpredictable work schedules than they might seem to offer initially?
3 Since a medical specialty is probably going to be a lifelong occupation, can you think of some ways to realistically choose your specialty before you begin serious education toward it?

Chapter highlights

This section answers the Objectives found at the beginning of the chapter.

1 Describe the roles of physician assistants.

- Physician assistants assist physicians in providing personal health services. They are specially trained to assist doctors of medicine or osteopathy, and are directly responsible for their own actions while working.

2 List the top five jobs in this chapter that have the highest projected growth.

- Industrial and organizational psychologist (53% job growth)
- Physician assistant (38%)
- Dental hygienist (36%)
- Physical therapist assistant (35%)
- Medical assistant (34%).

3 Differentiate between the job descriptions of dental hygienists and dental assistants.

- Dental hygienists educate patients about good oral hygiene, provide oral examinations, record findings, clean teeth, providing preventive dental care, take and develop X-rays, apply fluorides and other agents, and seal pits and fissures in the teeth.

- Dental assistants provide dental care for patients, and perform office and laboratory support work. They assist dentists, help patients to feel comfortable, prepare patients, access dental records, use suction and other devices, disinfect and sterilize equipment, prepare equipment trays, and educate patients about oral health care.

4 Describe the job duties of emergency medical technicians and paramedics.

- Emergency medical technicians and paramedics provide fast, life-saving care, and treat and transport patients to medical facilities. They are usually dispatched by 911 operators, and work with firefighters and police.

5 Explain the differences between chiropractors and physical therapists.

- Chiropractors treat neuromusculoskeletal problems affecting nerves, muscles, ligaments, tendons, and bones. They use spinal adjustments, manipulation, and other techniques to reduce back and neck pain.
- Physical therapists help to identify and correct dysfunctions of movement. They help restore and maintain overall health and fitness, and often work with patients who have or have had arthritis, stroke, heart disease, lower-back pain, cerebral palsy, fractures, and head injuries.

6 Outline the education required to become a psychologist.

- To be a psychologist, a Master's or doctoral degree, as well as a license, are required. Doctoral degrees include PhDs or Doctor of Psychology (PsyD) degrees. Doctoral degrees usually require five years of graduate study followed by a dissertation that utilizes original research.

7 Describe the duties of health care administrators and health information technicians.

- Health care administrators manage health care businesses and coordinate services of clinics, physician offices, hospitals, and nursing care facilities. Health information technicians manage health information provided by patients, physicians, and other health professionals.

8 Explain the roles of dietitians in the health care profession.

- Dietitians and nutritionists assist with selection and preparation of meals, promote healthy eating habits, evaluate patient diets, and suggest changes. They also research the best diets for individual patients and groups.

9 Describe the roles of clinical laboratory technologists.

- Clinical laboratory technologists assist pathologists in performing tests to determine presence of disease and to evaluate treatments. In the laboratory, they analyze body fluids, cells, and other media for microorganisms, chemicals, blood type, drug levels, and additional contents.

10 Explain the activities of various health educators.

- Health educators teach people about behaviors that promote wellness for individuals and communities. School health educators assist children and younger people to develop healthy living skills, working alongside school physicians and nurses, teachers, and other administrative personnel. They most often participate in community health programs.

Summary

The primary careers in health care are supported by many other areas of work. It is most important to understand the requirements of these primary careers. Physicians diagnose, prescribe, treat, examine, interview, counsel, and test patients. Their work is of primary responsibility in patient care, and physicians may specialize in diverse areas including anesthesiology, pediatrics, or gynecology. Registered or licensed practical nurses have hands-on job descriptions, and are responsible for a large amount of patient interaction and care. Medical assistants support many other health care professionals, including physicians and nurses. Dentists and orthodontists specialize in the teeth and oral tissues. Emergency medical technicians and paramedics deal with situations requiring immediate care and life support.

Pharmacists dispense medications prescribed by physicians, dentists, and other health professionals. Physical therapists and chiropractors focus on musculoskeletal therapies, while psychologists treat patients with mental and emotional conditions. Many diagnostic procedures involve the services of radiologists and radiologic technologists, while testing is performed by clinical laboratory technologists and technicians, which include phlebotomists. Together, this large, diverse group of medical personnel contribute to our health care system.

Review questions

1 What is holistic care?
2 Compare registered nurses with advanced practice nurses.
3 What is the difference between physician assistants and medical assistants?
4 What is telemedicine?
5 What is the role of the dental hygienist in health care?
6 Which technicians in health care are trained to perform endotracheal intubations?
7 What is the role of the pharmacist in a hospital?
8 List major types of dietitian.
9 Compare the physical therapist's responsibilities with those of a massage therapist.
10 What is industrial psychology?

Bibliography

AAPA. 2016. AAPA – Home Page. Available at: www.aapa.org. Alexandria: American Academy of PAs.

Academy of Nutrition and Dietetics. 2016. AND – Home Page. Available at: www.eatright. org. Chicago: Academy of Nutrition and Dietetics.

Accreditation Council for Pharmacy Education. 2016. ACPE – Home Page. Available at: www.acpe-accredit.org/default.asp. Chicago: Accreditation Council for Pharmacy Education.

Allicance for Cardiovascular Professionals. 2016. ACP – Home Page. Available at: www. acp-online.org. Midlothian: Alliance of Cardiovascular Professionals.

Amergican Dental Hygienists' Association. 2016. ADHA – Home Page. Available at: www. adha.org. Chicago: American Dental Hygienists' Association.

American Association for Respiratory Care. 2016. AARC – Home Page. Available at: www. aarc.org. Irving: American Association for Respiratory Care.

American Association of Bioanalysts. 2016. AAB – Home Page. Available at: www.aab.org. St. Louis: The American Association of Bioanalysts.

American Association of Colleges of Nursing. 2016. AACN – Home Page. Available at: www.aacn.nche.edu. Washington, D.C.: American Association of Colleges of Nursing.

American Association of Medical Assistants. 2016. AAMA – Home Page. Available at: www.aama-ntl.org. Chicago: American Association of Medical Assistants.

American Association of Orthodontists. 2016. AAO – Home Page. Available at: www. braces.org. St. Louis: American Association of Orthodontists.

American Board of Medical Specialties. 2016. ABMS – Home Page. Available at: www. abms.org. Chicago: American Board of Medical Specialties.

American Board of Professional Psychology. 2016. ABPP – Home Page. Available at: www. abpp.org. Chapel Hill: American Board of Professional Psychology.

American College of Surgeons. 2016. FACS – Home Page. Available at: www.facs.org. Chicago: American College of Surgeons.

American Dental Assistants Association. 2016. ADAA – Home Page. Available at: www. dentalassistant.org. Bloomingdale: American Dental Assistants Association.

American Dental Association. 2016. ADA – Home Page. Available at: www.ada.org. Chicago: American Dental Association.

American Dental Education Association. 2016. ADEA – Home Page. Available at: www. adea.org. Washington, D.C.: American Dental Education Association.

American Massage Therapy Association. 2016. AMTA – Home Page. Available at: www. amtamassage.org/index.html. Evanston: American Massage Therapy Association.

American Massage Therapy Association. 2016. Industry Fact Sheet. Available at: www. amtamassage.org/infocenter/economic_industry-fact-sheet.html. Evanston: American Massage Therapy Association.

American Medical Association. 2012. *Health Care Careers Directory 2012–2013, 40th Edition*. Chicago: American Medical Association. Print.

American Medical Association. 2016. AMA – Home Page. Available at: www.ama-assn. org/go/becominganmd. Chicago: American Medical Association.

American Medical Technologists. 2016. AMT – Home Page. Available at: www.american medtech.org. Rosemont: American Medical Technologists.

American Nurses Association. 2016. ANA – Home Page. Available at: http://nursingworld. org. Silver Spring: American Nurses Association.

American Nurses Association. 2016. NPR Series on Nurse Injuries. Available at: www. nursingworld.org/especiallyforyou/staff-nurses/staff-nurse-news/npr-series-on-nurse-injuries. html. Silver Spring: The American Nurses Association, Inc.

The American Occupational Therapy Association, Inc. 2016. AOTA – Home Page. Available at: www.aota.org. Bethesda: American Occupational Therapy Association.

American Optometric Association. 2016. AOA – Home Page. Available at: www.aoa.org. St. Louis: American Optometric Association.

American Osteopathic Association. 2016. American Osteopathic Association – Home Page. Available at: www.osteopathic.org. Chicago: American Osteopathic Association.

American Pharmacists Association. 2016. APhA – Home Page. Available at: www.pharmacist. com. Washington, D.C.: American Pharmacists Association.

American Physical Therapy Association. 2016. APTA – Home Page. Available at: www. apta.org. Alexandria: American Physical Therapy Association.

American Psychological Association. 2016. APA – Home Page. Available at: www.apa.org/ students. Washington, D.C.: American Psychological Association.

American Registry of Diagnostic Medical Sonographers. 2016. ARDMS – Home Page. Available at: www.ardms.org. Rockville: American Registry for Diagnostic Medical Sonography.

American Registry of Radiologic Technologists. 2016. ARRT – Home page. Available at: www.arrt.org. St. Paul: American Registry of Radiologic Technologists.

American Society for Clinical Laboratory Science. 2016. ASCLS – Home Page. Available at: www.ascls.org. McLean: American Society for Clinical Laboratory Science.

American Society for Clinical Pathology. 2016. ASCP – Home Page. Available at: www. ascp.org. Chicago: American Society for Clinical Pathology.

American Society for Cytopathology. 2016. ASC – Home Page. Available at: www.cytopathology.org. Wilmington, Delaware: American Society for Cytopathology.

American Society of Health-System Pharmacists. 2016. ASHP – Home Page. Available at: www.ashp.org. Bethesda: American Society of Health-System Pharmacists.

American Society of Radiologic Technologists. 2016. ASRT – Home Page. Available at: www.asrt.org. Albuquerque: American Society of Radiologic Technologists.

American Speech-Language-Hearing Association. 2016. ASHA – Home Page. Available at: www.asha.org. Rockville: American Speech-Language-Hearing Association.

ARC-PA. 2016. ARC-PA Home Page. Available at: www.arc-pa.org. Johns Creek: Accreditation Revie Commission on Education for the Physician Assistant.

Askew, J.P. 2010. *From Student to Pharmacist: Making the Transition*. Washington, D.C.: American Pharmacists Association. Print.

Association of American Medical Colleges. 2012. Estimating the number and characteristics of hospitalist physicians in the United States and their possible workforce implications. *Analysis in Brief* 12, no. 3.

Association of Schools and Colleges of Optometry. 2016. ASCO – Home Page. Available at: www.opted.org. Rockville: Association of Schools and Colleges of Optometry.

Association of Social Work Boards. 2016. ASWB – Home Page. Available at: www.aswb. org. Culpeper: Association of Social Work Boards.

Association of Surgical Technologists. 2016. AST – Home Page. Available at: www.ast.org. Littleton: Association of Surgical Technologists.

Audiology Foundation of America. 2016. AFA – Home Page. Available at: www.audfound. org. Mesa: Audiology Foundation of America.

Buchbinder, S.B., and Shanks, N.H. 2011. *Introduction to Health Care Management, 2nd Edition*. Burlington: Jones & Bartlett Learning. Print.

Bylsma, W.H., et al. 2010. Where have all the general internists gone? *Journal of General Internal Medicine* 25, no. 10: 1020–1023.

Cardiovascular Credentialing International. 2016. CCI – Home Page. Available at: www. cci-online.org. Raleigh: Cardiovascular Credentialing International.

Caudill, T., et al. 2011. Health care reform and primary care: Training physicians for tomorrow's challenges. *Academic Medicine* 86, no. 2: 158–160.

Center for Phlebotomy Education. 2016. CPE – Home Page. Available at: www.phlebotomy. com. Corydon: Center for Phlebotomy Education.

Commission on Dental Accreditation. 2016. ADA – CODA Home Page. Available at: www. ada.org/prof/ed/acred/commission/index.asp. Chicago: Commission on Dental Accreditation.

Commission on Dietetic Registration. 2016. CDRNet – Home Page. Available at: www.cdrnet.org. Chicago: Commission on Dietetic Registration.

Confluence Health. 2016. Optometry – Optometric Physicians Provide a Full Range of Primary Eye Health Care Service. Available at: www.confluencehealth.org/specialties/optometry/. Wenatchee: Confluence Health.

Cunningham, P.J. 2011. *State Variation in Primary Care Physician Supply: Implications for Health Reform Medicaid Expansions*. Research Brief No. 19. Washington, D.C.: Center for Studying Health System Change.

DeLaet, R. 2011. *Introduction to Health Care & Careers, Pap/Psc Edition*. New York: Lippincott, Williams, & Wilkins. Print.

Dental Assisting National Board, Inc. 2016. DANB – Home Page. Available at: www.danb.org. Chicago: Dental Assisting National Board.

Department of Health and Human Services (DHHS). 2012. *Health, United States, 2012*. Hyattsville: Department of Health and Human Services.

Dun & Bradstreet – First Research. 2016. Optometrists Industry Profile. Available at: www.firstresearch.com/industry-research/optometrists.html. Austin: Hoover's Inc.

Enelow, W.S., and Kursmark, L.M. 2010. *Expert Resumes for Health Care Careers, 2nd Edition*. St. Paul: Jist Works. Print.

Evergreen Nursing Services. 2014. Workplace Violence Prevention Policy. Available at: www.evergreennursing.ca/images/policy-pdf/workplace-violence-prevention-policy.pdf. Vancouver: Evergreen Nursing Services.

Freedman, J. 2012. 4 Bad Reasons Why Medical Students Choose A Specialty. Available at: www.kevinmd.com/blog/2012/12/4-bad-reasons-medical-students-choose-specialty.html. Nashua: KevinMD, LLC.

Freeman, B. 2012. *The Ultimate Guide to Choosing a Medical Specialty, 3rd Edition*. New York: McGraw-Hill Education/Medical. Print.

Goldberg, E.M. 2013. *So, You Want to Be a Physician: Getting the Edge in the Pursuit of Becoming a Physician or Other Medical Professional*. Seattle: CreateSpace Independent Publishing Platform. Print.

Gutkind, L. 2013. *I Wasn't Strong Like This When I Started out: True Stories of Becoming a Nurse*. Pittsburgh: In Fact Books. Print.

Jacobson, P.D. and Jazowski, S.A. 2011. Physicians, the Affordable Care Act, and primary care: Disruptive change or business as usual? *Journal of General Internal Medicine* 26, no. 8: 934–937.

Julian, K., et al. 2011. Creating the next generation of general internists: A call for medical education reform. *Academic Medicine* 86, no. 11: 1443–1447.

Keckley, P.H., et al. 2013. *Deloitte 2013 Survey of U.S. Physicians*. Washington, D.C.: Deloitte Center for Health Solutions.

Knapp, K.K. and Cultice, J.M. 2007. New Pharmacist Supply Projections: Lower Separation Rates and Increased Graduates Boost Supply Estimates. Available at: www.pharmacist.com/sites/default/files/files/new_pharmacist_supply_Knapp.pdf. Washington, D.C.: Journal of the American Pharmacists Association.

Mintz, M. 2016. Why Medical Students Aren't Choosing Primary Care (And Why They Should). Available at: www.primarycareprogress.org/blogs/16/394. Cambridge, Massachusetts: Primary Care Progress.

Moini, J. 2012. *Phlebotomy: Principles and Practice, Pap/Psc Edition*. Burlington: Jones & Bartlett Learning. Print.

National Academy of Sciences. 2010. *The Future of Nursing: Leading Change, Advancing Health*. Washington, D.C.: The Institute of Medicine.

National Registry of Emergency Medical Technicians. 2016. NREMT Data, Dashboard, and Maps. Available at: www.nremt.org/rwd/public/data/maps. Columbus: National Registry of Emergency Medical Technicians.

Neff, T., for UCHealth. 2016. CU Researchers Take Aim at PTSD, Burnout in ICU. Available at: www.uchealth.org/today/news/cu-researchers-take-aim-at-ptsd-burnout-in-the-icu. Denver: UCHealth.

Nelson, S., Tassone, M., and Hodges, B.D. 2014. *Creating the Health Care Team of the Future: The Toronto Model for Interprofessional Education and Practice*. Ithaca: ILR Press. Print.

Petterson, S.M., et al. 2012. Projecting US primary care physician workforce needs: 2010–2025. *Annals of Family Medicine* 10, no. 6: 503–509.

Public Health Online. 2016. A Guide to Becoming a Nutritionist – Teach Healthy Heabits with a Career as a Nutritionist. Available at: www.publichealthonline.org/nutrition/#context/api/listings/prefilter. Washington, D.C.: Public Health Online.

Redhead, C.S., and Williams, E.D. 2010. *Public Health, Workforce, Quality, and Related Provisions in PPACA: Summary and Timeline*. Washington, D.C.: Congressional Research Service.

Riegel, B., et al. 2012. Meeting global needs in primary care with nurse practitioners. *Lancet* 380, no. 9840: 449–450.

Schimpff, S.C. 2014. Why Is There A Shortage of Primary Care Physicians?. Available at: www.kevinmd.com/blog/2014/02/shortage-primary-care-physicians.html. Nashua: Medpage Today's KevinMD.com.

Schwartz, M.D. 2011. Health care reform and the primary care workforce bottleneck. *Journal of General Internal Medicine* 27, no. 4: 469–472.

Sheen, B. 2014. *Careers in Health Care (Exploring Careers)*. San Diego: Referencepoint Press. Print.

Starfield, B. 2011. Point: The changing nature of disease implications for health services. *Medical Care* 49, no. 11: 971–972.

Student Scholarships.org. 2016. Dietitians and Nutritionists – What They Do. Available at: www.studentscholarships.org/salary/594/dietitians_and_nutritionists.php?p=2. Washington, D.C.: StudentScholarships.org.

Su, D., and Li, L. 2011. Trends in the use of complementary and alternative medicine in the United States: 2002–2007. *Journal of Health Care for the Poor and Underserved* 22: 295–309.

Tomic, J., and Pesola, M. 2013. *Becoming a Physician Assistant*. Seattle: Amazon Digital Services, Inc. Electronic book.

U.S. Census Bureau. 2012. *Statistical Abstract of the United States, 2011*. Washington, D.C.: U.S. Census Bureau.

West, C.P., and Dupras, D.M. 2012. General medicine vs subspecialty career plans among internal medicine residents. *JAMA* 308, no. 21: 2241–2247.

Wilkins, A. 2014. *The Way of the Superior Dentist: Connecting with Patients, Creating Abundance, and Cultivating Your Passion*. Seattle: CreateSpace Independent Publishing Platform. Print.

Wischnitzer, S., and Wischnitzer, E. 2010. *Top 100 Health-Care Careers, 3rd Edition*. St. Paul: Jist Works. Print.

World Health Organization (WHO). 2010. *Primary Health Care*. Geneva, Switzerland: WHO.

Chapter 7

Professionalism in health care

After study of the chapter, readers should be able to:

1 Differentiate between the hard and soft skills required by health care professions.
2 Explain "professional distance."
3 Describe continuing education units.
4 Discuss how good judgment is related to critical thinking.
5 Explain cultural diversity and its importance in health care.
6 Outline how a patient advocate assists patients and their families.
7 List the steps that help to show empathy toward a patient.
8 Explain why behaving with integrity is so important in health care.
9 Explain what the concept of accountability in health care is based upon.
10 List examples of professional appearance.

Overview

A profession is an occupation that is based on specialized educational training. Professionalism is behavior that exhibits the features corresponding to the standards of that profession. In health care, professionalism is of the utmost importance, yet is not easy to explain simply. The meaning of professionalism in health care may be expressed as caring competence. Patients usually contact many different professionals as part of their health care, and each of these professionals plays a role in the patient's overall confidence that their treatment is being handled well. Each health care professional represents the entire facility they work in, as well as the services that are provided and their entire team of professionals.

There is a variety of areas that must be addressed, which together form the basis of a person's professional approach to his or her health care occupation. A professional in the health care field delivers consistent quality of care, regularly addresses quality improvement issues, and delivers the highest possible customer satisfaction.

Professionalism

Professionalism is developed when an individual has the skill, training, judgment, and behavior to perform a job well. In today's health care, professionalism includes the ability to communicate knowledge, diagnoses, and treatment options in a way that is easy to understand. Medical professionalism also involves confidentiality, continuity, compassion, honesty, and trust.

Health care professions require both *hard skills* and *soft skills*. Hard skills concern technical and operational abilities in your chosen field. Soft skills may also be called *people skills*, and are the things you bring to your profession that enhance your performance. Examples of hard skills in various health care fields include the ability to code, schedule, interview, manage records, assist other professionals, or take vital signs (see Figure 7.1). Examples of soft skills include integrity, dependability, respect, patience, good attitude toward your work, and ethics.

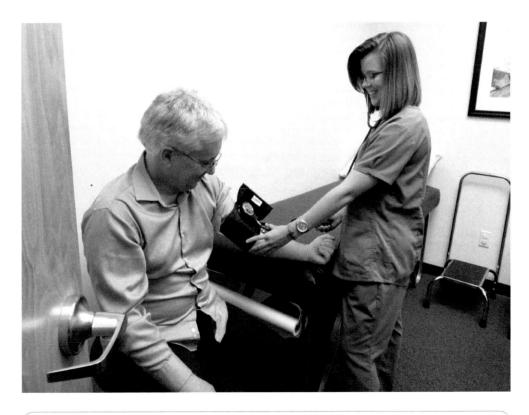

Figure 7.1 A medical assistant taking a patient's blood pressure (an example of "hard skills").

A true health care professional approaches his or her job positively and with enthusiasm. The patient is the focus of their work, and the daily goal is to provide excellent patient care, regardless of their actual job title. A professional attitude is shown by commitment to work and understanding its value to the patient. The health care professional's concern for the welfare of patients and providers is called altruism. Regarding patients, altruism involves understanding of beliefs, cultures, and perspectives. You should work for the benefit of patients and toward their positive experiences with your facility. It is important always to remain objective rather than *emotional* about situations involving patients who are upset, rude, angry, fearful, or experiencing pain. Every problem is an opportunity for you to take positive action. Develop self-discipline and practice it daily; this will help you to become more competent at your job and your self-confidence will increase.

Professional behavior

Professional behavior begins with your attitude, and demonstrates *caring competence*. Patients who are satisfied with their health care experience often say that their health care team really *cared* about their welfare. When patients are dissatisfied, poor outcomes are more likely to occur, including malpractice lawsuits. Good health care increases patient loyalty. It is important that health care professionals are dependable, complete their assignments, meet deadlines, perform all required duties, and are willing to help, comfortable with changing work functions, open to diversity, courteous, and considerate. A professional never complains about problems at work in an inappropriate situation, such as when a patient might overhear. It is important to be organized, have a well-designed work plan, always follow ethical guidelines, remain calm in all situations, encourage good health habits in others, and always try to improve.

Focus on professionalism

A health care provider who says, "It's not my job" while at work will probably not do well in their field. Health care professionals understand that their occupations require them to be willing to help, often in areas that may be outside their actual job description. The only exception is if they are asked to do something they are not trained for, or legally allowed to do.

Attending every scheduled day of work, and being on time, are crucial elements of professional behavior. Poor attendance often results in termination. Being absent or late may result in work not being completed, or may cause others to have to do the work that was assigned to you. In health care fields, patients may suffer because of these situations.

Communication

In order to communicate professionally, you must be careful when observing, listening, writing, and speaking. Good communication must occur regardless of whom you are exchanging information with, and it should always be done with politeness, respect, and tact. Poor communication skills result in information becoming misunderstood or perceived inaccurately. Both the giver and receiver of information must communicate well in order to ensure that the message was exchanged correctly. Good communication skills affect every health care profession.

Respect for patients

Patients have the right to *autonomy*, the capacity to make decisions based on their own reasons and motives, which is also described as *self-determination*. It is extremely important for health care professionals to respect the rights of patients to make their own health care decisions. This is accomplished by providing patients with information that allows them to make informed choices, honoring patient and family rights to make health care decisions, and assisting patients in planning their own health care.

Part of having respect for patients involves their dignity, worth, and uniqueness. This means designing patient care based on the patient's individual needs. Confidentiality of patient and provider information is crucial. The patient's privacy must always be protected. Also, care must be sensitive to the patient's culture, since people from so many different cultures are present in this country. Care must be provided to everyone, taking their cultural differences into account.

Health care professionals must be patient advocates. This is especially true for the most vulnerable patients. Regarding other health care providers, it is important to offer mentoring, and to take risks to assist your colleagues. Risks are also often taken on behalf of patients.

Focus on patient respect

In order to show respect to patients, you should always be courteous, validate their actions, and give them your honesty and sincerity. This is accomplished by remaining polite, keeping their information private, being non-judgmental, never allowing them to appear foolish, acknowledging needs, praising accomplishments, explaining delays or wait times, and letting them have control of their health care.

Comprehension

Comprehension involves the ways we learn information, process it, and remember what was communicated. Regardless of your chosen field, you must also be able to analyze information in order to use and remember it well. In health care, communication and understanding may be blocked by complex medical information and a lack of tools supporting education and comprehension. One effective education technique involves "teach-back" methods, which ensure that patient comprehension is achieved. This technique also works well between health care professionals.

There is a high level of skill that must be maintained in health care, so that tasks are performed correctly, carefully, and with close attention. Each patient deserves the best possible efforts. You should learn as much as you can about the theories behind your work and its required skills. Always observe and listen closely, and ask questions regularly. Read your employee manual and ask about policies and procedures if needed. Always attempt to perform your work as neatly and accurately as possible. Make sure to spend time continually educating yourself about your job.

> ## You should remember
>
> Good communication skills require self-awareness. You must understand your own personal style of communicating, which will help you to assess how others are receiving the information you send them. It is best to communicate assertively, rather than passively or aggressively.

Professional distance

Professional distance should be kept between health care workers and patients to demonstrate professionalism. Patients should not be viewed as personal friends, but as people you professionally serve. You may not always be able to please a patient, but you *should* always professionally serve them. The goal is to demonstrate caring while giving patients the best-quality, high-level health care possible. Steps to use in order to maintain professional distance are summarized in Table 7.1.

> ## Focus on professional distance
>
> Key factors concerning professional distance between health care professionals and patients include avoiding discussion of your personal life with patients and not accepting gifts from them. These sorts of behaviors may lead to possible breaches of ethics in the health care setting.

Table 7.1 Steps used in maintaining professional distance

Step	Explanation
Addressing the adult patient	Use only his or her last name (for example, Mrs. Jones, Mr. Smith) unless you have been given permission to use a first name
Addressing the pediatric patient	It is acceptable to use the first name of a child
Friendliness	Always be friendly, but avoid excessive friendliness
Humor	Use only if tasteful and appropriate
Meeting outside the health care office	Do not agree to meet a patient outside of the health care office unless you were previously acquainted before seeing the patient professionally
Money	Avoid giving or accepting money from the patient

Acceptance of constructive input

It is important to take responsibility for your own actions while working, and accepting *constructive input* properly in order to improve is a vital skill. When constructive input is given to you to help you improve in your work, you must understand it for what it is – an attempt to counsel or advise you, and not an attempt to insult or belittle you. You need to learn how to accept feedback about your work from a wide variety of individuals. Workplace evaluations of each health care professional are regularly conducted in order to optimize the effectiveness of health care organizations. A perfect evaluation of your work is rare, since there is always room to improve and grow in your skills and abilities. You are usually invited to offer your own suggestions about self-improvement. Remember never to be defensive about constructive input or feedback, and not to blame others, since the focus is on improving your own work.

Growth

Health care professionals are continually required to learn, improve, and become educated about the latest advancements in their field. Health care practices, standards, and regulations change often. It is wise to join several professional organizations related to your field. These organizations usually provide continuing education units (CEUs), of which you must earn a certain number over a specific time period in order to continue to practice. Continuing education may involve the reading of articles and other information, taking courses or seminars, and completing tested *modules* of the latest updates in your field. Adequate knowledge allows you to adjust to changes that may exist between specific areas of work, locations, and other situations. The memorization of "steps" does not constitute proper acquisition of knowledge, so it is important to learn everything about your chosen field, and not just the basic components.

Focus on continuing education

Continuing education is required for health care professionals in order to provide the best patient care, and gives them up-to-date knowledge and skills. Continuing education keeps us informed about the latest developments and technologies, fulfills licensing and certification requirements, helps to improve patient care, and addresses day-to-day challenges you may encounter on the job.

Judgment

In health care professions, good judgment is an essential skill. It requires evaluations, conclusions, and related actions. Therefore, judgment is often referred to as critical thinking, in which you make decisions based on analysis and evaluation. In health care professions, it is vital to apply good judgment in all situations, regardless of whether these situations annoy, distract, or upset you.

In order to perform your work efficiently and in a timely manner, you must be organized. Organization requires orderly planning and coordination. It uses time management skills, which allow you to prioritize workflow. When several work projects have almost the same importance, you must use your professional judgment, knowledge, and experience in order to prioritize them correctly. Table 7.2 lists the steps to take, beginning with simple problem-solving, and increasing in complexity toward critical thinking, as used in health care.

Persistence

To succeed in your health care profession, you must continue to work hard, remain determined, and overcome many obstacles. You must focus on completing your work correctly, regardless of anything that may make it difficult. Persistence means that you keep trying no matter what you must do to work effectively. Patients and other health care professionals rely on all members of the health care team to be persistent in their work.

In order to have a high quality of work, you must be proud of what you do and always try to achieve excellence. To do this, you may need additional help from others, more hours spent focusing on obstacles in your work, or even taking additional courses or receiving training that will help you improve. You should always strive to report risks that you come across, even if they are not directly related to your job. Alert other professionals who may be able to solve a problem that is outside your discipline – never just ignore the problem.

Teamwork

Teamwork requires workers to cooperate with and assist each other, which increases patient satisfaction and, ultimately, job satisfaction for all team members. Teamwork increases the likelihood of achieving a common goal. In a health care practice, the ultimate goal is excellent patient care. This requires cooperation between team members. All health care jobs

Table 7.2 Steps used in health care problem solving

Step	Situational example
Identifying the problem	Identify what is wrong with the patient
Identifying its effects	What effects are symptoms having upon the patient's health?
Identifying the desired outcome and objectives	What is the goal of treating these symptoms?
Identifying possible solutions	Which treatments are likely to be most effective for these symptoms?
Analyzing the possible solutions	What are the possible results of each treatment option?
Implementing the best solutions	Once choosing the best treatment option, how is it best implemented?
Evaluating the outcome	Was the chosen treatment totally, partially, or not effective? If not effective, what is the next treatment option?

depend on others doing their work properly and effectively. In order to achieve teamwork, all health care professionals must assist each other, avoid interpersonal conflict, be considerate of each other's responsibilities and duties, and perform extra responsibilities without complaining or questioning why this is needed.

You must be able to develop good working relationships with many different individuals at your workplace (see Figure 7.2). Avoid things like gossip, impatience, or rudeness. You should encourage the same from everyone around you. Regarding the relationship with patients: address them by their names in the way they expect to be referred to, avoid giving personal advice, keep humor tasteful and appropriate, avoid gifts of all types, and decline to meet patients outside of the workplace unless you knew them prior to being professionally involved with their health care.

Cultural diversity

Cultural diversity must also be respected, especially since health care professionals of today work with people from many diverse backgrounds. Respect is the key here, regardless of ethnicity. Every person has the right to be different, including his or her beliefs and lifestyle. Good communication will help you learn about differences and similarities. Avoid any bias

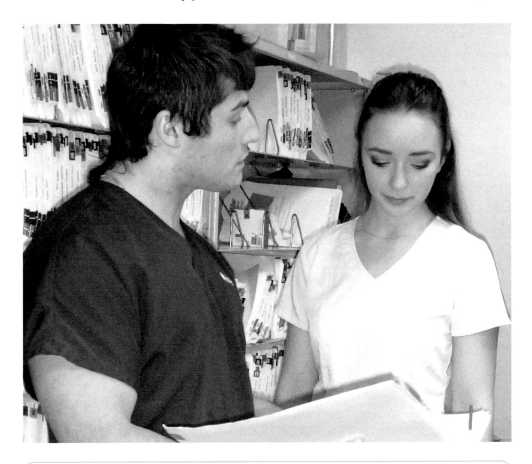

Figure 7.2 Two health care professionals working as a team.

or stereotypes – these only lead to poor communication, lack of respect, and a negative outcome. Everyone is an individual, and deserves the best health care that can be provided. You may sometimes need to act as a **patient advocate**, on behalf of a patient or a patient's family. Professional relationships with patients and good communications with them will help you in this regard.

A self-confident health care professional puts others at ease because this trait shows self-belief. Other professionals and patients will naturally integrate more effectively with you if you demonstrate **self-confidence**. Avoid projecting overconfidence or excessive self-confidence, however. Appearing to be "all-knowing" will not be respected by others, and will undermine your effectiveness at work. Tips for displaying acceptable self-confidence include remaining calm at all times, making eye contact, and smiling.

Empathy

Empathy is the ability to identify with another person's feelings, even though you may have never experienced the same situation in your own life. Empathy shows your sensitivity to the other person. It helps you to show another individual that you value their needs and support them regardless of ever having been in any similar situation yourself.

To better understand empathy, there are several key steps that the health care professional can take:

- Recognize the presence of fear, anger, disappointment, grief, and other strong feelings in the clinical setting
- Pause to imagine how the patient might be feeling
- Explain your perception of the feelings, using statements like "It sounds like you are upset about …," or "I can imagine that must be…."
- Give the patient your understanding that the feelings are legitimate
- Respect the patient's efforts to deal with his or her feelings
- Offer support and partnership, using statements like "Let's see what we can do together about this …," or "I am committed to working with you…."

> ### Focus on empathy
>
> Studies have shown that empathy is an important skill for health care providers, and is significantly related to improved clinical outcomes. By recognizing and empathizing with a patient's situation, the provider improves the odds of a successful health outcome.
>
> *Source:* http://healthaffairs.org/blog/2014/02/25/empathy-the-first-step-to-improving-health-outcomes/.

Flexibility

Flexibility in your work allows you to assist others in getting the overall job done correctly. You may be asked to assist another health care professional in something you have never done before. Always ask for instructions about anything you do not fully understand, and keep a positive attitude about being part of the team. Demonstrating flexibility in your work improves the overall success of your organization, which reflects well on everyone who is part of the team.

Self-motivation

In order to succeed in your health care profession, it is important to work with your own focused motivation, in order to achieve the goals of your employer. It is never wise to develop an attitude of simply waiting to be told what to do. Rather, successful individuals ask questions about what else can be done, where they can assist, and what materials they can study in order to become more skilled at a variety of employer needs. This self-motivation proves to health care employers that you care about the outcome of the organization as a whole, and makes you an especially valuable team member.

Integrity and honesty

At work, it is crucial always to show integrity and to be honest. *Integrity* means following appropriate codes of laws and ethics, as well as demonstrating honesty and trustworthiness. Integrity and honesty mean that items of all sizes are not removed from the workplace for any reason, the truth is always told, cheating is not tolerated, your time spent at work is accurately documented, and even that individuals you discover behaving dishonestly are reported.

Beyond the legal implications of behaving without integrity, ethics are involved, which consist of values that determine "right and wrong." When an individual lacks integrity or is dishonest, he or she loses the trust and respect of others. Actions that are dishonest may even result in patient harm or harm to coworkers. Respect the privacy of others, be loyal to your employer, and accept responsibility for your actions. When you have integrity, it means you do the right thing even when the conditions are difficult. If this means admitting a mistake that may result in consequences against you, or spending your own time correcting something that must be corrected, so be it. Integrity and honesty in health care are essential to your success, and to patients' well-being.

> ### You should remember
>
> The patient trusts in your honesty and integrity. Patients should never be misled into accepting treatments that are not required and must be made aware of treatment alternatives and informed of the risks and complications of each treatment option.

Enthusiasm

Showing enthusiasm for your health career is reflected in your daily activities. Health care professionals who are passionate about their jobs always try to do the best job possible. They remain actively interested in their duties. Enthusiasm about providing quality health care services to other people is essential for your success. Health care professionals who are enthusiastic about their work usually provide better care to the people they serve.

Part of the enthusiasm for your job involves showing *initiative*, meaning performing tasks that need to be done without being asked to by a supervisor. Initiative means doing things that help to improve the office's effectiveness, including cleaning, restocking, ordering, and many other tasks. It is important to anticipate what needs to be done and take steps to carry it out correctly. You should determine the most important task that needs to be completed, and take the initiative to carry it out.

Accountability

Maintaining integrity and honesty helps you to be perceived as accountable for your own actions. *Accountability* for your own actions is an extension of accepting constructive input, and even of being self-critical in order to improve. By remaining accountable, we improve in our skills and ability to work effectively, since there is no question that the workplace is held in regard and respect.

Accountability has become a major issue in health care. It involves procedures and processes by which a health care professional or team justifies and takes responsibility for actions. The concept of accountability is based on the parties involved, the activities involved, and the procedure used to evaluate them. Accountability may involve individual patients or physicians, non-physician health care providers, hospitals, managed care plans, professional associations, employers, private payers, the government, investors and lenders of capital, lawyers, and courts. Accountability consists of domains such as professional competence, legal and ethical conduct, financial performance, adequacy of access, public health promotion, and community benefit. To evaluate accountability, the two basic procedures are evaluation of compliance with criteria for specific content areas and dissemination of this evaluation, and responses or justifications by the accountable party or parties.

Appearance

Your professional appearance communicates your seriousness about work as well as your professional attitude. It ensures confidence and respect in patients and coworkers. You may be required to wear a particular uniform. Otherwise, conservative clothing and grooming is essential (see Figure 7.3). Trends such as tattoos and piercings are not encouraged, though these have become slightly more acceptable. It is best to cover tattoos with clothing and remove excessive skin piercings, as directed by the policies and procedures manual.

Your skin, fingernails, hair, clothing, and shoes should always be clean. The use of deodorant or antiperspirant is encouraged. You should practice good dental hygiene. Avoid perfumes and other personal products with strong odors, since these may cause allergic responses, bother a patient with nausea, or trigger asthmatic attacks. Also, odors such as cigarette smoke must not be present. Dangling earrings, open-toed shoes, and excessively long hair can all be potential hazards in the workplace. Jewelry should be kept to a minimum, and should not have any distasteful images or wording. Your hair should be styled appropriately, pulled back from the face and collar, and only dyed in natural colors. Fingernails should be trimmed, of a natural color, and acrylic nails must be avoided because they are risks for infection.

Stress management

It is vital for health care professionals to manage their stressors so that their work is unaffected. Stress is a normal part of everyday life and work, but it must be managed appropriately. In health care, stress may be caused by a variety of physical, emotional, and chemical factors. Illness and disease may occur as a result of physical and emotional tension. The way you manage your stress determines how you will react – positively or negatively – in stressful situations.

Good stress, or *eustress*, leads to positive reactions. It often occurs on a daily basis, and low levels of stress result in motivation, the solving of problems, meeting deadlines, and

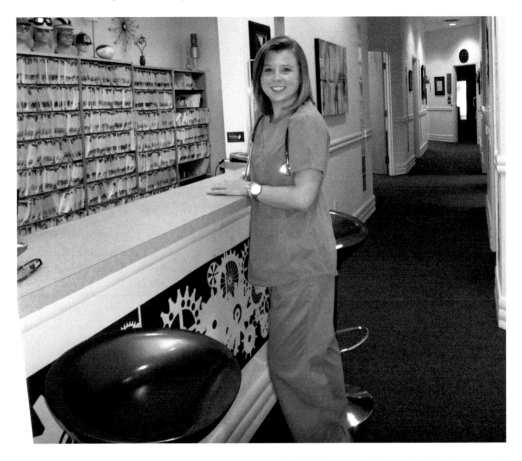

Figure 7.3 A professional appearance projects competence and increases the patient's confidence.

completing tasks. Therefore, eustress is helpful when it results in a person completing necessary activities. Bad stress, or *distress*, leads to negative reactions. It can make it hard to participate in normal activities and to enjoy everyday life. High levels of stress often affect the appetite, causing excessive eating or an inability to eat, and lead to nervousness as well as an inability to focus on what you need to do.

You should remember

The average health care worker spends so much time caring for and supporting patients that he or she often neglects personal stress levels. It is not selfish for you to take care of yourself and reduce your stress. Tips to accomplish stress reduction include addressing your stress at work by communicating, balancing your professional and personal life, and making "peaceful" moments during your day.

Causes of stress

Your personality influences the things that cause you stress. What "stresses you out" may not be perceived as being very stressful by another person. Common daily causes of stress include:

- Excessive demands
- An inability to say "no" to others
- A lifestyle that is disorderly or chaotic
- Carrying unrealistic expectations
- Being inflexible
- Self-doubt
- Taking constructive input or problems personally.

Many health care workers feel that excessive demands are placed on their time and skills too regularly. Emergencies may be a regular part of their work. Regular life-and-death situations can stress out even the strongest individuals, and are extreme causes of stress. Physical signs of stress include agitation, anxiety, or depression, which other people often can easily detect. When stress causes a health care worker to have a negative attitude, this may be harmful to the worker as well as the people on his or her health care team. Significant causes of stress in an average person's lifetime include:

- Death of a spouse or family member
- Divorce or separation
- Marriage or reconciliation from a separation
- Hospitalization due to injury or illness, of yourself or a family member
- Loss of a job or retirement, or a job change
- Significant personal success, such as a job promotion
- Problems at work that may put your job at risk
- Sexual problems
- Having a baby
- Children leaving or returning home
- Significant financial status improvement or worsening
- Substantial debt, including credit cards and mortgages
- Moving or remodeling your home.

Focus on causes of stress in health care professions

The most significant causes of stress in health care professions include heavy patient loads, overly high expectations from superiors and patients, and professional activities intervening on personal life. It is okay to ask for help with your patient loads when you need it, communicating when you can't meet all expectations, and plan your schedule to have enough time where work is not allowed to intrude.

Coping with stress

In emergencies, dealing with patient deaths, and when patients become angry, your goal is to remain calm and professional. Emotional responses to these situations may reduce your effective treatment of patients. Show that you care, but remain objective. Learn to recognize occurrences that trigger your own reactions. You should learn to control your temper if you find yourself easily angered on a regular basis. You may have to "unlearn" something that has been a lifelong behavior in order to become more professional and, therefore, more effective.

It is hard to focus on the needs of patients and other people when you are dealing with excessive stress. Coping strategies are needed to handle stress so that you can continue to provide good patient care. If stress is not handled, it may lead to *overload* or *burnout*. You must identify the actual causes of your stress, and avoid behaviors that may temporarily "handle" them, such as drinking, using drugs, or overeating. These behaviors eventually will produce *more* stress.

Methods of coping with stress include the following:

- Simplifying your life and your work – use time management techniques and avoid procrastination; learn to say "no" to non-important activities
- Setting priorities by making lists of what you need to do, and determining which are necessary, somewhat necessary, and not necessary
- Identifying and then reducing what causes you stress – make lists of what you feel stress from, and devise ways to simplify or eliminate them
- Shifting your thinking to divert focus away from stressful thoughts – learn to look at stressful situations as opportunities
- Asking for social support from friends, family members, colleagues or coworkers, students, classmates, members of religious groups, people with common hobbies or interests
- Taking time to relax and renew yourself – allow yourself time during each day for some enjoyable activities and take a break from stressful activities.

You should remember

Remaining calm during emergencies, stressful situations, or when someone else is angry requires a group of learned skills and behaviors. These include recognizing signs of anger before it reaches its climax, showing empathy, expressing concern, allowing others time to calm down, using statements that focus on "I" instead of "You," suggesting activities that may divert stress or anger, respecting personal space, interpreting non-verbal communication, and keeping your requests "soft" by using a steady and calm tone of voice.

Personal health

You can also help to reduce your stress by taking proper care of your own health. Your personal health must be good in order to provide quality care to other people. You can be a good role model for patients, family, and friends by maintaining your own health. This means you must have adequate nutrition, exercise, and sleep.

Adequate nutrition means appropriate and regular meals, especially breakfast. Healthy, balanced foods will go a long way in providing you the energy you need to maintain personal health. Good nutrition combats stress, keeps your weight within acceptable parameters, and promotes overall good health. Breakfast is extremely important, since it prepares the body for daily functions. Your diet must contain healthy foods, which aid in stress reduction, maintaining proper weight, and better health.

Regular exercise increases energy, reduces stress, maintains a healthy body weight, and improves self-esteem. Aerobic activities can strengthen your heart as well as provide many other health benefits. These activities include running, cycling, and swimming. Non-aerobic exercises are of shorter duration and do not require significant oxygen to accomplish, such as weight lifting or climbing a flight of stairs.

You should make exercise something you enjoy so that you will look forward to it being a regular part of your life. Exercising with a friend or a group of people is often very motivational (see Figure 7.4). You should work out at least three times per week, for between 20 and 30 minutes. It is acceptable to exercise up to six times per week, with one day spent resting in order for the body to rejuvenate and repair.

Sleep is essential for increasing your ability to be efficient in your activities. Tiredness actually increases stress and can even result in illness. You should always allow yourself time to rest when you feel tired. Most adults require eight hours of sleep every night. You should set a regular, reasonable time to go to bed, and avoid the following, all of which can interfere with normal sleep:

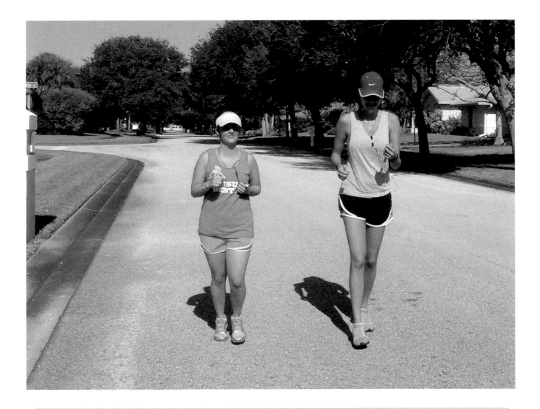

Figure 7.4 Group exercise.

- Drinking caffeinated beverages in the afternoon or evening
- Smoking – nicotine withdrawal can occur during the night, disrupting sleep
- Drinking alcohol with dinner can disrupt sleep patterns
- Eating foods that cause heartburn may disrupt sleep; also, a large amount of food consumed at dinner can affect quality of sleep.

Sleep quality is improved by regular diet and adequate nutrition, and these two factors may be enough to balance the negative factors to a certain degree. Chronic sleep problems must be discussed with a physician. Without treatment, poor sleep quality, over time, can affect emotional, mental, and physical health.

You should remember

Fatigue is a constant part of overworked health care professionals. Changing work schedules and the need to work longer hours than usual are primary contributors to fatigue. It is of the utmost importance to avoid sleep deprivation and fatigue – both of these conditions can seriously harm your ability to serve your patients, and may also result in significantly poor overall health.

Once physiologic needs are satisfied, attending to psychological needs is essential for personal health. According to psychiatrist Abraham Maslow, psychological needs begin with physical safety and emotional security, followed by love and belonging. After these, esteem and recognition are required. The ultimate psychological need is achieving self-actualization, which is the fulfillment of a person's own potential.

Focus on staying healthy

Health care professionals recommend several simple ways to remain healthy so that they can continue to provide great patient care. These include regular hand washing, keeping all surfaces clean, having regular vaccinations, drinking enough water and healthy fluids, taking appropriate medications when sick, and keeping your medicine cabinet stocked with medications you rely on.

Personal hygiene

Health care professionals must exhibit excellent personal hygiene since patients' first impressions are important. You should always be clean, well groomed, and properly dressed in order to be perceived as capable and qualified. Normal dress codes in the health care facility include clothing that is clean, intact, and well pressed. Shoes should be clean, appropriate, and well polished. Jewelry should be plain and simple.

> ### CASE STUDY
>
> Professionalism in health care encourages patients and other people who visit health care facilities to believe that their well-being is taken seriously. It is never advisable to behave unprofessionally while working. Not everyone understands this, however. One day in his job as a pharmacy technician, Brian processed a prescription for a friend whom he "owed a favor," even though he knew the medication was actually for his friend's brother. When later confronted by his supervising pharmacist, Brian responded with anger and hostility. The pharmacist, an older woman, was afraid of Brian's outburst and did not take any other action.
>
> 1 Was Brian's action of trying to "help" his friend a violation of the law?
> 2 How should Brian have responded when questioned by the pharmacist?
> 3 What should the pharmacist have done about Brian's response?

Chapter highlights

This section answers the Objectives found at the beginning of the chapter.

1 Differentiate between the hard and soft skills required by health care professions.

- In health care, hard skills concern technical and operational abilities. They include ability to code, schedule, interview, manage records, assist other professionals, or to take vital signs.
- Soft skills (people skills) are things you bring to your profession that enhance your performance. They include integrity, dependability, respect, patient relationships, good attitude toward your work, and ethics.

2 Explain "professional distance."

- Professional distance is the amount of physical or social interaction that is considered appropriate between a professional and the people he or she serves, and should be maintained between health care workers and patients to demonstrate professionalism. Patients should not be viewed as personal friends, but as people you professionally serve. You should try to please them, *always* professionally serve them, and demonstrate caring while giving them the best care possible.
- Avoid discussing your personal life with patients or accepting gifts from them.

3 Describe continuing education units.

- Continuing education units (CEUs) are provided by various professional organizations related to your chosen health care field. You must earn a certain amount of CEUs over a specific time period in order to continue to practice. This may involve reading articles and other information, taking courses or seminars, and completing tested modules of the latest updates. Continuing education provides up-to-date knowledge and skills, keeps you informed about latest developments and technologies, fulfills licensing and certification requirements, helps improve patient care, and addresses day-to-day job challenges.

4 **Discuss how good judgment is related to critical thinking.**

● Good judgment is essential in health care, and requires evaluations, conclusions, and related actions. Judgment is often referred to as critical thinking, in which you make decisions based on analysis and evaluation. It is vital to apply good judgment even when a situation may annoy, distract, or upset you.

5 **Explain cultural diversity and its importance in health care.**

● Cultural diversity (multiculturalism) is the quality of diverse or different cultures throughout the societies of the world. It must be respected, regardless of ethnicity, especially since health care professionals work with people from many diverse backgrounds. Good communication helps here, and you must avoid any bias or stereotypes – everyone deserves the best health care that can be provided.

6 **Outline how a patient advocate assists patients and their families.**

● A patient advocate is a health care professional that works on behalf of patients and their families during medical treatment or hospitalization. They must have professional relationships with patients, and good communications with them as well. Patient advocates should show self-confidence and self-belief, but avoid projecting overconfidence or excessive self-confidence. They must remain calm at all times, make eye contact, and smile.

7 **List the steps that help to show empathy toward a patient.**

● Recognize fear, anger, disappointment, grief, and other strong feelings
● Pause to imagine how the patient might be feeling
● Explain your perception of the patient's feelings
● Give the patient your understanding that the feelings are legitimate
● Respect the patient's efforts to deal with his or her feelings
● Offer support and partnership.

8 **Explain why behaving with integrity is so important in health care.**

● In health care, when an individual lacks integrity or is dishonest, he or she loses the trust and respect of others. Dishonest actions may result in harm to patients or coworkers. You must do the right thing even when the conditions may be difficult. Integrity (and honesty) are essential to success in health care, and to the well-being of patients. Your patients trust in your honesty and integrity.

9 **Explain what the concept of accountability in health care is based upon.**

● Accountability in health care is based on the parties involved, the activities involved, and the procedure used to evaluate them. It may involve individual patients or physicians, non-physician health care providers, hospitals, managed care plans, professional associations, employers, private payers, the government, investors and lenders of capital, lawyers, and courts. Activities include professional competence, legal and ethical conduct, financial performance, adequacy of access, public health promotion, and community benefit. Evaluation involves compliance with criteria for specific content areas, dissemination of this evaluation, and responses or justifications by the accountable party or parties.

10 **List examples of professional appearance.**

- Professional appearance may include uniforms, conservative clothing and grooming, covering of excessive tattoos, removal of excessive skin piercings, overall cleanliness of your body and clothing, use of deodorant or antiperspirant, good dental hygiene, avoiding perfumes and other personal products, avoiding smoking cigarettes during work hours, minimal jewelry, use of closed-toed shoes, acceptable length and styling of hair, and trimmed fingernails of a natural appearance.

Summary

In health care, professionalism is the core of a successful career. It is important not only to know your job well, but also to know how you can best interact with patients, family members, and other professionals. You must maintain a respectful, positive, and caring approach, which are the basic components of overall professionalism. Your communication skills must be excellent. You must always maintain confidentiality and respect privacy. The true professional is able to handle difficult situations and constructive input with ease. Healthy lifestyles must be practiced in order to optimize patient care. This includes adequate exercise, balanced nutrition, and uninterrupted sleep. Stress management is crucial.

The health care profession requires you to be open to learning, possess good judgment, and maintain a high degree of organization. Though it can be extremely difficult work, the rewards of establishing yourself as a health care professional are excellent.

Review questions

1 Why is professional behavior an important quality for health care workers?
2 What is critical thinking?
3 Why is teamwork essential for health care professionals?
4 What is cultural diversity?
5 What is self-motivation?
6 How should health care professionals manage stress?
7 Why is personal health so important for health care professionals?
8 What is the ultimate goal of Abraham Maslow's hierarchy of needs?
9 What is the difference between hard skills and soft skills?
10 Why is continuing education important for health care professionals?

Bibliography

Annals of Internal Medicine. 1996. What is Accountability in Health Care?. Available at: http://annals.org/article.aspx?articleid=709376. Philadelphia: American College of Physicians.

Apesoa-Varano, E.C., and Varano, C.S. 2014. *Conflicted Health Care: Professionalism and Caring in an Urban Hospital*. Nashville: Vanderbilt University Press. Print.

Auerbach, D.I., et al. 2007. Better late than never: Workforce supply implications of later entry into nursing. *Health Affairs* 26, no. 1: 178–185.

Boulet, J.R., et al. 2006. The international medical graduate pipeline: Recent trends in certification and residency training. *Health Affairs* 25, no. 6: 469–477.

Buchbinder, S.B., and Shanks, N.H. 2014. *Introduction to Health Care Management, 2nd Edition*. Burlington: Jones & Bartlett Learning. 2014. Print.

Coyne, J.S., et al. 2009. Hospital cost and efficiency: So hospital size and ownership type really matter? *Journal of Healthcare Management* 54, no. 3: 163–174.

Cross, G.M. 2004. What does patient-centered care mean for the VA? *Forum* (November 2004), Academy Health.

Damberg, C.L., et al. 2009. Taking stock of pay-for-performance: A candid assessment from the front lines. *Health Affairs* 28, no. 2: 517–525.

Davis, C.M. 2011. *Patient Practitioner Interaction: An Experiential Manual for Developing the Art of Health Care, 5th Edition*. Thorofare: Slack Incorporated. Print.

Ericksen, K. 2016. Healthcare Insiders Expose the Pros and Cons of Working in a Hospital. Available at: www.rasmussen.edu/degrees/health-sciences/blog/working-in-hospital-pros-and-cons. Bloomington: Rasmussen College.

The European Food Information Council. 2016. Motivating Change Tips for Health Care Professionals. Available at: www.eufic.org/article/en/artid/motivating-change-tips-for-health-careprofessionals. Brussels: EUFIC.

Ficarra, B. 2013. Empathy in Health Care. Available at: www.healthworkscollective.com/barbara-ficarra/114336/empathy-health-care. New York: Health Works Collective.

Fortin, A.H., Dwamena, F.C., Frankel, R.M., and Smith, R.C. 2012. *Smith's Patient Centered Interviewing: An Evidence-Based Method, 3rd Edition*. New York: McGraw-Hill Education/Medical. Print.

Garber, A.M. 2005. Evidence-based guidelines as a foundation for performance incentives. *Health Affairs* 24, no. 1: 174–179.

Ginter, P.M. 2013. *The Strategic Management of Health Care Organizations, 7th Edition*. St. Paul: Jossey-Bass. Print.

Health and Care Professions Council. 2014. Professionalism in Healthcare Professionals. Available at: www.hpc-uk.org/assets/documents/10003771professionalisminhealthcareprofessionals.pdf. London: Health and Care Professions Council.

Health Care Careers Now. 2016. Qualities of A Good Health Professional. Available at: www.healthcarecareersnow.com/qualities-of-a-good-health-professional.html. Washington, D.C.: Health Care Careers Now.

Hebeck, E. 2002. Key Personality Traits Essential for Health Care Jobs. Available at: http://usatoday30.usatoday.com/money/jobcenter/workplace/healthcare/2002-11-19-personality_x.htm. McLean: USA Today / Gannett Co., Inc.

Hill, A. 2014. Empathy: The First Step to Improving Health Outcomes. Available at: http://healthaffairs.org/blog/2014/02/25/empathy-the-first-step-to-improving-health-outcomes/. Bethesda: Health Affairs Blog.

Institute of Medicine (IOM). 2000. *To Err Is Human: Building a Safer Health System*. L.T. Kohn, J.M. Corrigan, and M.S. Donaldson, eds. Washington, D.C.: National Academy Press.

Institute of Medicine (IOM). 2004. *Rewarding Provider Performance: Aligning Incentives in Medicare*. Washington, D.C.: National Academy Press.

Jha, A.K., et al. 2012. The long-term effect of premier pay for performance on patient out-comes. *New England Journal of Medicine* 366: 1606–1615.

Kramer, M., et al. 2011. Clinical nurses in Magnet hospitals confirm productive, healthy unit work environments. *Journal of Nursing Management* 19, no. 1: 5–17.

Lee, T.H. 2015. *An Epidemic of Empathy in Healthcare: How to Deliver Compassionate, Connected Patient Care That Creates a Competitive Advantage*. New York: McGraw-Hill Education. Print.

Leebov, W. 2012. *Resolving Complaints for Professionals in Health Care: Communication Skills for Effective Service Recovery*. Seattle: CreateSpace Independent Publishing Platform. Print.

Lighter, D. 2011. *Basics of Health Care Performance Improvement: A Lean Six Sigma Approach*. Burlington: Jones & Bartlett Learning. Print.

Love Your Patients! 2016. What Can We Do To Show Our Respect For Our Patients?. Available at: www.loveyourpatients.org/respect.htm. Morrison: Scott Louis Diering, M.D.

Makary, M. 2013. *Unaccountable: What Hospitals Won't Tell You and How Transparency Can Revolutionize Health Care, Reprint Edition*. New York: Bloomsbury Press.

Makely, S. 2012. *Professionalism in Health Care: A Primer for Career Success, 4th Edition*. Upper Saddle River: Prentice Hall. Print.

McCausland, C. 2007. When Doctors Get Sick – What Happens When Physicians Fall Ill? Here Are Three Local Doctors Who Ended Up on the Other Side of the Examination Table. Available at: www.baltimoremagazine.net/2007/11/when-doctors-get-sick. Baltimore: Baltimore Magazine.

McCausland, C. 2007. When Doctors Get Sick – What Happens When Physicians Fall Ill? Here Are Three Local Doctors Who Ended Up on the Other Side of the Examination Table. Available at: www.baltimoremagazine.net/2007/11/when-doctors-get-sick. Baltimore: Baltimore Magazine.

Miller, W.R., and Rollnick, S. 2012. *Motivational Interviewing: Helping People Change, 3rd Edition*. New York: The Guilford Press. Print.

Mitchell, D., and Haroun, L. 2011. *Introduction to Health Care, 3rd Edition*. Boston: Delmar Cengage Learning. Print.

Morrison-Valfre, M. 2008. *Foundations of Mental Health Care, 4th Edition*. Maryland Heights: Mosby. Print.

Nburge.com. 2011. Principles Of Health Care Science – You Are The Future of Healthcare – Personal Qualities of the Health Care Professional – Part 1. Available at: www.nburge.com/phs/?p=227. Birmingham: Nburge.com.

O'Donnell, M. 2015. 8 Vital Traits Every Allied Health Professional Should Have. Available at: www.healthecareers.com/article/8-vital-traits-every-allied-health-professional-should-have/170541. Centennial: Health Ecareers.

Purtilo, R.B., Haddad, A.M., and Doherty, R.F. 2013. *Health Professional and Patient Interaction, 8th Edition*. Philadelphia: Saunders. Print.

Real Balance Global Wellness Services Inc. 2016. The Role of Empathy in Healthcare. Available at: https://realbalance.com/the-role-of-empathy-in-healthcare. Fort Collins: Real Balance.

Rosner, F. 2004. Informing the patient about a fatal disease: From paternalism to autonomy – The Jewish view. *Cancer Investigation* 22, no. 6: 949–953.

Sahler, O.J., Carr, J.E., Frank, J., and Nunes, J. 2012. *The Behavioral Sciences and Health Care, 3rd Edition*. Boston: Hogrefe Publishing. Print.

Schoen, C., et al. 2012. A survey of primary care doctors in ten countries shows progress in use of health information technology, less in other areas. *Health Affairs* 31, no. 12: 2805–2816.

Segal, S. 2012. When It Comes to Medical Care, Honesty is Essential. Available at: www.kevinmd.com/blog/2012/04/medical-care-honesty-essential.html. Nashua: MedPage Today's KevinMD.com.

Stanfield, P.S., et al. 2009. *Introduction to the Health Professions, 2nd Edition*. Sudbury, MA: Jones and Bartlett Learning.

Topol, E. 2015. *The Patient Will See You Now: The Future of Medicine Is in Your Hands*. New York: Basic Books. Print.

U.S. Department of Labor. 2016. Healthcare Wide Hazards – Stress. Available at: www.osha.gov/SLTC/etools/hospital/hazards/stress/stress.html. Washington, D.C.: U.S. Department of Labor.

University of Alabama at Birmingham. 2016. Department of Anesthesiology and Perioperative Medicine. Available at: http://services.medicine.uab.edu/publicdocuments/anesthesiology/jc0414art2.pdf. Birmingham: UAB School of Medicine.

University of Massachusetts Medical School. 2001. Guidelines for Professional Behavior. Available at: www.umassmed.edu/uploadedfiles/Professionalism.pdf. Worcester: UM Medical School.

USDA ChooseMyPlate.gov. 2016. Resources For You. Available at: www.ChooseMyPlate.gov. Washington, D.C.: U.S. Department of Agriculture.

Vogt, W.B., and Town, R. 2006. *How Has Hospital Consolidation Affected the Price and Quality of Hospital Care?* Princeton: The Robert Wood Johnson Foundation. Print.

Wicks, R.J. 2005. *Overcoming Secondary Stress in Medical and Nursing Practice: A Guide to Professional Resilience and Personal Well-Being*. New York: Oxford University Press. Print.

Patient populations

Contents

8 Health care for special populations 187

Overview 189
Children 190
Women 191
Ethnic minorities 193
Elderly 196
People with disabilities 199
HIV and AIDS 200
Chronically ill 202
Homeless 202
Uninsured 203
Illegal immigrants 204
Case study 205
Chapter highlights 205
Summary 207
Review questions 207
Bibliography 207

9 Introduction to global health issues 210

Overview 210
Concepts of global health 211
Concepts of public health and community-based care 211
Smallpox eradication 212
The effects of disease on life expectancy 213
Risk factors for disease 214
Ethical and human rights concerns 216
Universal health coverage 216
Culture and health 217
Nutrition and global health 220
Case study 225

Chapter highlights   225
Summary   227
Review questions   228
Bibliography   228

10 Global health: communicable and non-communicable diseases   230

Overview   230
Communicable diseases   231
Non-communicable diseases   241
Case study   251
Chapter highlights   251
Summary   253
Review questions   253
Bibliography   254

11 Emergencies   256

Overview   256
Emergency and urgent care   257
Triage   258
Natural and man-made disasters   258
Health care during natural disasters   261
Emergency procedures   263
Case study   276
Chapter highlights   276
Summary   278
Review questions   278
Bibliography   279

Chapter 8

Health care for special populations

After study of the chapter, readers should be able to:

1 Explain the three divisions of child health care programs.
2 Detail the Women's Health Initiative and its findings.
3 Identify the ethnic minority group most likely to be uninsured or underinsured than other Americans.
4 List the most prevalent chronic conditions affecting the elderly.
5 Discuss barriers to health care for people with disabilities.
6 Explain the varieties of care required by AIDS patients.
7 List the four modifiable risk factors that result in chronic disease.
8 Identify the organizations that assist more than 1.1 million homeless patients.
9 Explain how costs of giving medical treatment to the uninsured are absorbed.
10 List where the majority of migrant workers in the United States are originally from.

Overview

In the United States, certain special populations have a more difficult time accessing health care services, and therefore are at higher risk of having poor health. These underprivileged people may have arrived at their current situations because of varying conditions, including not only health, but also economic, geographic, and social conditions. These special populations include children, women, minorities, the elderly, HIV/AIDS patients, the chronically ill, homeless people, and the uninsured. These populations also may experience barriers to financing of health care and acceptance on a cultural or racial basis. The impact of the Affordable Care Act upon these populations is also significant, and will be discussed along with the health needs and challenges that they face.

Poor health includes physical, psychological, and social health. These are often inter-related, occurring at the same time. An individual's vulnerability is determined by predisposing and enabling factors, as well as needs. All of these factors influence illness and recovery from illness. In general, the more risk factors an individual has, the less access to care they have.

Children

The majority of children in the United States are covered by private insurance (more than 53%) or Medicaid (more than 38%). Children living below the poverty level receive less overall health care, including recommended vaccinations. With less access to health care, poorer children are impacted in their education, since they often stay home to recuperate over a longer period of time. Often, a poor child who is sick attends school regardless of how they feel, because of lack of health care or lack of parental ability to take leave from work to care for them. This increases the likelihood that they will expose other children to illnesses.

There are several unique factors concerning the health care of children. These include *dependency*, *developmental vulnerability*, and *new* morbidities. The health needs of children require adults (not only their parents) to assist. These relationships concerning their dependency may change, may become quite complicated, and may affect how health services are utilized for the care of children. Also, physical and emotional changes of children are described as developmental vulnerability. The lives of children can be greatly impacted by illnesses, injuries, social circumstances, and disruption of the family unit. New morbidities consistently develop that affect children. These may include emotional disorders, learning difficulties, alcohol or drug abuse, and violence in families and neighborhoods.

Traditional methods of health care may not be sufficient to address childhood dependency, developmental vulnerability, and new morbidities. Instead, there may be a requirement for multi-discipline health care services, and prevention strategies provided by the community. Also, there are three million or more disabled children in the United States, and approximately one million with severe, chronic illnesses. These conditions may be related to birth or congenital conditions, resulting in unique forms of health care specifically designed for them.

Demographics and socioeconomic factors greatly impact the area of oral health care in children. While more than three out of four white American children are described as having "excellent" oral health, other groups are much lower, with Hispanic children having less than half of their population ranked in the same way. There is a distinct relationship between childhood oral health and family income. Children above the poverty level have up to four times better oral health than those below the poverty level. Poor oral health often results in the child missing school, having to visit the emergency department more often, and ultimately, lessening overall quality of life over the long term.

There are many diverse programs of child health care that, unfortunately, do not work well together. There are three broad divisions:

● Personal medical and preventive services – primary and specialty services, mostly funded by private health insurance, out-of-pocket payments, and Medicaid

- Population-based community health services – disease prevention and community health promotion services, such as immunizations, lead screening, and child abuse and neglect prevention. Other examples include rehabilitation, case management, referral programs, and monitoring for developmental disabilities. These are mostly funded by federal programs such as Medicaid, which provides the Early Periodic Screening, Diagnosis, and Treatment program, and the Title V (Maternal and Child Health) part of the Social Security Act
- Health-related support services – nutrition education, family support, early intervention, and rehabilitation programs. These may include HIV education and psychotherapy for children, and parental education about developmental delays. These are mostly funded by the Department of Agriculture in the Supplemental Food Program for Women, Infants, and Children, and the Department of Education's Individuals with Disabilities Education Act.

Focus on health care for children

According to the CDC, 5.5% of American children under 18 years of age do not have health insurance. Also, 3.8% of American children under age 18 do not have a usual source of health care.

Sources: www.cdc.gov/nchs/data/nhis/earlyrelease/insur201506.pdf; www.cdc.gov/mmwr/preview/mmwrhtml/mm6442a8.htm.

Women

American women are expected to live, on average, 4.8 years longer than men, but have increased morbidity and poorer health outcomes. For example, more than one in three women have chronic conditions that need continued medical treatment, while only 30% of men require the same. In all stages of life, women have higher percentages of *deaths from heart disease and stroke*. Though men have an overall higher *occurrence*, one in three women die from heart disease, but only one in four men do. Strokes are fatal in three out of five women, but only fatal in two in five men. Also, more than four out of ten women who have a heart attack die within the following year, while only one in four men have the same outcome.

While 88% of women visit a health care provider in a calendar year, only 80% of men do the same. Women also have higher annual charges for all types of care, and receive more intensive services (see Figure 8.1). Women are more likely to delay seeking or receiving needed health care in comparison to men. Certain conditions, such as mental disorders, affect women two to three times as often as men. For example, major depression affects about 7% of American men, but affects 12% of American women – almost double. With regard to eating disorders, nine out of ten cases occur in younger women.

Death related to alcohol abuse in women is 50% to 100% higher than in men. Older women also experience much higher degrees of Alzheimer's disease than men. Significantly, new cases of HIV are highest in minorities, with black women having the highest rates in comparison to all other females in minority groups. Diabetes mellitus affects female American Indians or Alaska Natives significantly more than any other female minorities.

The Public Health Service's Office on Women's Health coordinates a strong agenda concerning female health care. It implemented the National Action Plan on Breast Cancer, and has programs concerning the prevention of physical and sexual violence against women,

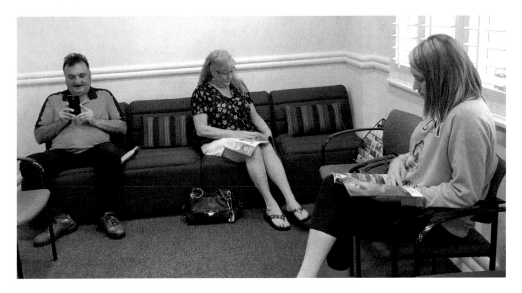

Figure 8.1 A waiting room with more female patients than male patients.

promotion of breastfeeding, encouragement of women's health education and research, heart health, and girl and adolescent health. The Advisory Committee for Women's Services, part of the Substance Abuse and Mental Health Services Administration, targets many areas of women's health care. The largest clinical trial in U.S. history concerning female health care was the Women's Health Initiative, focusing on major causes of death and disability, including heart disease, cancer, and osteoporosis. It found that postmenopausal hormone therapy was linked to invasive breast cancer, coronary heart disease, stroke, and pulmonary embolism.

Because women are more likely than men to work part time, with more work interruptions, and receive lower wages, they are more often covered as dependents under their husbands' plans. More women than men are covered by Medicaid, while more men than women are uninsured. Though contraceptives are often not covered by health care plans, women are more likely than men to use them. More than 62% of American women use some form of contraception, with birth control pills being most common at 31%. The Affordable Care Act requires private insurance to cover, without cost sharing, many preventive services for women, including contraceptives approved by the Food and Drug Administration (FDA), screening for domestic violence, breastfeeding support, and testing for the human papillomavirus (HPV).

Focus on health care for women

The percentage of American women under the age of 65 who lack health insurance coverage is 11.9%.

Source: www.cdc.gov/nchs/data/nhis/earlyrelease/
earlyrelease201609_01.pdf.

Ethnic minorities

In the United States, there are 15 recognized racial categories, which include white, black, American Indian or Alaska Native, Asian Indian, Chinese, Filipino, Japanese, Korean, Vietnamese, other Asian, Native Hawaii, Guamanian or Chamorro, Samoan, other Pacific Islander, and a category called "some other race." As of 2010, ethnic minorities make up more than 36% of the population of the United States. Table 8.1 breaks down the largest minority groups.

Culturally competent care

Culturally competent care can be explained as providing health care that is sensitive to the values of patients that are based on their particular ethnic or religious backgrounds. It involves specificity involving cross-cultural clinical interactions between patients and health care professions. The degree to which health care professionals can understand and accommodate patient expectations and practices helps to determine the success of health care for patients of all cultures.

> ### You should remember
>
> A lack of culturally competent care directly contributes to poor patient outcomes, reduced patient compliance, and increased inequality of health care.

Hispanics or Latinos

Hispanics or Latinos are the fastest-growing segment of the minority population of the United States. While the overall population increased by 10% between 2000 and 2010, the Hispanic/Latino population increased by 43%. In total, this population is expected to reach 57 million in the year 2015. Significantly, approximately one in four Hispanics live below the federal poverty level. Of those who experience barriers in accessing medical care, Hispanics from Central or South America report the greatest difficulty, compared to those from Mexico or Spain. The inability of many Hispanic people to speak English is also associated with having less access to medical services.

Table 8.1 Percentages of larger minority groups in the USA

Hispanics or Latinos	16.3
Blacks (African Americans)	12.3
Asians	4.7
Identifying as two or more races	1.9
American Indians and Alaska Natives	0.7
Native Hawaiians and other Pacific Islanders	0.2

Sources: www.massmed.org/continuing-education-and-events/conference-proceeding-archive/wch2012vivaldipres-(pdf)/; www.census.gov/prod/2001pubs/c2kbr01-5.pdf; www.infoplease.com/ipa/a0762156.html.

Higher unemployment among Hispanics is linked to low education levels. In general, Hispanics are more likely to be semi-skilled and work in non-professional occupations. They are also more likely to be uninsured or underinsured than other Americans. Of Hispanics, Mexicans had the highest amount of uninsured (33%), followed by Cubans (28.1%), and Puerto Ricans (15.8%). However, those listed as "other Hispanics" have 31.8% of their populations uninsured. Hispanics share the highest murder rates, along with blacks, of all races in America. Another significant health factor in adult Hispanics is the consumption of five or more alcoholic drinks per day, which is higher in this group than in blacks or Asians. However, fewer Hispanics smoke than people of other groups.

Focus on health care for Hispanics and Latinos

The percentage of Hispanic or Latino Americans who lack health insurance coverage is 30.4%, which is higher than a number of other groups.
Source: www.houstontx.gov/health/chs/HispanicHealthDepBooklet.pdf.

Blacks (African Americans)

In comparison to white Americans, blacks are generally less economically advantaged, have poorer health statuses and shorter life expectancies, increased age-adjusted death rates for most leading causes of death, increased age-adjusted maternal mortality rates, and also increased mortality rates for infants and younger children. Blacks have much higher percentages of low-birth-weight babies than all other minorities. The top five causes of death among blacks are ranked as follows:

1 Heart disease
2 Cancer
3 Cerebrovascular disease
4 Diabetes mellitus
5 Accidents.

Focus on health care for blacks

The percentage of black Americans under the age of 65 who lack health insurance coverage is 17.8%.
Source: https://hit.health.tn./gov/reports/surveyreports/brfss_factsheet/
healthcareaccess BRFSS factsheets TN 2005.pdf.

Asians

There are only about 14 million Asians in the United States, but they are experiencing significant population growth. By 2015, the Asian American population will have reached approximately 16.5 million. In general, they have higher education levels than other minorities and earn higher wages. A smaller percentage live below the poverty level than blacks or Hispanics. There are some significant Asian cultural beliefs that result in Asian women receiving less than adequate preventive health care compared to other minorities. Rates of obesity range widely among Asians. They also have the overall lowest smoking rates, except for Korean Americans, who have a higher smoking rate than blacks or Hispanics. Asian Indians are more than twice as likely to have diabetes mellitus than white Americans.

> ## You should remember
>
> Asian Americans are the highest-income, best-educated, and fastest-growing racial group in the United States. At least 83% of this population is made up of people from the following countries: China, the Philippines, India, Vietnam, Korea, and Japan.
>
> *Source:* www.pewsocialtrends.org/asianamericans-graphics/.

American Indians and Alaska Natives

American Indians or Native Americans are among the lowest socioeconomic classes of people in the United States. Part of this concerns geography. More than three out of four of these individuals live in areas outside of reservations or off-reservation trust lands. This population is growing at 26.7% per year, yet this group experiences significantly high rates of diabetes mellitus, hypertension, chemical dependency, AIDS/HIV mortality, and infant mortality and morbidity. Native Americans, compared to other groups, have much higher rates of death from alcoholism (519% higher), tuberculosis (500% higher), diabetes mellitus, homicide, injuries, and suicide.

Fortunately, the health of Native Americans is improving. However, life expectancy is still 4.6 years lower than the U.S. population as a whole. Since 1832, the American government has provided health services to American Indians. These services have been expanded in recent years to allow better choices, development, and administration of health care. Traditional Native American medicine is allowed by several related laws, alongside current Western medicine. The Indian Health Care Improvement Act has helped Native Americans experience reduced prejudice, higher levels of trust, and increased self-responsibility. The Indian Health Service has improved levels of health care availability, but in general, Native Americans still experience barriers to accessing treatment. Though there are 161 service units managed by various tribes, lack of geographic accessibility has slowed their efforts.

> ## Focus on health care for American Indians and Alaska Natives
>
> The percentage of American Indians and Alaska Natives under age 65 who lack health insurance coverage is 27%.
> *Source:* https://kaiserfamilyfoundation.files.wordpress.com/2013/01/7977.pdf.

Native Hawaiians and other Pacific Islanders

For Native Hawaiians, health care centers receive funding through the Health Resources and Services Administration or HRSA. This provides medical services, education, health promotion, and disease prevention services, including nutrition programs, screening for hypertension and diabetes, immunizations, and basic primary care services. Native Hawaiians may experience cultural, financial, geographic, and social barriers preventing access to health services. Also, services may be unavailable in certain Hawaiian communities. There are more than 1.4 million people classified as "Native Hawaiians and other Pacific Islanders." People classified as "other Pacific Islanders" include those from Guam, American Samoa, Tahiti, Fiji, and other Pacific islands.

In these groups, there are some important health disparities, such as higher cancer death rates, lower five-year cancer survival rates, and higher infant mortality rates. Diabetes is three times more prevalent than in non-Hispanic whites, and obesity, smoking, and alcohol consumption all occur more commonly as well. Native Hawaiians and other Pacific Islanders are 21.5% more likely to live in poverty than the total U.S. population (source: http://newsok.com/article/3771773).

> ## You should remember
>
> Native Hawaiians and other Pacific Islanders predominantly live in Hawaii. Significant health problems among this group include smoking, excessive alcohol consumption, and obesity.

Elderly

Of elderly Americans, chronic diseases play an important part in future disabilities and related health care. Chronic diseases may be linked to emotional as well as physical causes. They can only be managed, not cured, requiring continued health care services from a variety of professionals. Severe chronic diseases may require increasing amounts of assistance. Often, chronic conditions accumulate, resulting in additional services being needed with increased aging.

Generally, the most prevalent chronic conditions affecting the elderly include hypertension, arthritis, heart disease, cancer, and diabetes (see Figure 8.2). After the age of 85, most people (60%) have hearing impairment and 28% have visual impairment. In the elderly, the conditions that result in most cases of functional impairment include dementia, stroke, and hip fractures. People over age 85 are five times more likely to have dementia, and 10–15 times more likely to have a hip fracture than a person aged between 60 and 65. After age 85, dementia affects 20% of people. In nursing homes, 40% of residents have dementia.

Among the *oldest-old* Americans, 66% report excellent health and 40% or more report having no limits in their daily activities. These people do not visit a physician any more often than people classified as *youngest-old*. However, hospital and nursing home stays are much more common. After age 65, about 1.6 million Americans live in institutional settings. Of these, 1.4 million live in nursing homes, with about 66% being 85 or older. Care is often required for daily living activities, or these individuals have cognitive impairment related to Alzheimer's disease or another type of dementia.

Medicare is responsible for covering many elderly people, and Part A of Medicare offers automatic enrollment for all elderly beneficiaries. Most elderly Americans purchase Medicare Part B, even though its supplemental medical coverage is voluntary. A large number of the elderly also purchase Part C (Medicare Advantage) from a private insurance company. Medicare Advantage Plans provide all of Parts A and B, and may offer additional coverage, including hearing, vision, dental, and/or health and wellness programs. Most Advantage plans also offer Part D (prescription drug coverage). Medicare pays a fixed amount to private insurers who offer Advantage plans to cover costs of Part B premiums and additional services.

For the elderly, as well as the disabled, Medicaid covers many services that are not covered by Medicare. It also pays Medicare premiums, offers cost-sharing, and covers pre-

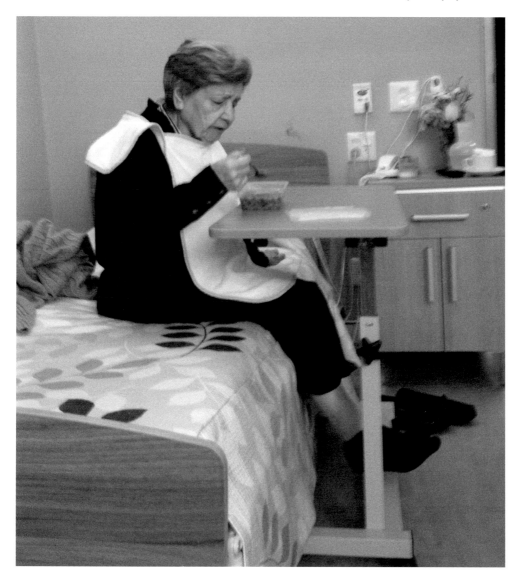

Figure 8.2 An elderly woman.

scription drugs. Often, elderly people do not utilize Medicaid since they cannot deal with the complexities of its organization. For long-term health care, Medicaid is the primary payer, but only covers this type of care if the applicant is low-income. Often, elderly people use up all of their savings, becoming eligible for long-term care under Medicaid. Medicaid payments are well below market rates in most cases. This often results in managed care organizations and physicians not accepting Medicaid patients.

Long-term care covers the elderly as well as children and adults under age 65 who have health impairments. The need for long-term care is increasing, with significant cost escalations, in relation to the population over age 65, and especially people over age 80. There are not enough personnel to provide long-term care for the rapidly aging population. Often, elderly people who cannot live on their own have no family or friends to assist them regarding care.

There are more than seven million elderly or disabled Americans who are eligible for both Medicare and Medicaid. The costs of caring for these people are double those for other Medicare patients and eight times higher than for children on Medicaid. The Program of All-Inclusive Care for the Elderly (PACE) provides comprehensive services to older people requiring chronic care. It helps them to remain living in their communities.

PACE originated to cover long-term care for elderly immigrants, and is now present in 30 states, offering adult day care, physical therapy, occupational therapy, recreational therapy, nutrition counseling, personal care, social services, medical care, and meals. It also offers home care, hospital care, and nursing home care. Medicare and Medicaid covers PACE programs with capitation payments; PACE coverage is available for people 55 years of age or older who are state-certified as requiring nursing home care, yet still able to live safely in their communities. The average PACE participant is 80 years old, has more than seven medical conditions, has a 50% chance of having dementia, and has three limited daily living activities. However, more than 90% of these individuals are able to continue living in their communities.

Another consideration is the problem of *elder abuse*. This refers to any intentional harmful or negligent act by a caregiver or any other person that causes harm or serious risk of harm to a vulnerable elderly adult. Each state has passed some form of elder abuse prevention laws, covering physical, sexual, exploitative, and emotional abuse, as well as neglect and abandonment. Health care professionals should be aware of the warning signs of elder abuse. These include:

- Bruises, broken bones, abrasions, burns, or pressure marks
- Unexplained withdrawal from normal activities, sudden changes in alertness, or unusual depression
- Sudden changes in financial situations
- Bedsores, unattended medical needs, poor hygiene, or unusual weight loss
- Behaviors of spouses that involve threats or other uses of power and control
- Strained or tense relationships, or frequent arguments between the elderly individual and the caregiver.

Elder abuse forensic centers are being established in various parts of the United States, which investigate elder abuse cases. These centers combine professionals from legal, medical, social services, and law enforcement agencies. Their case reviews involve checking in-home medical and mental statuses of patients, performing investigations that utilize warning signs as evidence of abuse, recording interviews with possible victims of abuse, educating people about elder abuse, and researching cases throughout the country.

The Administration on Aging (AoA) is the principal agency of the U.S. Department of Health and Human Services designated to carry out the provisions of the Older Americans Act of 1965. This Act promoted the well-being of elderly individuals by providing services and programs designed to help them live independently, and empowered the federal government to distribute funds to the states for supportive services for individuals over the age of 60. The Office of Elder Justice and Adult Protective Services handles elder abuse cases. Federal funding to combat elder abuse is, however, very poor in comparison with other areas of law. Less than $15 million is currently budgeted by the federal government to combat this growing problem, and more attention as well as financial resources need to be allocated.

> ### You should remember
>
> Americans age 65 and older make up about 95% of all hospice patients, about 94% of all residential care patients, and about 85% of all nursing home residents.
>
> *Source:* Sulz and Young, 2014.

People with disabilities

Throughout the world, about 15% of the population has some form of disability. Disability rates are increasing because of the aging population, increased prevalence of chronic conditions, and other causes. Disabled people generally have less access to health care services, yet they have the same basic health care needs as all other individuals. The disabled have a higher vulnerability to secondary, co-morbid, and age-related conditions because of this lack of access.

Barriers to health care for people with disabilities include excessive costs, limited availability of services, physical barriers, and inadequate skills of health care workers. Transportation is perhaps the most significant cost consideration. Services that may be uniquely required by the disabled are often not available in all areas. Physical barriers may include inadequate access to health care facilities, medical equipment that does not adjust for people with disabilities, inadequate signs and posted instructions, doorways that are too narrow for wheelchairs, steps instead of ramps, lack of proper bathroom facilities, and poorly designed parking areas. Levels of disability are listed in Table 8.2.

Most disabled people are under age 65 and in their working years. However, the elderly are more likely to have a disability, and that disability is usually severe. The risk of disability increases greatly with increased age. The five most common conditions that cause work limitations include:

- Mental retardation
- Absence of a leg or legs
- Lung or bronchial cancer
- Blindness in both eyes
- Multiple sclerosis.

Health care options for the disabled include Social Security Disability Insurance (SSDI), Supplemental Security Income (SSI), Veterans' Disability Pensions, Medicare, and Medicaid. About two out of every three people with Level I through V disabilities receive private health insurance, while about one in five have public health coverage. About 17% of the disabled have no insurance coverage.

> ### You should remember
>
> According to the CDC, about 16% of adult Americans are hearing-disabled, while about 9% are visually disabled.
>
> *Source:* www.cdc.gov/nchs/fastats/disability.htm.

Table 8.2 Levels of disability

Level	Description	Percentage of affected people
I	Unable to perform basic activities of daily living (ADLs) without another person's help. Examples of ADLs include walking, eating, dressing	2% of adults
II	Unable to perform instrumental activities of daily living (IADLs) without another person's help. Examples of IADLs include mobility outside the home, performing light housework, preparing meals	3% of adults
III	Unable to perform more than one activity (such as hearing, seeing, lifting 10 pounds, climbing a flight of stairs, or walking three city blocks), or having difficulty with two ADLs, but not needing another person's assistance	4% of adults
IV	Able to perform, but with difficulty, two or more activities (hearing, seeing, etc., as listed in Level III)	5% of adults
V	Able to perform, but with difficulty, only one of the same activities as listed in Level III above	8% of adults
VI	No functional limitations. This is the majority of the population, listed as "no disabilities"	78% of adults
Childhood	Long-lasting physical conditions that limit ability to walk, run, play; or a long-lasting mental or emotional condition that limits ability to learn or perform regular schoolwork	4% of children

Source: www.ncbi.nlm.nih.gov/pmc/articles/pmc3422022/table/T1/.

HIV and AIDS

The human immunodeficiency virus or HIV is responsible for the development of acquired immune deficiency syndrome or AIDS. Though the numbers of reported AIDS cases per year fluctuates, deaths are fortunately decreasing. This is because of the development of new and better treatments. However, the number of AIDS patients is increasing, with more than 487,000 patients documented with the disease in 2010. Table 8.3 shows the numbers of various groups of people who have AIDS.

Males have a much higher rate of contracting AIDS than females, and black males are the highest of all groups with the disease. In this group, AIDS is a leading cause of death. The racial component of HIV/AIDS infections is linked to behavioral, economic, social, and other factors. In rural areas, newly diagnosed AIDS patients are mostly younger females,

Table 8.3 Reported AIDS cases in various groups, in the United States (as of 2010)

Males, 13 and older	810,676
Females, 13 and older	198,544
Children under 13	9,209
Ethnic groups	–
Black	473,229
White	429,804
Hispanic	197,449
Asian	8,759
American Indian/Alaska Native	3,721
Native Hawaiian or other Pacific Islander	870

Sources: http://continuingcosmetology.com/onlinecourses/florida/pdf/fl12hrbw.pdf; www.coursehero.com/file/p2 lheg/race-or-ethnicity-estimated-of-aids-diagnoses-2010-cumulative-estimated-of-aids/.

non-white, who contracted the disease through heterosexual contact. They are often from poorer socioeconomic classes.

Without specific therapy, an HIV-positive mother has a 20% chance of transmitting the virus to her baby. Fortunately, antiretroviral therapy has been effective in reducing mother-to-fetus transmission. This is significant because most children with HIV contracted it in this manner. Overall, women are a quickly growing population in relation to HIV/AIDS. It is one of the top ten causes of death in black American women age 15–44, and of Hispanic American women age 25–44. The top two methods of exposure are heterosexual contact and injected drug use. Together, black and Hispanic women make up 79% of all AIDS cases reported in American women.

Homosexual men, inner-city young adults, poorer women, and substance abusers who have left treatment are among the highest risk groups. Also, tuberculosis is linked to HIV since it is an opportunistic infection, and is the worldwide leading cause of death among HIV-positive individuals. HIV-positive people also are likely to develop multidrug-resistant tuberculosis, which is hard to treat and often fatal.

Unfortunately, because of homophobia, a fear and/or hatred of gay men and lesbians, there was a slow overall response to the HIV epidemic. Also, testing may not limit its spread since many people do not change their behavior once learning they have the virus. The virus cannot be cured, and its transmission is not affected by current treatments. Government policies have been rather discriminatory against HIV/AIDS patients, in conjunction with Social Security disability claims.

As AIDS persists in an individual, there is a slow decline in physical, cognitive, and emotional function. The patient requires a variety of types of care, including supervised living, mental health support, and eventually hospice care. Many patients eventually require public entitlement or private disability programs, such as SSDI and SSI. Medicare and Medicaid are primary payers currently. The Affordable Care Act prohibits health insurance from being denied because of pre-existing medical conditions, including HIV/AIDS.

Chronically ill

In the United States, seven out of ten deaths, annually, are from chronic diseases. They are now the leading cause of death, with heart disease, cancer, and stroke making up more than 50% of annual deaths. More than one in four adults has one chronic illness or more, totaling 80 million Americans. More than $153 billion per year is spent caring for people who are overweight or obese, or have other chronic illnesses.

Diabetes mellitus alone costs more than $116 billion to treat every year, and heart disease costs are more than $475 billion. There are four modifiable risk factors that result in chronic disease:

- Physical activity – only about one in five Americans gets adequate aerobic and muscular exercise
- Nutrition – less than one in four Americans eats five or more servings of fruits and vegetables per day, yet most Americans eat more than the recommended amount of saturated fat
- Smoking – approximately one out of every five Americans still smokes tobacco cigarettes, though this number is much lower than it was in previous decades. Younger people are among the groups most likely to smoke
- Alcohol – while approximately three out of four adult Americans consume alcoholic beverages, only about 6% are actually alcoholics. Alcoholism is the number one drug problem in America.

In the United States, more than 56 million people are disabled, and of these, more than 38 million are severely disabled. Disability increases in prevalence with age, and more than 70% of adults age 80 or older have a disability. The majority of disabilities are linked to chronic conditions such as arthritis, asthma, back problems, diabetes, and heart disease. The disabled are more likely to carry private health insurance or be covered by Medicare and Medicaid.

Physical disability concerns a person's mobility and performance of basic activities of daily living. *Mental disability* involves emotional and cognitive states. *Social disability* may be the most severe of all, since it encompasses physical and mental factors.

> ### You should remember
>
> It may be hard to believe, but statistics show that nearly one in two Americans has a chronic condition or illness. Also, about 96% of Americans live with an *invisible illness* – one that does not require any special assistive devices – and may appear perfectly healthy.
>
> *Sources:* www.cdc.gov/chronicdisease/overview;
> www.disabled-world.com/disability/types/invisible/.

Homeless

It is estimated that there are 3.5 million homeless people in the United States. Of these, about 1.35 million are children. The majority of homeless people are found in major urban areas, but more than 27% are in suburban and rural areas. The majority of homeless people in this country are men, followed by families with children. However, women are more likely than men to live below the poverty level, and this increases their risk for becoming homeless.

A significant primary cause of homelessness is domestic violence, linked to 18% of families, and one in four homeless women state this as the main reason they became homeless.

Homelessness is related to personal, social, and economic factors. The economic factors mean that the homeless have poor access to health care. Education is also a primary contributor, with most mothers who have been homeless not completing high school. The majority of the homeless are uninsured, partially because federal institutions that could otherwise help require a physical street address in order for them to qualify. Causes of homelessness also include lack of low-income housing, unemployment, family or personal crises, excessive rent increases, reduced public benefits, illness, release from public mental hospitals, substance abuse, and overcrowding of jails and prisons.

Homelessness itself leads to additional health problems linked to use of alcohol, drugs, and cigarettes, as well as poor sleeping conditions, poor footwear and extensive walking, inadequate nutrition, assault and other forms of victimization, increased exposure to illnesses, and exposure to the elements. Homeless adults often have a variety of medical conditions or illnesses. Homeless children are twice as likely to die than children who live in a home.

The homeless are more likely to be hospitalized and to receive outpatient care. They lack transportation, have reduced ability to follow treatment plans, are often emotionally or mentally incapacitated, lack adequate sanitation, may not have the ability to safely store medications, and are impacted by poor diets. The Health Care for the Homeless program and community health centers have attempted to assist. More than 1.1 million homeless patients are served by various community health centers, offering walk-in appointments. Often, services are available free of charge.

For homeless veterans, services are available through the Department of Veterans Affairs (VA). Mentally ill veterans are treated through the Homeless Chronically Mentally Ill Veterans Program. Those with psychiatric conditions and alcohol or drug abuse problems are treated through the Domiciliary Care for Homeless Veterans Program. Additionally, they may receive help from the Salvation Army, including supplemental housing.

> ### You should remember
>
> As of 2014, of every five homeless people, three were individuals and two were part of a family. About 15% of the homeless are considered "chronically homeless," and tragically, about 9% of the homeless are U.S. military veterans.
>
> *Source:* www.hudexchange.info/resources/documents/2014-AHAR-part1.pdf.

Uninsured

While children in the United States have experienced declining rates of uninsurance, mostly due to the Children's Health Insurance Program, adult Americans in general have higher levels of uninsurance today. Minorities are more likely to lack health insurance than white Americans. Table 8.4 breaks down the percentages of uninsured Hispanics, blacks, Asians, and whites in America.

Overall, the majority of uninsured people are younger members of the workforce, most prevalently in the Western and Southern United States, who do not have a college degree. Uninsured people are usually in poorer health than those who have health insurance. More

Table 8.4 Uninsured percentages of various Americans

Hispanics or Latinos	30.4
Blacks (African Americans)	17.8
Asians	16.2
Whites	14.9

Sources: https://hit.health.tn.gov/reports/surveyreports/brfss_factsheet/healthcareaccess BRFSS factsheets tn 2005. pdf; https://aspe.hhs.gov/report/affordable-care-act-and-asian-americans-and-pacific-islanders; www.episcopalhealth. org/files/5714/6844/7140/Issue_Brief_22_FINAL.pdf.

than half (53%) of the uninsured report having no regular health care source. Often, the uninsured go to the emergency department of a hospital when treatment is needed, where they are treated regardless of their ability to pay, impacting the overall health care system at a rate of more than $57 billion annually. These costs are mostly absorbed by Medicaid, charitable organizations, and federal grants given to non-profit hospitals. Nearly one in three uninsured people postpone seeking medical care because of its cost. It is estimated that 29.8 to 31 million Americans still remain uninsured today, even after the implementation of the Affordable Care Act.

Focus on the uninsured

Even under the Affordable Care Act, many uninsured people say that the high cost of insurance is the primary reason they lack coverage. Today, most uninsured people are in low-income working families.

Illegal immigrants

There are special considerations for people who come to the United States intending to establish a new life in this country. Often, illegal immigrants are poorer people who seek better opportunities in the United States than in their home countries. An example would be farmworkers, many of whom are not legal citizens as they begin working in the United States. The actual number of illegal immigrants is unknown but estimated to be approximately 12 million. Of migrant workers, approximately 75% have been documented as being born in Mexico or Central America.

Most migrant worker families earn less than $22,000 per year. This includes migrant workers allowed by the U.S. government into the country for specific job situations. While these individuals are not considered "legal" by the government, they are in a slightly better situation since they are working in jobs of which the government is aware. Their activities and behaviors can be monitored to a certain degree, while illegal immigrants who enter the country and begin working outside of migrant worker programs are harder to find.

More than half of all migrant workers receive public assistance of some kind. Most are uninsured, and often avoid accessing health care services when they need them. For example, while about 76% of American women seek prenatal care during their first trimester, only about 42% of female migrant workers do the same. Significant health problems among migrant workers include obesity, which usually increases the longer they remain in the United States, tuberculosis, and HIV/AIDS. Individual states as well as the federal Health Resources and Services Administration (HRSA) Migrant Health Program offer health care services to migrant workers and their families.

You should remember

Most immigrants come to the United States for employment, not health care. However, they are much more likely to be uninsured than U.S. citizens. Usually, undocumented immigrants and recent legal immigrants are kept from receiving Medicaid and CHIP coverage by federal law.

CASE STUDY

Health care for the homeless is a regular consideration of today's health care system. Ann is a U.S. Army veteran who became homeless after returning to this country and being unable to hold down a steady job due to post-traumatic stress disorder. Eventually, she sought help from a social worker who connected her to a program that helps veterans to rebuild their lives.

1　Use the Internet to find organizations that help homeless veterans.
2　Are there any organizations that specialize in helping homeless females?
3　Which organizations help to provide health care for the homeless?

Chapter highlights

This section answers the Objectives found at the beginning of the chapter.

1 Explain the three divisions of child health care programs.

- Personal medical and preventive services – primary and specialty services, mostly funded by private health insurance, out-of-pocket payments, and Medicaid
- Population-based community health services – disease prevention and community health promotion services, such as immunizations, lead screening, and child abuse and neglect prevention. Other examples include rehabilitation, case management, referral programs, and monitoring for developmental disabilities.
- Health-related support services – nutrition education, family support, early intervention, and rehabilitation programs, including HIV education and psychotherapy for children, and parental education about developmental delays.

2 Detail the Women's Health Initiative and its findings.

- The largest clinical trial in U.S. history concerning female health care was the Women's Health Initiative, focusing on major causes of death and disability, including heart disease, cancer, and osteoporosis. It found that postmenopausal hormone therapy was linked to invasive breast cancer, coronary heart disease, stroke, and pulmonary embolism.

3 Identify the ethnic minority group most likely to be uninsured or underinsured than other Americans.

- Hispanics are more likely to be uninsured or underinsured than other Americans. Of Hispanics, Mexicans had the highest proportion of uninsured (33%), followed by Cubans (28.1%), and Puerto Ricans (15.8%). However, those listed as "other Hispanics" have 31.8% of their populations uninsured.

4 List the most prevalent chronic conditions affecting the elderly.

- Generally, the most prevalent chronic conditions affecting the elderly include hypertension, arthritis, heart disease, cancer, and diabetes. After the age of 85, most people (60%) have hearing impairment, and 28% have visual impairment.

5 Discuss barriers to health care for people with disabilities.

- Barriers to health care for people with disabilities include excessive costs, limited availability of services, physical barriers, and inadequate skills of health care workers. Transportation is perhaps the most significant cost consideration. Services that may be uniquely required by the disabled are often not available in all areas.

6 Explain the varieties of care required by AIDS patients.

- AIDS patients require a variety of types of care, including supervised living, mental health support, and eventually hospice care. Many patients eventually require public entitlement or private disability programs, such as Social Security Disability Income and Supplemental Security Income.

7 List the four modifiable risk factors that result in chronic disease.

- Physical activity
- Nutrition
- Smoking
- Alcohol.

8 Identify the organizations that assist more than 1.1 million homeless patients.

- More than 1.1 million homeless patients are served by various community health centers, offering walk-in appointments. Often, services are available free of charge.

9 Explain how costs of giving medical treatment to the uninsured are absorbed.

- Often, the uninsured go to the emergency department of a hospital when treatment is needed, where they are treated regardless of their ability to pay. The costs are mostly absorbed by Medicaid, charitable organizations, and federal grants given to non-profit hospitals.

10 List where the majority of migrant workers in the United States are originally from.

- Approximately 75% of migrant workers in the United States have been documented as being born in Mexico or Central America.

Summary

Special populations in the United States often have poorer health as well as greater difficulty in accessing needed health care services. Poorer children are greatly impacted by lack of health care and inadequate immunizations. Women have increased morbidity and poorer health outcomes than men, in general, and often require continued medical treatment for chronic conditions. The 15 recognized minorities in the United States require culturally competent care that is sensitive to their ethnic or religious backgrounds. The elderly make up a larger segment of the U.S. population than ever before, and usually require significantly more health care for one or more chronic conditions. Those who are disabled have the same basic needs regarding health care as the rest of the population, but often have less access. The chronically ill, such as people with HIV/AIDS, require billions of dollars of health care per year. The U.S. health care system is also impacted by the homeless, whose health care costs are often absorbed by the government and various organizations, uninsured people who require health care services, and illegal immigrants.

Review questions

1 What factors are unique concerning the health care of children?
2 What are the differences concerning heart disease and stroke between men and women?
3 What is "culturally competent care"?
4 What are the top five causes of deaths among blacks?
5 Which ethnic group has much higher rates of death from alcoholism and tuberculosis than other groups?
6 Which part of Medicare offers automatic enrollment for all elderly beneficiaries?
7 How would you describe the average participant in the PACE program?
8 What are the five most common conditions that cause work limitations?
9 What group makes up the majority of uninsured Americans?
10 What are some of the significant health problems of migrant workers?

Bibliography

Agency for Healthcare Research and Quality. 2016. Priority Populations. Available at: www.ahrq.gov/health-care-information/priority-populations/index.html. Rockville: Agency for Healthcare Research and Quality.

American Academy of Family Physicians. 2016. Care of Special Populations. Available at: www.aafp.org/afp/topicModules/viewTopicModule.htm?topicModuleId=45. Hasbrouck Heights: American Academy of Family Physicians.

Ansari, Z., et al. 2003. A public health model of the social determinants of health. *Social and Preventive Medicine* 48, no. 4: 242–251.

BRFSS. 2010. Fact Sheet: Health Care Access. Available at: https://hit.health.tn.gov/reports/surveyreports/brfss_factsheet/healthcareaccess BRFSS factsheets TN 2005.pdf. Nashville: Tennessee Department of Health.

Brody, S., and Brody, J.K. 2013. *The Voice of Experience: Stories about Health Care and the Elderly*. New York: Samuel and Jane Brody Publishers. Print.

Burkholder, M., and Bremer-Nash, N. 2013. *Special Populations in Health Care*. Burlington: Jones & Bartlett Learning. Print.

CDC. 2014. National Health Interview Survey Early Release Program – Health Insurance Coverage: Early Release of Estimates From the National Health Interview Survey, 2014. Available at: www.cdc.gov/nchs/data/nhis/earlyrelease/insur201506.pdf. Atlanta: U.S. Centers for Disease Control and Prevention.

CDC. 2015. Morbidity and Mortality Weekly Report – QuickStats: Percentage of Children and Adolescents Aged 0–17 with No Usual Place of Health Care, by Race and Hispanic Ethnicity. Available at: www.cdc.gov/mmwr/preview/mmwrhtml/mm6442a8.htm. Atlanta: U.S. Centers for Disease Control and Prevention.

CDC. 2016. Chronic Disease Prevention and Health Promotion – The Leading Causes of Death and Disability in the United States. Available at: www.cdc.gov/chronicdisease/overview. Atlanta: U.S. Centers for Disease Control and Prevention.

CDC. 2016. Disability and Functioning (Noninstitutionalized Adults 18 Years and Over). Available at: www.cdc.gov/nchs/fastats/disability.htm. Atlanta: U.S. Centers for Disease Control and Prevention.

CDC. 2016. Lack of Health Insurance Coverage and Type of Coverage. Available at: www.cdc.gov/nchs/data/nhis/earlyrelease/earlyrelease201609_01.pdf. Atlanta: U.S. Centers for Disease Control and Prevention.

Contnuing Cosmetology. 2016. Continuing Cosmetology – Course Home Page. Available at: http://continuingcosmetology.com/onlinecourses/florida/pdf/FL12HRBW.pdf. Orlando: Continuing Cosmetology.com.

CourseHero. 2010. Race or Ethnicity Estimated Of AIDS Diagnoses. Available at: www.coursehero.com/file/p2lheg/race-or-ethnicity-estimated-of-aids-diagnoses-2010-cumulative-estimated-of-aids/. Redwood City: Course Hero, Inc.

Disabled World. 2016. Invisible Disabilities List and Information. Available at: www.disabled-world.com/disability/types/invisible/. New York: Disabled World.

Episcopal Health Foundation. 2016. New Evidence Shows Additional Benefits of Medicaid Expansion in Texas. Available at: www.episcopalhealth.org/files/5714/6844/7140/Issue_Brief_22_FINAL.pdf. Houston: Episcopal Health Foundation.

Feldman, H. 2013. *Redesigning Health Care for Children with Disabilities*. Baltimore: Paul H. Brookes Publishing Co. Print.

Health Resources and Services Administration. 2016. HRSA – Home Page. Available at: www.hrsa.gov. Rockville: Health Resources and Services Administration.

HoustonTexas.gov. 2016. Hispanic Health Profile. Available at: www.houstontx.gov/health/chs/HispanicHealthDepBooklet.pdf. Houston: HoustonTx.gov.

HRSA Health Center Program. 2016. Policy for Special Populations – Only Grantees Requesting a Change in Cscope to Add a New Target Population. Available at: http://bphc.hrsa.gov/about/specialpopulations/index.html. Rockville: Health Resources and Services Administration.

Infoplease. 2010. Population of the United States by Race and Hispanic/Latino Origin – Census 2000 and 2010. Available at: www.infoplease.com/ipa/a0762156.html. San Mateo: Sandbox Networks, Inc.

Institute of Medicine, National Academy of Sciences (IOM). 1988. *The Future of Public Health*. Washington, D.C.: National Academies Press.

Joint Commission International. 2016. JCI – Home Page. Available at: www.jointcommissioninternational.org. Oak Brook: Joint Commission International.

KFF.org. 2009. A Profile of American Indians and Alaska Natives and Their Health Coverage. Available at: https://kaiserfamilyfoundation.files.wordpress.com/2013/01/7977.pdf. Menlo Park: Kaiser Family Foundation.

KFF.org. 2015. Community Health Centers: Recent Growth and the Role of the ACA. Available at: http://kff.org/uninsured. Menlo Park: Kaiser Family Foundation.

Lowdermilk, D.L., Perry, S.E., and Cashion, M.C. 2015. *Maternity and Women's Health Care, 11th Edition*. Maryland Heights: Mosby. Print.

Mahan Buttaro, T., et al. 2012. *Primary Care: A Collaborative Practice, 4th Edition*. Maryland Heights: Mosby. Print.

NCBI.NLM.NIH.gov. 2016. Instructions for Activities of Daily Living Stage Assignment. Available at: www.ncbi.nlm.nih.gov/pmc/articles/pmc3422022/table/T1/. Bethesda: National Center for Biotechnology Information.

O'Neill, J.E. and O'Neill, D.M. 2009. *Who Are the Uninsured? An Analysis of America's Uninsured Population, Their Characteristics and Their Health*. New York: Employment Policies Institute.

Peterson-Iyer, K. 2016. Culturally Competent Care in U.S. Clinical Health Care Settings. Available at: www.scu.edu/ethics/practicing/focusareas/medical/culturally-competent-care/introduction.html. Santa Clara: Santa Clara University.

PewResearchCenter. 2010. Meet the New Immigrants: Asians Overtake Hispanics. Available at: www.pewsocialtrends.org/asianamericans-graphics/. New York: Pew Research Center.

Purnell, L.D. 2008. *Guide to Culturally Competent Health Care, 2nd Edition*. Philadelphia: F.A. Davis Company. Print.

Shi, L., and Johnson, J., eds. 2014. *Public Health Administration: Principles for Population-Based Management, 3rd Edition*. Burlington: Jones & Bartlett Learning.

Shi, L., and Singh, D.A. 2014. *Delivering Health Care in America: A Systems Approach, 6th Edition*. Burlington: Jones & Bartlett Learning. Print.

Shi, L., and Stevens, G. 2010. *Vulnerable Populations in the United States, 2nd Edition*. San Francisco: Jossey-Bass. Print.

Smart Traveler Enrollment Program. 2016. What is STEP?. Available at: https://step.state.gov/step. Washington, D.C.: U.S. Department of State.

The University of Iowa – Public Policy Center. 2016. Health Policy – Populations with Special Health Care Needs (SHCN). Available at: http://ppc.uiowa.edu/health/research/populations-special-health-care-needs-shcn. Iowa City: The University of Iowa – Public Policy Center.

U.S. Census Bureau. 2001. The Black Population: 2000 – Census 2000 Brief. Available at: www.census.gov/prod/2001pubs/c2kbr01-5.pdf. Washington, D.C.: U.S. Department of Commerce / Census Bureau.

U.S. Department of Health and Human Services. 2012. *A Guide to Primary Care of People with HIV/AIDS*. Seattle: CreateSpace Independent Publishing Platform. Print.

U.S. Department of Health and Human Services. 2012. The Affordable Care Act and Asian Americans and Pacific Islanders. Available at: https://aspe.hhs.gov/report/affordable-care-act-and-asian-americans-and-pacific-islanders. Washington, D.C.: U.S. Department of Health and Human Services.

U.S. Department of Housing and Urban Development. 2014. The 2014 Annual Homeless Assessment Report (AHAR) to Congress October 2014. Available at: www.hudexchange.info/resources/documents/2014-AHAR-part1.pdf. Washington, D.C.: U.S. Department of Housing and Urban Development.

Vivaldi, M.T. 2010. Myths, Heart Disease and the Latino Population. Available at: www.massmed.org/continuing-education-and-events/conference-proceeding-archive/wch-2012vivaldipres-(pdf)/. Waltham: Massachusetts Medical Society.

World Health Organization. 2016. Media Centre – Disability and Health. Available at: www.who.int/mediacentre/factsheets/fs352/en. Washington, D.C.: Pan American Health Organization.

Chapter 9

Introduction to global health issues

After study of the chapter, readers should be able to:

1 Explain the goal of public health and what it involves.
2 Identify how public health differs from traditional medicine.
3 Describe the eradication of smallpox.
4 Explain the possible outcome when a person spends a longer period of time sick or disabled.
5 Identify the significantly important risk factors for disease.
6 Explain the elderly support ratio.
7 Identify the goal in limiting human rights when a disease outbreak occurs.
8 Define universal health coverage.
9 Explain the terms "culture," "subculture," and "society."
10 Explain the global health problem of obesity.

Overview

Global health concerns are health-related issues across national boundaries that may best be solved by worldwide cooperation. To do this, principles of public health may be applied to international health problems. Global health involves many different disciplines of the health sciences and beyond. It utilizes clinical care on the individual level to prevent health issues in the worldwide population. To achieve better global health, there must be a global perspective about public health. Important examples of global health concerns include pregnancy-related deaths and *malnutrition*. Better global health can be achieved by improving organization and management of health care while technologies evolve that will help to better implement health strategies.

Concepts of global health

Today's global health issues include antimicrobial resistance, the emergence or re-emergence of infectious diseases, HIV and AIDS, malaria, tuberculosis, the eradication of polio, and the increasing prevalence of cancer, diabetes, and cardiovascular disease. There are many questions concerning global health, as follows:

- What determines health?
- How is health status measured?
- How does disease relate to global health care?
- How important are cultures in relation to health care?
- How are health systems organized, and how do they function?
- What transitions are occurring related to demographics and epidemiology?
- What are the most important risk factors for various health conditions?
- What are the links between health, development, education, health care balance or equity, and poverty?

Regarding global health, key health issues include health during childhood, environmental health, injuries, nutrition, and reproductive health. Communicable and non-communicable diseases are also important health issues globally, and are discussed in detail in Chapter 10. Global cooperation helps to address key health issues, as well as what must be done when conflicts or natural disasters and other emergencies occur. Many different people must work together in order to solve global health problems, not only in health care, but also in science and technology.

Concepts of public health and community-based care

Public health is concerned with the prevention of disease and preservation of life via the promotion of physical and mental health through efficient, organized community efforts. This involves control of community-wide infections, sanitary conditions, education about hygiene, health care organization to ensure earlier diagnosis and treatment, and the improvement of community living standards.

A key factor in improving public health is the immunization of children against communicable diseases. Other factors include regular hand washing, smoking cessation, healthier diets, supplementary feeding for the malnourished, exercise programs, HIV and AIDS education, screening for hypertension and diabetes, screening of eyesight in children, prophylactic measures against worms in children, and the use of seat belts in automobiles and helmets when biking or cycling. Public health functions include disease surveillance and the operation of public health clinics and laboratories.

The American Public Health Association publishes, as part of its code of ethics, the following principles:

- Disease prevention
- Respect for individual patient rights
- Community-wide health promotion
- Focus on disenfranchised individuals and communities
- Evidence-based public health efforts
- Cooperation between different disciplines

- Appreciation of diverse beliefs, cultures, and values
- Enhancement of physical and social environments to increase outreach.

Public health differs from traditional medicine in that it focuses on the population rather than just individuals. Public health bases its ethics on public versus personal service. It emphasizes disease prevention and health promotion for communities. Public health targets the environment and human behaviors and lifestyles, as well as medical care. The branch of public health known as epidemiology studies the patterns and causes of disease in specific populations. Then, information can be applied to controlling public health problems. By mobilizing communities, improvements in health behaviors can be made.

Smallpox eradication

One of the greatest accomplishments in the history of public and global health was the eradication of smallpox. As recently as 1966, smallpox was responsible for the deaths of nearly two million people worldwide, or 30% of those affected, every year, reaching 50 different countries. When a patient survived the disease, there were often long-term complications such as blindness or severe scarring.

The smallpox vaccine was developed by Edward Jenner in 1798. However, only in the 1950s was the vaccine able to be mass-produced and refrigerated. In 1965, the United States, through the Centers for Disease Control and Prevention (CDC), assisted with financial and technical support to implement the World Health Organization (WHO) plan for compulsory smallpox vaccinations. All WHO member countries were required to manage funds effectively, report cases of smallpox, encourage research, and be flexible in vaccinations per local area needs.

Widespread vaccinations worked extremely well. In 1977, the last endemic case of smallpox was recorded in the country of Somalia. By 1980, the disease was declared by WHO to have been eradicated worldwide, though it was previously eliminated in Latin America (1971) and Asia (1975).

Between 1967 and 1979, $23 million per year were spent to eradicate smallpox. Before the campaign began, low- and middle-income countries such as India suffered total economic losses in relation to smallpox of approximately $1 billion per year. Part of the success of this campaign was due to the assigning of a single individual in each country who was responsible for smallpox eradication.

Focus on smallpox

Smallpox was more easily eradicated than many other diseases because it was passed directly between individuals, without any carriers or reservoirs. It had a distinctive rash that made diagnosis easy.

The effects of disease on life expectancy

Across the world, each country has variances in how long a male or female is expected to live. This is because of differences in the prevalence of disease, environmental conditions, and other factors. A system called health-adjusted life expectancy *(HALE)* was created to calculate life expectancy of people of all nations, while considering how many years would be spent in good health. The projected years of poor health of an individual are "weighted" based on severity of likely diseases and conditions, and then subtracted from overall life expectancy. A comparison of selected countries' life expectancies, using 2013 data, is shown in Table 9.1. To summarize this information, the longer a person of a specific country is likely to spend sick or disabled, the greater the difference will be between the life expectancy at birth and the health-adjusted life expectancy.

Another important indicator of life expectancy is the disability-adjusted life year *(DALY)*. It defines the total of years lost because of premature death and years lived with disability. Another way to understand DALYs is "years of healthy life that are lost."

Some basic differences emerge when considering the leading causes of death and the leading causes of DALYs. In high-income countries, the *top three causes of death* are ischemic heart disease, stroke, and cancers of the trachea, bronchus, and lungs. In low- and middle-income countries, the top three causes of death are stroke, ischemic heart disease, and chronic obstructive pulmonary disease (COPD).

Table 9.1 Life expectancy at birth and health-adjusted life expectancy (HALE) for various countries

Country	Life expectancy at birth (male)	HALE (male)	Life expectancy at birth (female)	HALE (female)
Australia	80	71	85	74
Brazil	72	63	79	68
Canada	80	71	84	73
China	74	67	77	69
Iran	72	63	76	65
Israel	**81 (highest)**	71	84	74
Italy	80	71	85	74
Japan	80	**72 (highest)**	**87 (highest)**	**78 (highest)**
Kenya	60	52	**63 (lowest)**	**54 (lowest – tie)**
Peru	76	66	79	68
Russian Federation	63	55	75	66
South Africa	**57 (lowest)**	**49 (lowest)**	64	**54 (lowest – tie)**
United Kingdom	79	69	83	72
United States	76	68	81	71

Source: http://data.un.org/data.aspx?q=HALE&d=WHO&f=MEASURE_CODE%3aWHOSIS_000002.

> ## You should remember
>
> When considering disability-adjusted life years (DALYs) for a specific population, remember that periods in which people are living with disabilities are taken into account. Causes of death and DALYs have been divided into three groups:
>
> I – communicable, maternal, perinatal, and nutritional
> II – non-communicable diseases
> III – injuries of all types.

Risk factors for disease

Risk factors for various diseases may include personal behaviors, lifestyles, environmental exposures, or inherited characteristics. Health risks are probabilities of adverse outcomes, or factors that increase these probabilities. In low- and middle-income countries, risk factors may also include the lack of safe drinking water, inappropriate sanitation, poor cooking techniques that increase household smoke levels, unsafe working conditions, and the existence of wars and other conflicts. Significantly important risk factors may include hypertension, high cholesterol, lack of physical exercise, high body mass index (BMI), and high-fasting plasma glucose. Other factors include *underweight* children, smoking, air pollution, iron deficiencies, and less-than-adequate breastfeeding practices.

In high-income countries, risk factors are also mostly related to diet, exercise, smoking, and pollution. Another risk factor in these countries is the presence of lead in the environment. For people who have DALYs, additional factors include drug use. High-income countries also have more people who are overweight or obese, as well as significant numbers of smokers. The top ten risk factors for death, in various types of countries, are shown in Table 9.2.

Table 9.2 Top 10 risk factors for deaths in various types of countries

High-income countries	Low- and middle-income countries
1. Dietary risks	1. Dietary risks
2. Hypertension	2. Hypertension
3. Smoking	3. Smoking
4. High body mass index	4. Household air pollution
5. Physical inactivity	5. Ambient particulate matter pollution
6. High-fasting plasma glucose	6. High-fasting plasma glucose
7. High total cholesterol	7. Physical inactivity
8. Ambient particulate matter pollution	8. High body mass index
9. Alcohol use	9. Alcohol use
10. Lead	10. High total cholesterol

Source: www.sciencedaily.com/releases/2015/09/150911094941.htm.

Population growth and aging

Population growth and aging are highly important to global health. The current worldwide population is just under 7.3 billion, and growing. Trends show that overwhelming population growth is occurring in low- and middle-income countries. Fertility rates are generally higher in these countries than in high-income countries, though fertility rates are falling in many of them. The growing populations of these countries will result in more sanitation and water supply infrastructure improvements. As a result, there may be negative health and even education impacts.

The worldwide population is also aging, primarily in high-income countries that have lower fertility rates. The *elderly support ratio* describes the imbalance of people aged 65 years or more in comparison to those between the ages of 15 and 64. This factor greatly impacts how disease affects health costs. People are living longer and experiencing more time with morbidities and disabilities in relation to non-communicable diseases. Health care costs are therefore rising, and the elderly support ratio means that it will be more difficult to finance these costs because there are more and more elderly in comparison to the numbers of working age people.

As of 2010, 15.9% of the populations of high-income countries were over age 65, while only 5.8% of the populations of low- and middle-income countries were over this age. The predictions for 2050 are as follows:

- High-income countries: 26.2% of the population over age 65
- Low- and middle-income countries: 14.6% of the population over age 65.

Poverty and the economy

The costs of health care are very important to most people, but especially to those near the poverty level. For them, large health expenditures can seriously harm their financial status and lead to poverty. Illness may lead to reduced income, plus costs to cover transportation to and from health care facilities. Certain diseases lead to disabilities such as paralysis or deformities. Mental health conditions or chronic diseases such as diabetes or stroke often result in long-term disabilities. When a person has a long-term disability, the costs of health care over time can be significant.

Health and education

The health and education of families are interconnected, in that they lead to multigenerational changes in behaviors related to good health. Children are affected by malnutrition and various diseases, which affect their schooling as well as their cognitive development. Better education about health allows people to fight illness more successfully. Malnutrition and illnesses of parents often lead to the same in their children. These conditions may affect school enrollment, attendance, concentration, and performance.

Education about appropriate health measures improves likely health outcomes. For example, parents who are better educated about health are more likely to make sure their children receive all appropriate immunizations. Better health education also discourages unhealthy behaviors and lifestyles. Women with better schooling have been shown to have children whose mortality rates are decreased. Also, women of better economic development have children with reduced mortality rates, though this is not as significant as mothers with better education.

Ethical and human rights concerns

Throughout the world there are conventions and treaties that recognize access to health services and information as basic human rights. Unfortunately in many countries, poorer people often are not afforded these rights. People with serious conditions such as tuberculosis often do not receive prompt or adequate care because health care workers are afraid to interact with them. This may lead to the infection and death of many people.

Other ethical and human rights issues are related to new or emerging diseases such as Severe Acute Respiratory Syndrome (SARS) or Ebola. Individuals have rights, but so does society in its protection of the mass population. Research upon human subjects is another challenging ethical area, wherein individuals are at risk of the results of research carried out in order for other people to be treated against disease. In low- or middle-income countries, decisions are continually made to determine which populations and *disease groups* receive priority for treatment.

Limits to human rights

Human rights are temporarily limited in certain situations, such as during epidemics of infectious diseases. For example, when SARS or Ebola has affected the public sufficiently, governments have suspended travel, the ability to go to work, and even the ability to leave your own home. Sports events and other gatherings have been postponed. Though governments have the obligation to protect public health, there is controversy about their ability to control the movements of the people they govern. The goal in limiting human rights should be to minimize the likelihood of a disease outbreak affecting too many people. Therefore, when these temporary limits must be imposed, they should follow due process of law. The rights of the people should be monitored during these times, and all rights should be reinstated as quickly as possible.

Universal health coverage

Universal health coverage or universal coverage is defined by WHO as ensuring that everyone can receive needed promotive, preventive, curative, rehabilitative, and palliative health services. These services must have enough quality to be effective, and their use must not expose the user to financial hardship. Universal health coverage should help people obtain the appropriate services they need without suffering financial hardship to pay for them. Universal health coverage should provide basic health care services free or so inexpensively that access is not restricted and hardship is not caused.

A universal health coverage system would be affordable, have a well-trained and highly motivated workforce, offer fair access to needed medicine and technologies, and offer integrated basic services for the following:

- Maternal and child health
- Non-communicable diseases
- Control of communicable diseases such as HIV, tuberculosis, malaria, and neglected tropical diseases (NTDs).

The provision of insurance is more difficult for low-income countries. Most countries help to insure their people through various combinations of payroll taxes, general taxes, and contributions called *premiums* from insured individuals. In countries where only a small portion of the population pays taxes, financing for health care is more difficult. It is also difficult to collect contributions from poor, rural populations.

The best way to pay health care providers is also in question, and a variety of methods may be used. Various countries choose nationalized health insurance, various methods handled by different organizations, or methods based on certain types of beneficiary. Insurance may cover the public, private individuals, or both. Today, there is a global movement focused on universal health coverage for all countries. Those moving toward or already offering universal coverage include Mexico, Nigeria, Korea, Thailand, China, Vietnam, and many others.

Culture and health

A **culture** is a societal group made up of accepted knowledge, beliefs, morals, customs, and laws. It usually shares standards or rules among its members, which produce behaviors they consider acceptable or proper. A culture may also be a group of people with defined behaviors and beliefs that are learned and shared. There may be cultures within families, social groups, economic groups, the arts, religion, and even languages. *Subcultures* are smaller cultural groups that may have more specified differences in language, foods, music, interpersonal relationships, and art. In the United States, there are numerous subcultures. A society consists of groups of people within a certain locality that share the same cultural traditions. Societies are held together by relationships between the groups of people they contain. The United States is unique in the number of different large foreign subcultures it contains, including people originally from Africa, Asia, Europe, Central and South America, the various Pacific islands, and the Middle East. Within each of these, many unique smaller subcultures also exist.

Culture helps to determine health status in many ways. It is related to health behaviors such as attitudes toward diet, childbirth, breastfeeding, hygiene, and others. Culture also helps to determine perceptions about illness, including the meanings of "good health" and "illness." People of various cultures also use health services in different ways: some very quickly when they feel sick, and others only when they become extremely ill. There are also different practices concerning medical treatment among various cultures.

Some cultural values improve health outcomes, while others do not. Those that believe in safer sex, better diets, and more regular exercise generally have healthier populations. Certain cultural practices may adapt better or worse to various settings or lifestyles. People outside of cultural groups may not be able to understand certain practices within the groups. The term *cultural relativism* specifies that the uniqueness of each culture means that it can be evaluated only according to its own values and standards. Individuals who are interested in global health must understand that each individual culture is unique, and as a result, must understand what behavioral changes will be needed in order to improve the health of various cultural groups.

Health beliefs and practices

Health beliefs and practices differ throughout the many cultures of the world. Some cultures, for example, view certain diseases as normal components of everyday life, while others may view the same diseases as severe conditions. Examples include malaria, considered normal in large parts of South Africa, and schistosomiasis in Egypt.

Diseases are considered to be biological and psychophysiologic malfunctions or maladaptations. Common examples of diseases include AIDS, pneumonia, or polio. *Illnesses* are defined as reactions to disease or discomfort that may be personal, interpersonal, or cultural. When a person feels ill, he or she often describes the feeling or the symptoms, often with a specific name for the perceived illness. There may be no actual *disease*, yet perceptions of disease have wide cultural variations.

In the United States and other high-income countries, the causes of disease are explained by using the Western medical paradigm. For example, *type 2 diabetes* occurs because of obesity, or may be genetically linked, while colds and influenza are caused by viruses. Heart disease may be caused by high cholesterol, obesity, or smoking.

However, in many low- and middle-income countries, illness may be perceived as being caused by other factors, according to the biomedical model. If a patient's body is perceived as being *out of balance*, such as being too hot or too cold, illness is believed to occur as a result (see Table 9.3). Imbalance may be linked to unhealthy behaviors or diets. Some people even believe that disease has a supernatural cause, including possession of the soul, behaviors that offend "gods," or being bewitched by another person. Others believe that illness is a sign that a person needs to re-evaluate his or her life, or that it is caused by the efforts of enemies, ancestors, and natural or hereditary causes.

Some cultures believe that extreme emotional stress causes illness, and others link illness to forbidden or excessive sex practices. Folk illnesses are those believed to have been caused by non-physiologic factors such as inappropriate diet or eating habits. These illnesses are often treated by "healers" who use natural substances, massage, and other techniques.

As a result of so many different cultural beliefs about illness, practices required to avoid illness also vary. For example, many Nigerian people believe that pregnant women must avoid sweets, eggs, or snails in their diet in order to have healthy babies. In Brazil, pregnant women should not eat fish or game meat, such as venison. Some cultures believe that traditional potions, jewelry, or techniques such as scarification are needed to remove bad or evil spirits, thus preventing illness. Other rituals are practiced to prevent self-harm, inflict harm on others, or to prevent infertility and deaths of infants.

Many cultures use home remedies to first treat an illness, and then visit a local healer. They may avoid seeking Western medical help until the illness has become severe, but often continue to use their own local remedies simultaneously. Poorer cultures often pay for

Table 9.3 Conditions and treatments based on theories of "hot" and "cold"

"Hot" conditions	"Cold" medical remedies	"Cold" food remedies
Constipation, fever, infections, sore throat, ulcers	Bicarbonate of soda, milk of magnesia, orange flower water, sage	Chicken, dairy products, honey, lima beans, milk, raisins, vegetables
"Cold" conditions	"Hot" medical remedies	"Hot" food remedies
Cancer, colds, headache, pneumonia, tuberculosis	Aspirin, cinnamon, cod liver oil, garlic, penicillin	Beef, cereals, eggs, oils, spicy foods, wine

medical treatments with whatever they have instead of money – including animals, fruits, vegetables, and small gifts. People usually prefer local healers who are similar to them in language, respectability, and beliefs. One common factor among most cultures is that an illness is usually first treated at home prior to seeking outside treatment. Health care providers also differ greatly throughout the world's cultures (see Table 9.4).

Health behaviors

While many health behaviors are good, others contribute to leading risk factors for illness and premature death. In low- and middle-income countries, this can be better understood by looking at their top ten causes of death each year, as of 2010:

- Stroke
- Ischemic heart disease
- Chronic obstructive pulmonary disease
- Lower respiratory infections
- Diarrhea
- HIV and AIDS
- Malaria
- Injuries occurring in relation to roadways
- Tuberculosis
- Diabetes.

Notice that the primary risk factors for this list include undernutrition or obesity, use of tobacco, air pollution, unsafe sex practices, contaminated water, and poor sanitation.

In low- and middle-income countries, there is a higher than normal number of premature deaths of underweight infants, which may be linked to certain food taboos for pregnant women. Undernutrition is also linked to poor breastfeeding techniques, and incorrectly timed introduction of other foods to infants.

Sanitary practices are also of vital concern in these countries, and people may need to be taught the importance of hygiene. They may be unaware of the need to wash their hands regularly with soap and water, the safe use of water, and the disposal of human waste. Air pollution, whether outdoor or indoor, is another major risk factor for disease. Cooking indoors without proper ventilation may allow pollutants from certain fuel sources to accumulate to dangerous levels. Education about the dangers of smoking may be able to slow or eradicate the habit from these countries, which many people take up in their early teenage

Table 9.4 Examples of health care providers in various cultures

Western biomedical health service providers	Physicians, nurses, nurse practitioners, pharmacists, dentists, etc.
Eastern medical providers	Chinese practitioners, acupuncturists, chemists, herbalists, Indian *ayurvedic* practitioners
Indigenous providers	Healers, bone-setters, diviners, midwives, priests, shamans, sorcerers, spiritualists, witches

years. Regardless of the income level of each country, behaviors are related to culture, and often do not result in good health.

The ecological perspective

The concept of *ecological perspective* attempts to explain why people behave in certain ways concerning their health. The ecological perspective is based on individual, interpersonal, institutional, community, and public policy areas. Individual behaviors are influenced by attitudes, beliefs, knowledge, and personality. Family members, friends, and peers form interpersonal processes and primary groups that influence behavior. Institutional policies, regulations, rules, and informal structures also have behavioral influences. Regarding communities, formal or informal social standards exist among individuals and groups of people, including organizations. Finally, public policies at the local, state, and federal levels encourage healthy actions and practices about health practices.

Nutrition and global health

Nutrition is vital for the growth and development of children. Therefore, the importance of nutrition and global health cannot be minimized. Large numbers of people are undernourished: for example, poor women and children in low-income countries in regions such as Southern Asia and some parts of Africa. Children under age five who are underweight make up the group that has the highest risk for death. Another important risk factor concerns infant deaths because of less than adequate breastfeeding. When an infant is correctly and sufficiently breastfed, immunity against infectious disease is strongly developed. However, when breastfeeding is less than adequate, an infant is at much higher risk of death from infectious disease.

Goals related to nutrition and global health have been established under the name Millennium Development Goals. These include the eradication of poverty and hunger, achieving universal primary education about nutrition, promoting gender equality and empowering women, reducing child mortality, improving maternal health, and battling HIV and AIDS, malaria, tuberculosis, and other diseases.

> ## You should remember
>
> Approximately 45% of childhood deaths are related to malnutrition. Therefore, to decrease these mortality rates, nutritional problems must be solved.
> *Source:* www.who.int/mediacentre/factsheets/fs178/en/.

Undernutrition

The term *undernutrition* is used for a type of malnutrition caused by an inadequate food supply, or an inability to use the nutrients in food. Undernutrition in children is based on three factors: height-for-age, weight-for-age, and weight-for-height. Approximately 16% of children under age five throughout the world are underweight, and most of these live in low-income countries. More than three million child deaths every year can be linked to poor nutrition – this is more than 8,000 nutrition-related deaths *daily*.

For adults, undernutrition is measured by a *BMI* less than 18.5. In many poorer countries, men and boys are less undernourished than women and girls, partly because of cultural reasons. Basic causes of malnutrition include inadequate education, poor resources and controls, and political and economic factors and structures. Malnutrition leads to weakening of a person's body, illness, infection, and chronic conditions that eventually develop.

The good news concerning undernutrition is that it has been decreasing over at least the past 20 years. Many countries in Asia and South America have greatly reduced undernutrition in children under the age of five. In poorer countries, vitamin A supplements have increasingly been added to children's diets, decreasing blindness.

> ### Focus on vitamin A
>
> Vitamin A deficiency leads to atrophy of the epithelial tissue, resulting in keratomalacia, xerophthalmia, night blindness, and lowered resistance to infection of the mucous membranes.

However, undernutrition still is significant in many pregnant women and children. Globally, approximately 165 million children have growth stunting, 100 million are underweight, and 50 million are wasted. Poorer women across the globe also are often underweight. Micronutrients in the diet are often lacking, in varied amounts over different locations. For example, the prevalence of vitamin A deficiency in children is highest in Africa, but in pregnant women, it is highest in Asia. The prevalence of zinc deficiency in all groups is highest in Africa. The prevalence of iodine deficiency in all groups is highest in Europe. The prevalence of iron deficiency in all groups is also highest in Africa.

Obesity

The term *obesity* refers to an abnormal increase in the proportion of fat cells, mainly in the viscera and subcutaneous tissues of the body. Obesity manifests as excess body weight in comparison to height. A person is considered obese when the BMI exceeds 30. There is a formula for determining obesity. It is calculated by dividing a person's weight in kilograms by the square of the person's height in meters. An adult with a BMI of 25 to 29.9 is considered *overweight*. A BMI of 30 or greater indicates obesity. Body mass index calculations are as follows:

Underweight = < 18.5
Normal weight = 18.5 to 24.9
Overweight = 25 to 29.9
Obese = > 30

The formulas used for these calculations are as follows:

$$BMI = \frac{Weight\ (lb) \times 703}{Height\ (inches)^2} \text{ or } BMI = \frac{Weight\ (kg) \times 703}{Height\ (m^2)}$$

To estimate an individual's body fat percentage, a professional uses a tool called a *caliper* to measure the thickness of a fold of skin (see Figure 9.1).

Throughout the world, nearly 37% of people are overweight or obese, and this rate has increased 28% since 1980. Also, nearly 7% of children under age five are overweight.

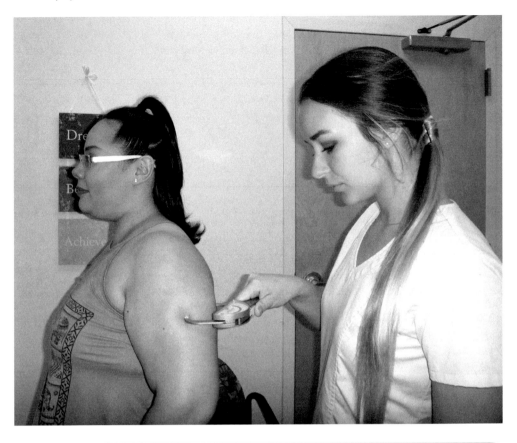

Figure 9.1 Using a caliper to measure BMI in an obese patient.

In nearly every country, the percentage of people who are overweight or obese is increasing. These conditions are closely linked to hypertension, hyperlipidemia, coronary artery disease, heart attack, type 2 diabetes, gallbladder disease, osteoarthritis, sleep apnea, and breast and colon cancer. Prevention of obesity is aimed at reinforcement of long-term lifestyle changes, including a balanced diet and regular exercise.

The primary cause of being overweight or obese is an increase in total energy intake and a decrease in total energy expenditure. While some people may be genetically predisposed, most individuals who are overweight or obese develop these conditions because of their chosen lifestyles. Genetic variations may influence behavior, metabolism, and digestion. However, unhealthy behaviors play the predominant role in being overweight or obese. In some cultures, being overweight is actually considered to be a sign of wealth, success, and prosperity.

The global increases in people who are overweight or obese are based on increased wealth, socioeconomic status, and urbanization. Drinks with more sugar and highly processed, less nutritional foods have become extremely popular due to their convenience. Lifestyles that favor reduced exercise have become prevalent. People have become used to sitting in front of computers or televisions for many hours.

It is interesting to note that countries which maintain their traditional food cultures, and resist modernization of available foods, have less obesity. Urbanization, however, has caused many countries to lose farmland, meaning fewer farmers and less local fresh produce. This type of healthy food has been replaced, as a result, by denser, less nutritional, highly processed animal-based foods. Also, *fast food* has become prominently linked to obesity since it has high caloric content and highly processed ingredients, along with extreme levels of fat, sugar, and salt.

The marketing of food products also favors poor nutrition, and unfortunately, children are frequently targeted by this type of marketing. Over the past 40 years, the process of adding various types of sugar to processed foods and sweetened beverages has greatly contributed to obesity rates. In the United States, for example, sugar-sweetened drinks contain the largest sources of added sugars in comparison with all types of foods.

The intake of red and processed meat has been proven to be linked to weight gain, heart disease, type 2 diabetes, certain cancers, and death. Along with the global increase in meat-related foods, there has been a large decrease in consumption of fruits, vegetables, and whole grains. Partly because of jobs that require less physical activity, the prevalence of television and video games, and the availability of motor vehicles, people across the globe sit still for more hours of the day than ever before. So, by adding to this scenario foods that greatly increase energy intake, it is easy to understand the epidemic of obesity.

Focus on meat in the diet

Recent studies recommend that red meat, bacon, or sausage should only be consumed once per week, in order to reduce the likelihood of heart disease. Other meat sources, such as fish and chicken, are healthier choices.

Not nearly enough people follow the recommended guidelines of 30 or more minutes of moderate physical activity for most days of each week. In urban settings, people often avoid exercise outside due to limited exercise areas and fear of crime. With industrialization, there are fewer jobs such as farming or mining, which require high energy expenditure, and more jobs such as those based in offices and manufacturing plants, which require less energy expenditure. Urbanization also means less walking and more use of motorized transportation. Other factors for obesity include decreased sleep, increased stress, and increased indoor forms of entertainment.

Being overweight or obese is linked to 44% of worldwide diabetes, 23% of ischemic heart disease cases, and up to 41% of some types of cancer. Obese or overweight people are mostly found in North and South America (27%), followed by Europe (23%) and the Eastern Mediterranean area (19%). Women have higher rates of obesity than men. Individual rates of obesity among various populations of the United States are listed in Table 9.5.

You should remember

In the United States, more than one-third of adults are obese. This makes up 34.9% of the adult population of the country, or 112.7 million people. Approximately one out of every five deaths are linked to obesity.
Sources: www.cdc.gov/obesity/data/adult.html; www.medscape.com/viewarticle/809516.

Table 9.5 Rates of U.S. obesity in individual populations

Population group	Percentage of obese people in this population
Blacks	47.8
Hispanics	42.5
Whites	32.6
Asians	10.8

Source: www.cdc.gov/obesity/data/adult.html.

Childhood obesity is another serious problem, since it often continues into adulthood. Worldwide, the percentage of obese or overweight children has increased more than 47% since 1980. The critical part of this scenario is that the problem has increased much faster in children than in adults in more than three decades. In children under five years of age, Europe leads with these conditions (12.5%), followed by the Eastern Mediterranean area (8.9%) and Africa (7.9%).

In high-income countries, increases in obesity have begun to slow down. Today, the largest increases are predicted to occur in low- to middle-income countries. It is critical to reverse this situation since being obese or overweight is among the greatest risks for death worldwide. More than 2.8 million adult deaths occur every year in relation to being obese or overweight.

Nutrition and pregnancy

During pregnancy, nutrition is absolutely essential for the health of both the mother and the baby. Folic acid, iron, and calcium are very important for pregnant women. Deficiencies of folic acid are linked to neural tube defects in babies, such as spina bifida. Pregnant women must get enough protein and energy from their diets. It is recommended that a pregnant woman eat 300 calories per day more than usual while carrying a baby.

Nutritional needs during infancy and childhood

A child's development in infancy requires proper nutrition in order to avoid, potentially, a lifetime of physical or mental growth problems. Inadequate nutrition during this period may mean that throughout life, the child will not be able to battle infections normally. Young children must consume enough protein, carbohydrates, and fats from their diets, as well as adequate vitamins and minerals. Sufficient amounts of vitamin A, iodine, iron, and zinc are essential. Evidence shows that infants grow better and stay healthier if breastfed, without consuming any supplemental nutrition, for the first six months of life.

When a child finishes breastfeeding, replacement nutrition must be adequate in order to avoid infections and illnesses. Stunted children are not likely to ever catch up to normal growth status, and any physical or mental developmental damage will probably be permanent.

All adolescents, male and female, go through *growth spurts*, but those who are stunted in childhood cannot make up their growth during adolescence. Adolescents of both sexes also have needs for adequate calcium, folic acid, iodine, and iron.

Nutritional needs during adulthood and old age

During adulthood and old age, adequate nutrition is just as important for normal health. In these ages, the diet may be harmful if not managed closely. Excessive amounts of cholesterol, fat, salt, and sugar must be avoided. In old age, dietary requirements are highly specialized. Unfortunately, many older people have poor diets because of financial situations or lack of support from other people. To avoid becoming obese, especially because of reduced amounts of physical activity, the diet must supply the correct amounts of protein, energy, and iron. Calcium and vitamin D are crucial dietary supplements in order to reduce risks of *osteoporosis*.

CASE STUDY

Issues of poor food quality plague many countries. Education about better ways to safeguard the food supply has been proven to increase health standards and decrease related diseases. For example, in Thailand, there is a struggle to grow enough food because of factors such as low rainfall, poor soil quality, and lack of forest lands to supplement food shortages. This has resulted in low protein levels in the diets of Thai citizens. A new fish-farming project, in which tilapia are raised using safe, secure, and healthy methods, is helping to eradicate this problem.

1 Why is buying fish from markets difficult for many Thai citizens?
2 How can training people in Thailand and other countries improve their self-sufficiency regarding food production?
3 How can "fish farms" offer higher-quality protein supplies?

Chapter highlights

This section answers the Objectives found at the beginning of the chapter.

1 **Explain the goal of public health and what it involves.**

- Public health is concerned with the prevention of disease and preservation of life via the promotion of physical and mental health through efficient, organized community efforts.
- This involves control of community-wide infections, sanitary conditions, education about hygiene, health care organization to ensure earlier diagnosis and treatment, and the improvement of community living standards.

2 **Identify how public health differs from traditional medicine.**

- Public health differs from traditional medicine in that it focuses on the population rather than just individuals. Public health bases its ethics on public versus personal service. It emphasizes disease prevention and health promotion for communities. Public health targets the environment, human behaviors and lifestyles, as well as medical care.

3 **Describe the eradication of smallpox.**

- The smallpox vaccine was developed by Edward Jenner in 1798. In the 1950s, mass-production and refrigeration of the vaccine were developed. In 1965, compulsory smallpox vaccinations were introduced, which encouraged cooperation between countries. Vaccines and specimen kits were supplied, and by 1977, the last endemic case of smallpox was recorded – in the country of Somalia. By 1980, the disease was declared "eradicated" worldwide. An average of $23 million per year had been spent to eradicate smallpox, and in each country, a single individual had been designated as responsible for smallpox eradication. Smallpox was more easily eradicated than other diseases since it was passed directly between individuals, and had a distinctive rash that made diagnosis easy. Anyone who survived smallpox was immune for life. Affected people became bedridden, meaning they were unlikely to infect others.

4 **Explain the possible outcome when a person spends a longer period of time sick or disabled.**

- To summarize, the longer a person of a specific country is likely to spend sick or disabled, the greater the difference will be between the life expectancy at birth and the health-adjusted life expectancy.

5 **Identify the significantly important risk factors for disease.**

- Hypertension
- High cholesterol
- Lack of physical exercise
- High body mass index (BMI)
- High-fasting plasma glucose.

6 **Explain the elderly support ratio.**

- The *elderly support ratio* describes the imbalance of people aged 65 or more in comparison to those between the ages of 15 and 64. This factor greatly impacts how disease affects health costs. People are living longer and experiencing more time with morbidities and disabilities in relation to non-communicable diseases. Health care costs are therefore rising, and the elderly support ratio means that it will be more difficult to finance these costs because there are more and more elderly in comparison to the numbers of working age people.

7 **Identify the goal in limiting human rights when a disease outbreak occurs.**

- The goal in limiting human rights should be to minimize the likelihood of a disease outbreak affecting too many people. Therefore, when these temporary limits must be imposed, they should follow due process of law. The rights of the people should be monitored during these times, and all rights should be reinstated as quickly as possible.

8 **Define universal health coverage.**

- Universal health coverage means that everyone can receive needed promotive, preventive, curative, rehabilitative, and palliative health services. These services must have enough quality to be effective, and their use must not expose the user to financial hardship. There should be fair access to services regardless of ability to pay.

9 **Explain the terms "culture," "subculture," and "society."**

- A culture is a societal group made up of accepted knowledge, beliefs, morals, customs, and laws. It usually shares standards or rules among its members, which produce behaviors they consider acceptable or proper.

- Subcultures are smaller cultural groups that may have more specified differences in language, foods, music, interpersonal relationships, and art.
- A society consists of groups of people within a certain locality that share the same cultural traditions. Societies are held together by relationships between the groups of people they contain.

10 **Explain the global health problem of obesity.**

- Throughout the world, nearly 37% of people are overweight or obese, and nearly 7% of children under age five are overweight. The primary cause is an increase in total energy intake and a decrease in total energy expenditure, because of a lifestyle that favors reduced exercise. Increases in body mass index are based on increased wealth, socioeconomic status, and urbanization. Drinks with more sugar and highly processed, less nutritional foods have become extremely popular due to their convenience. However, countries that maintain their traditional food cultures, and resist modernization of available foods, have less obesity. Urbanization has caused many countries to lose farmland, meaning fewer farmers and less local fresh produce. Not nearly enough people get the recommended 30 or more minutes of moderate physical activity for most days of each week. Obesity is also linked to decreased sleep, increased stress, and increased indoor forms of entertainment. It often causes diabetes, ischemic heart disease cases, and certain types of cancer. Women have higher rates of obesity than men. Childhood obesity is serious, since it often continues into adulthood. The problem has increased much faster in children than in adults in the last three decades. More than 3.4 million adult deaths occur every year in relation to being obese or overweight.

Summary

Global health issues can only be adequately addressed by establishing a worldwide perspective concerning public health. Cooperation between countries helps to improve how we combat disease, benefiting everyone. A great example is shown by the various countries that contributed to the battle and eventual eradication of smallpox. With the growing elderly population, global health initiatives are being refocused on issues that address longer lifespans, medical costs, and the burdens that health care for the elderly will place upon younger generations. Universal health coverage is a global movement designed to offer care to all people, regardless of their ability to pay for services. Increased knowledge about adequate nutrition and healthier lifestyles is benefiting people from all countries, and today's younger people are better educated about health than at any time in history. This increased education in health matters is encouraging people to resist highly processed, less nutritional foods, and change their diets and habits to include more healthy choices.

> ### Review questions
>
> 1 What principles make up the code of ethics of the American Public Health Association?
> 2 What are risk factors for disease?
> 3 What is the relationship between education and health?
> 4 What are ethical and human rights issues concerning new diseases?
> 5 What is universal health coverage?
> 6 What are the various subcultures in the United States?
> 7 What is the Western medical paradigm?
> 8 What is the relationship between nutrition and global health?
> 9 What are the outcomes of obesity?
> 10 Why is nutrition essential for the health of the body during pregnancy?

Bibliography

Benatar, S., and Brock, G. 2011. *Global Health and Global Health Ethics*. New York: Cambridge University Press. Print.

Bic, Z. 2014. *Nutrition and Global Health*. San Diego: Cognella Academic Publishing. Print.

Biehl, J., and Petryna, A. 2013. *When People Come First: Critical Studies in Global Health*. Princeton: Princeton University Press. Print.

CDC. 2016. Adult Obesity Facts – Obesity Prevalence Maps. Available at: www.cdc.gov/obesity/data/adult.html. Atlanta: U.S. Centers for Disease Control and Prevention.

Center for Strategic and International Studies. 2016. Universal Health Coverage. Available at: http://csis.org/files/publication/140109_bristol_globalactionuniversalhealth_web.pdf. Washington, D.C.: CSIS.

Cotlear, D., Nagpal, S., Smith, O., Tandon, A., and Cortez, R. 2015. *Going Universal: How Twenty-Four Countries Are Implementing Universal Health Coverage from the Bottom Up*. Washington, D.C.: World Bank Publications. Print.

Edberg, M. 2012. *Essentials of Health, Culture, and Diversity: Understanding People, Reducing Disparities*. Burlington: Jones & Bartlett Leaning. Print.

Farmer, P., Kleinman, A., Yong Kim, J., and Basilico, M. 2013. *Reimagining Global Health: An Introduction*. Oakland: University of California Press. Print.

GHEC. 2016. GHEC – Home Page. Available at: http://globalhealtheducation.org. New York: GlobalHealthEducation.org.

Gilbert, G.G., Sawyer, R.G., and McNeil, E.B. 2014. *Health Education: Creating Strategies for School and Community Health, 4th Edition*. Burlington: Jones & Bartlett Learning. Print.

Glanz, K., Rimer, B.K., and Viswanath, K. 2015. *Health Behavior: Theory, Research, and Practice, 5th Edition*. San Francisco: Jossey-Bass. Print.

Global Citizen. 2016. Global Povery Project – Home Page. Available at: www.globalpovertyproject.com. New York: GlobalPovertyProject.com.

Global Health and Human Rights. 2016. GHHR – Home Page. Available at: www.globalhealthrights.org. Washington, D.C.: GlobalHealthRights.org.

Harlan, C. 2014. *Global Health Nursing: Narratives from the Field*. New York: Springer Publishing Company. Print.

Henderson, D.A., and Preston, R. 2009. *Smallpox: The Death of a Disease – The Inside Story of Eradicating a Worldwide Killer*. Amherst: Prometheus Books. Print.

Lancet, The. 2012. *Technologies for Global Health*. London: The Lancet. Print.

Medscape. 2016. Obesity's Toll: 1 in 5 Deaths Linked to Excess Weight. Available at: www.medscape.com/viewarticle/809516. New York: Medscape.

Minkler, M., and Wallerstein, N. 2008. *Community-Based Participatory Research for Health: From Process to Outcomes, 2nd Edition*. San Francisco: Jossey-Bass. Print.

Pinto, A.D., and Upshur, R.E.G. 2013. *An Introduction to Global Health Ethics*. London: Routledge. Print.

Project Guardian. 2016. RB Health Hygiene Home – Project Guardian. Available at: www.globalnutritionhealth.org. Slough: Reckitt Benckiser Group plc.

RAND Corporation. 2015. Community-based Health Care. Available at: www.rand.org/topics/community-based-health-care.html. Santa Monica: RAND Corporation.

Schneider, M.J. 2013. *Introduction to Public Health, 4th Edition*. Burlington: Jones & Bartlett Learning. Print.

ScienceDaily. 2015. Poor Diet and High Blood Pressure now Number One Risk Factors for Early Death. Available at: www.sciencedaily.com/releases/2015/09/150911094941.htm. Rockville: ScienceDaily.

Skolnik, R. 2015. *Global Health 101 (Essential Public Health), 3rd Edition*. Burlington: Jones & Bartlett Learning. Print.

Stein, N. 2014. *Public Health Nutrition: Principles and Practice in Community and Global Health*. Burlington: Jones & Bartlett Learning. Print.

U.S. Department of Health and Human Services. 2016. Office of Global Affairs (OGA). Available at: www.globalhealth.gov. Washington, D.C.: U.S. Department of Health and Human Services.

UBC-MJ. 2016. Culture and Health. Available at: www.ubcmj.com/pdf/ubcmj_2_2_2011_19-20.pdf. Vancouver: UBC Medical Journal.

UNData. 2014. Healthy Life Expectancy (HALE) at Birth (Years). Available at: http://data.un.org/data.aspx?q=HALE&d=WHO&f=MEASURE_CODE%3aWHOSIS_000002. New York: UNData.

Wolff, J. 2013. *The Human Right to Health (Norton Global Ethics Series)*. New York: W.W. Norton & Company. Print.

World Economic Forum. 2012. Global Population Ageing: Peril or Promise?. Available at: www.weforum.org/reports/global-population-ageing-peril-or-promise. New York: World Economic Forum.

World Health Organization. 2016. Children: Reducing Mortality. Available at: www.who.int/mediacentre/factsheets/fs178/en/. New York: World Health Organization.

World Health Organization. 2016. Last Cases of Smallpox – 1979. Available at: www.who.int/csr/disease/smallpox/en. New York: World Health Organization.

Chapter 10

Global health
Communicable and non-communicable diseases

After study of the chapter, readers should be able to:

1 Describe various causes of communicable diseases.
2 Describe the important link between tuberculosis and human immunodeficiency virus (HIV).
3 List the five species of *Plasmodium* that cause malaria.
4 Describe schistosomiasis and Chagas disease.
5 Describe the symptoms of trypanosomiasis.
6 Identify the risk factors for cardiovascular disorders.
7 List the risk factors for cancer.
8 Differentiate between the most common types of diabetes.
9 Outline the four major mental health disorders throughout the world.
10 Describe fetal alcohol syndrome.

Overview

Many communicable and non-communicable diseases are increasing in prevalence throughout the world. The world has made great progress against some of the leading causes of communicable diseases. However, even though there has been substantial gains made against diseases such as measles, almost 115,000 children still die of measles every year. The number of new HIV infections globally is also falling. Worldwide life expectancy, at birth, is at its highest point ever. Unfortunately, these gains are not seen by the world's poorest people, regardless of whether they live in industrialized or developing countries. Emerging and re-emerging infectious diseases such as the Ebola virus, which has caused a major epidemic in Western Africa, continue to occur.

Resistance to certain medicines that treat bacterial, viral, and parasitic infections still occurs in large amounts. There is a great need to develop new medicines to replace those that are becoming less effective and to develop vaccines that can prevent many different infections. A growing proportion of the world's population is at risk for developing non-communicable diseases. With increased lifespans, many people also live longer with disabilities. Non-communicable diseases such as cardiovascular disease, cancer, and mental disorders are more prevalent than ever before.

Communicable diseases

Communicable diseases *(infectious diseases)* are directly transmitted from one person or animal to another, by contact with excretions or other body discharges. They are also indirectly transmitted by means of other substances or inanimate objects, such as contaminated drinking glasses, toys, or water, or by means of vectors. Examples of vectors include flies, mosquitos, ticks, and other insects. Communicable diseases may be caused by bacteria, chlamydia, fungi, parasites, rickettsiae, and viruses. Examples of communicable diseases include diphtheria, herpes simplex, influenza, and meningitis. Table 10.1 lists examples of how various communicable diseases are spread.

In young children, communicable diseases such as lower respiratory infections, malaria, and AIDS are still prevalent in terms of deaths.

Communicable diseases play a greater role in disability in low- and middle-income countries than they do in deaths. Today, communicable diseases cause approximately 40% of worldwide disability-adjusted life years (DALYs) in low- and middle-income countries, as well as approximately 31% of deaths in these countries. In 2013 alone, AIDS and tuberculosis *each* killed about 1.5 million people. Diarrheal diseases were responsible for the deaths of nearly 800,000 children under the age of five, and malaria killed another 550,000 people. Newly emerging infections, re-emerging infections, and antimicrobial resistance are present threats to global health.

In sub-Saharan Africa, communicable diseases cause nearly half of total DALYs. In South Asia, they cause approximately 22% of total DALYs. More poor people are affected by communicable diseases because of lack of knowledge about protection against unsafe water and other factors. Overcrowding among the poor increases the spread of tuberculosis, while

Table 10.1 Methods of spreading communicable disease

Diseases	Method
Entamoeba histolytica, *Escherichia coli*, Salmonella	Food-borne
Influenza, meningitis, tuberculosis	Inhalation
Anthrax	Non-traumatic contact
Hepatitis, HIV	Sexual or bloodborne
Rabies	Traumatic contact
Malaria, onchocerciasis	Vector-borne
Cholera, rotavirus	Water-borne

lack of protection against vectors increases cases of malaria. People of higher income also vaccinate their children in much higher numbers than those of lower income.

Fortunately, many communicable diseases can be easily prevented or treated, and childhood vaccinations are readily available (see Figure 10.1). Risk of diarrhea and various parasitic diseases can be reduced from the proper use of water and the presence of good sanitation. Treatments for malaria, many parasitic infections, and tuberculosis are effective, inexpensive, and safe – yet many poorer people in low- and middle-income countries do not have adequate access to them. Better use of antibiotics has the potential to reduce antimicrobial resistance. Table 10.2 lists how many communicable diseases may be controlled.

The leading causes of death from communicable diseases worldwide are lower respiratory conditions, AIDS, diarrheal diseases, tuberculosis, malaria, and measles, in order of prevalence. However, in low- and middle-income countries, diarrheal diseases are more prevalent than AIDS, and malaria is more prevalent than tuberculosis. The regions of the world with the highest prevalence of deaths from communicable diseases are summarized in Table 10.3.

Also in low- and middle-income countries, among children between the ages of five and 14, the three leading causes of death are diarrheal diseases, AIDS, and road injuries. In people from the ages of 15 to 49, the three leading causes of death are AIDS, road injuries, and tuberculosis.

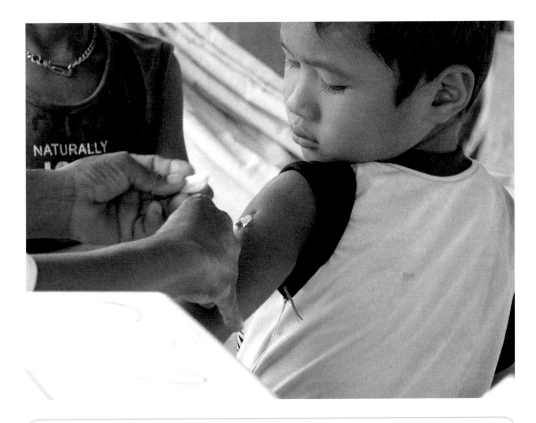

Figure 10.1 Immunization of a child.

Table 10.2 Methods of controlling communicable diseases

Diseases	Methods of control
Ebola virus, HIV, Guinea worm, sexually transmitted infections	Behavioral changes
Diarrheal disease, HIV and AIDS, respiratory disease, tuberculosis	Case management (treatment) and better care
Avian influenza, cholera, meningitis	Case surveillance, reporting, and containment
Diarrheal disease, maternal health, neonatal health, respiratory disease	Improved care seeking, disease recognition
Diarrheal diseases	Improved water, hygiene, and sanitation
Hookworm, lymphatic filariasis, onchocerciasis	Mass chemotherapy
Diphtheria, hepatitis B, influenza, measles, meningitis, pertussis, polio, smallpox, tetanus, yellow fever	Vaccinations
Dengue, malaria, onchocerciasis, West Nile virus, yellow fever	Vector control

Table 10.3 Prevalence of deaths from communicable diseases

Region	Percentage of total deaths in this region
Sub-Saharan Africa	49
South Asia	21
Middle East and North Africa	10
Latin America and the Caribbean	10
East Asia and Pacific	9
High-income countries	6
Europe and Central Asia	5

Source: www.bcm.edu/departments/molecular-virology-and-microbiology/emerging-infections-and-biodefense/introduction-to-infectious-diseases.

Focus on Zika virus

As of January 2016, the Zika virus had spread from Africa, Southeast Asia, the Pacific islands, and Brazil to the United States because of travelers who had been bitten by infected *Aedes* mosquitos. Up to November 2016, there were 37,100 confirmed cases in the United States and its territories. A unique case occurred in the state of Utah, in which a man contracted Zika from an unknown source – he had not traveled outside of the country, but did care for his father, an international traveler, who died from the disease. This indicates more mystery about the Zika virus, in that there may be other, unknown modes of transmission. The most common signs and symptoms are fever, rash, joint pain, and conjunctivitis (red eyes). This virus can be dangerous for pregnant women in any trimester, since it can be transmitted to the fetus and cause microcephaly. Complications of microcephaly include seizures, developmental delays, feeding problems, hearing loss, and vision problems. There are no vaccines or medications available to prevent or treat Zika infections. Up to November 2016, the CDC had monitored more than 3,600 pregnant women in the United States and its territories with the Zika virus. Every state in the country has now had a travel-associated case of Zika. The three states with the most cases are New York, Florida, and California.

Source: www.cdc.gov/zika/index.html.

Influenza

Influenza is a viral infection of the respiratory tract. The infection usually lasts for about one week. The influenza virus is easily transmitted between individuals via droplets and small particles that are produced when an infected individual coughs or sneezes. Influenza usually spreads rapidly, in seasonal epidemics. Most people infected with influenza recover within one to two weeks, and do not require medical treatment.

Seasonal influenza viruses circulate worldwide, affecting people of all age groups, with epidemics peaking in the winter in *temperate* regions, which are those that experience only moderate temperature changes between seasons. These viruses pose a serious public health problem since severe illness and death can occur. The most effective way to prevent infection is with an influenza vaccination. There are three types of seasonal influenza viruses. Type A influenza includes many subtypes such as H1N1 and H3N2. The Type A and B influenza viruses are much more common globally than Type C. Worldwide, about 5 to 10% of adults and 20 to 30% of children are affected every year. These annual "flu" epidemics result in three to five million cases of severe illness and between 250,000 and 500,000 deaths.

Focus on influenza

In young children, the elderly, and people with other serious medical conditions, influenza can lead to severe complications of underlying conditions, pneumonia, and even death.

HIV and AIDS

There are now more than 35 million people living with HIV throughout the world. People with the highest risk of acquiring HIV include females, uncircumcised males, and anyone who has another sexually transmitted disease. HIV and AIDS are covered in detail in Chapter 13.

Tuberculosis

Tuberculosis (TB) is caused by the bacterium known as *Mycobacterium tuberculosis*, which is spread through aerosol droplets. When an infected individual transmits these droplets into the air and another individual breathes them in, TB is transmitted. It affects the lungs in 80% of cases, but can also affect some other body organs. Exposure is more likely when individuals encounter infected people in close proximity such as prisons or poor conditions such as slums. Therefore, the homeless are more likely to be infected with TB. Active disease is more prevalent in individuals with an already-weakened immune system.

There are about 11 million people living with tuberculosis, while the number of new cases annually is about 9.6 million, and deaths number 1.5 million. Global areas with the highest prevalence for TB are Africa (28%), India (23%), Indonesia (10%), and China (10%).

An untreated individual who has active pulmonary TB may infect 10–15 others within a year. Without proper treatment about 70% of these individuals will die. Fortunately, people with TB in other organs usually do not spread the disease. The active form of TB is signified by a persistent cough lasting for more than three weeks, general weakness, decreased appetite, and profuse night sweats. However, not every person infected with TB becomes ill, and the disease remains latent in 90% of these individuals and cannot be spread.

Focus on tuberculosis

Approximately 30% of the world's population is infected with tuberculosis, yet active TB will only occur in about 10% of these people, primarily in those who are immunocompromised.

Source: www.who.int/mediacentre/factsheets/fs104/en/.

There is an important relationship between TB and HIV. In a person's lifetime, the risk of developing active TB when you are not infected with HIV is only 10%. However, if HIV-positive, the *annual* risk of developing active TB is much higher – 30%. HIV is associated with a higher proportion of non-pulmonary TB compared to TB that is not related to HIV.

The Bacillus Calmette-Guerin (BCG) vaccine is prescribed most commonly for immunization against tuberculosis. It is rarely administered in the United States as an immunizing agent, but is often given in other countries to infants and to caregivers who are at high risk for intimate and prolonged exposure to people with active tuberculosis. The World Health Organization (WHO) recommends a six-month drug regimen for TB, including isoniazid, rifampin, pyrazinamide, and ethambutol for the first two months, and then isoniazid and rifampin for the final four months. Patients should be supported to follow their drug regimens by health care workers and other individuals outside family members, in order to better assure compliance.

Malaria

Malaria is a severe infectious illness caused by one of five species of the protozoan genus *Plasmodium*. These include *Plasmodium falciparum*, *P. vivax*, *P. ovale*, *P. malariae*, and *P. knowlesi*. An Anopheles mosquito first bites a human who has malaria, then bites another human, thus transferring the disease. Malarial infection can also be spread by a blood transfusion from an infected patient, or through the use of a contaminated hypodermic needle. The endemic disease is mostly limited to tropical areas of South and Central America, Africa, and Asia. However, a number of new cases are introduced into the United States by refugees, military personnel, and travelers returning from malarial areas of the world. As of 2013, there were an estimated 207 million cases worldwide, and 627,000 people died – mostly children in Africa.

As of 2014, 97 countries had continuing transmission of malaria, with about 50% of the world's population living in areas at risk. There may have been as many as 200 million cases of malaria in 2014, with 80% in Africa, 12% in Southeast Asia, and 5% in the Eastern Mediterranean region. Most deaths occurred in Africa, and most of these were children under the age of five. Malaria is the tenth leading cause of death globally for all ages and both sexes, but for children under five years of age, it is the third leading cause of death.

For pregnant women, malaria is linked to low-birthweight children, spontaneous abortion, premature delivery, stillbirth, and severe anemia. Up to 15% of African mothers suffer severe anemia, leading to 10,000 malaria-related anemia deaths annually.

Diarrheal diseases

Diarrhea is the frequent passage of loose, watery stools, which may also contain mucus, pus, blood, or excessive amounts of fat. Diarrhea is usually a symptom of some underlying disorder. Conditions in which diarrhea is an important symptom include dysenteric disorders, malabsorption syndrome, irritable bowel syndrome, and inflammatory bowel disease. Diarrhea may also be transmitted by bacteria, viruses, and parasites. Transmission is often through contaminated water or food via the fecal–oral route. Microorganisms that cause diarrhea may be spread by flies, by lack of proper hand washing, or by using dirty cooking utensils.

Diarrheal diseases resulting from infections are most common in low- to middle income countries and usually affect poor children. Disease is linked to overcrowding, poor-quality housing, lack of sanitation and clean water, presence of domestic animals, lack of refrigerated food storage, poor general hygiene practices, and poor nutrition. Because of dehydration, diarrhea kills infants and young children in a short period of time.

However, death from diarrheal diseases has decreased greatly over the past 30 years, due to improved nutrition, better disease treatment, improved health care standards, and oral rehydration therapies. Diarrheal diseases still affect about 1.7 billion people annually, with low- and middle-income countries reporting children under three years of age acquiring three of these diseases every year. These diseases cause about 10% of all deaths in these children. Prevention of diarrheal diseases includes the following basic strategies:

- Exclusive breastfeeding for the first six months of life
- Improved complementary feeding introduced with breastfeeding after six months
- Immunization
- Clean water
- Appropriate sanitation
- Proper hand washing.

To reduce the severity of diarrheal diseases and possible deaths, oral rehydration therapy is recommended, along with zinc supplementation during acute diarrheal episodes, and antibiotics for bloody diarrhea.

Neglected tropical diseases

There are also 12 *neglected tropical diseases* that infect more than one billion people around the world every year. Extremely poor people are most affected. These diseases include:

- Ascariasis (roundworm) – The most common parasitic infection in the world, caused by a parasitic worm, *Ascaris lumbricoides*, which migrates through the lungs in its larval stage (see Figure 10.2). The eggs are passed in human feces, contaminating the soil and allowing transmission to the mouths of others via the hands, water, or food. After hatching in the small intestine, the larvae travel through the wall of the intestine and are carried by the lymphatics and blood to the lungs. The parasites can each be more than one foot in length in their adult stages. This condition affects more than one billion people worldwide.

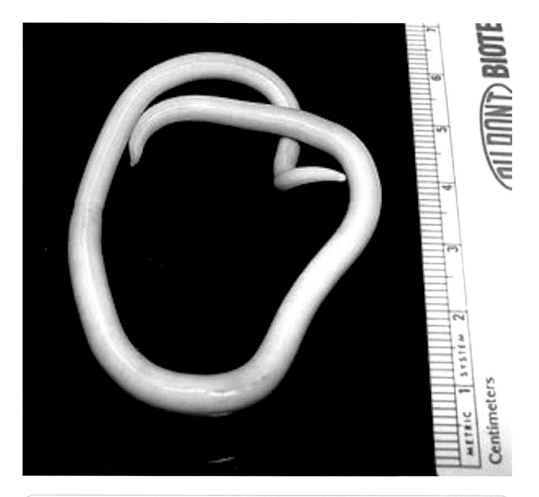

Figure 10.2 *Ascaris lumbricoides*, which causes ascariasis.

- **Hookworm** disease – A roundworm infestation that may involve either of two important intestinal parasites in humans: *Ancylostoma*, which causes ancylostomiasis, and *Necator*, which causes necatoriasis. They can cause abdominal pain, iron deficiency anemia, premature birth, low birthweight, and a variety of developmental abnormalities. Hookworm disease affects over 800 million people globally.
- Trichuriasis – Infestation with the roundworm *Tricuris trichiura*. The condition is usually asymptomatic, but heavy infestation may cause abdominal pain, nausea, bloody diarrhea, and anemia. The worms may live 15 to 20 years. This condition affects over 700 million people worldwide.
- Schistosomiasis (snail fever) – A parasitic infection caused by the genus *Schistosoma*. It is transmitted to humans by contact with water containing the infective stage of the parasite. Symptoms depend on the part of the body infected. *Schistosoma* may be found in the bladder, rectum, liver, lungs, spleen, intestines, and portal venous system. The disease causes abdominal pain, diarrhea, bloody stools, blood in the urine, liver damage, kidney failure, infertility, bladder cancer, poor growth, and learning difficulties. It affects more than 200 million people worldwide, and is the most deadly of all of these diseases.
- **Filariasis** – A disease caused by the presence of filariae or microfilariae in body tissues. Filarial worms are round, long, and threadlike, and are common in most tropical and subtropical regions. They tend to infest the lymph nodes, lymphatics, subcutaneous tissues, and skin after entering the body as microscopic larvae through the bite of a mosquito, blackfly, or midge. The infection is characterized by occlusion of the lymphatic vessels, with swelling of the arms, legs, or genitals; skin thickening; and pain. It affects more than 120 million people worldwide, and is also called elephantiasis (see Figure 10.3).

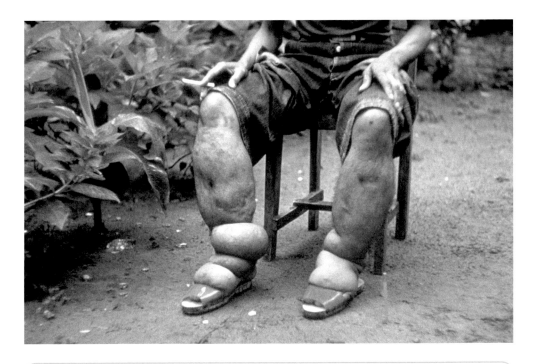

Figure 10.3 Elephantiasis (Filariasis).

- Trachoma – A chronic infectious disease of the eye caused by the bacterium *Chlamydia trachomatis*. It is characterized initially by inflammation, pain, photophobia, and lacrimation (see Figure 10.4). It affects more than 40 million people worldwide.
- Onchocerciasis – A form of filariasis common in Central and South America and Africa. It is characterized by subcutaneous nodules, pruritic rash, and eye lesions. Onchocerciasis is transmitted by the bites of black flies under the skin. It affects more than 26 million people worldwide, and is also known as *river blindness*.
- Leishmaniasis – Infection with any species of protozoan of the genus *Leishmania*. The diseases caused by these organisms may be cutaneous, mucocutaneous, or visceral. Leishmaniasis affects more than 12 million people worldwide.
- Chagas disease – A protozoal infection caused by *Trypanosoma cruzi*, transmitted to humans by certain insects that are found only in the Americas, and mainly in poorer areas of Latin America. It may occur in acute or chronic form, both of which can be asymptomatic or life-threatening. The most recognized sign of acute infection, which is common in children but rare in adults, is swelling of the eyelids on the side of the face nearest the bite. The acute form is also marked by a lesion at the site of the bite. Symptoms include fever, swollen lymph nodes, headache, enlargement of heart ventricles, heart failure, and enlarged esophagus or colon. Chagas disease affects more than seven million people worldwide. It is also referred to as *American trypanosomiasis* or *Brazilian trypanosomiasis*.
- **Leprosy** – A chronic communicable disease caused by *Mycobacterium leprae*, which may take either of two forms, depending on the degree of immunity of the host. Tuberculoid

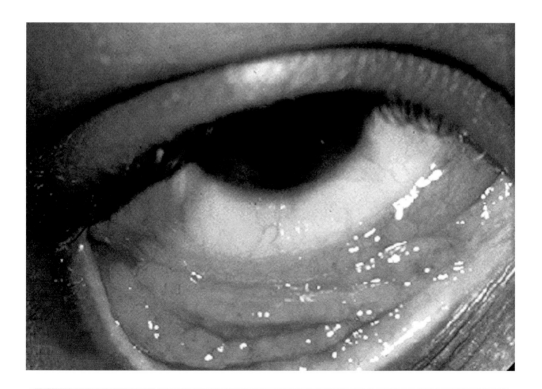

Figure 10.4 Trachoma.

leprosy, seen in those with high resistance, presents as thickening of the cutaneous nerves and non-painful, saucer-shaped skin lesions. Lepromatous leprosy, seen in those with little resistance, involves many body systems, with widespread plaques and nodules in the skin, inflammation of the iris (*iritis*), keratitis, destruction of nasal cartilage and bone, testicular atrophy, and peripheral edema. Blindness may result. Children are more susceptible than adults. It affects more than 230,000 people worldwide, and is also called *Hansen's disease* (see Figure 10.5).

- **Trypanosomiasis** – An infection by an organism of the *Trypanosoma* genus. *African trypanosomiasis* is transmitted to humans via the bite of the tsetse fly, and occurs only in Central and East Africa, where these flies are found. Symptoms of central nervous system involvement include lethargy, sleepiness, headache, convulsions, and coma. The disease is fatal unless treated, though it may be years before the patient reaches the neurologic phase. It affects more than 30,000 people worldwide, and is also called sleeping sickness.
- **Buruli ulcer** – An ulcer of the skin with widespread necrosis of subcutaneous fat, caused by a species of *Mycobacterium ulcerans*. It is manifested by a small, firm, painless, movable subcutaneous nodule that enlarges and ulcerates. It occurs principally in Central Africa, but has been seen in other tropical areas, and affects more than 5,000 people worldwide.

The majority of these diseases are transmitted by ingesting worm eggs, coming into contact with contaminated water, being bitten by various insects, and coming into contact with

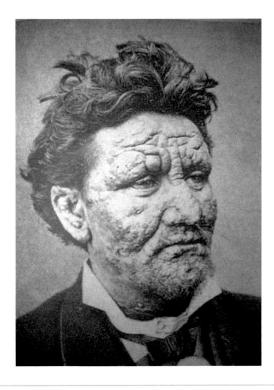

Figure 10.5 Leprosy.

bacterial discharges causing person-to-person transmission. These neglected tropical diseases may worsen the effects of other infectious diseases, or make individuals more susceptible to them. The financial cost of managing these diseases can also be very large. Several of these diseases have been combatted with good results, including onchocerciasis, trachoma, and lymphatic filariasis.

Viral hepatitis

Viral hepatitis is a viral inflammatory disease of the liver caused by one of the hepatitis viruses: A, B, C, D, E, or G. All have chronic forms except for hepatitis A. Speed of onset and probable course of the illness vary with the type and strain of the virus. The characteristics of the disease and its treatment are, however, the same. The various types of viral hepatitis are covered in detail in Chapter 13.

Non-communicable diseases

The most common non-communicable diseases are cardiovascular disease, cancer, diabetes mellitus, mental disorders, musculoskeletal disorders, and chronic respiratory disease. The prevalence of non-communicable diseases has been increasing over the last few decades, partially due to a reduction in communicable diseases and the aging of populations. About 58% of deaths in low- and middle-income countries are from non-communicable causes, followed by 31% due to communicable diseases and 11% from injuries. Non-communicable diseases are the leading causes of deaths in high-income countries for all age groups and both sexes.

In low- and middle-income countries, the leading causes of death are ischemic heart disease and stroke. In high-income countries, the leading causes of death are cardiovascular disease and cancer. Differences in causes of disability in countries of different economic levels are shown in Table 10.4.

Risk factors

Leading risk factors for non-communicable diseases are related to lifestyle and health behaviors. For example, use of alcohol or tobacco, physical activity, and diet are important risk factors for non-communicable diseases. The majority of these diseases are very expensive to treat. By quitting smoking, for example, the likelihood of developing lung cancer can be significantly reduced. This is much less expensive choice when compared to the costs of treatment for lung cancer.

Table 10.4 Causes of disability

High-income countries	Low- and middle-income countries
Non-communicable diseases – 85%	Non-communicable diseases – 49%
Communicable diseases – 5%	Communicable diseases – 40%
Injuries – 10%	Injuries – 11%

Source: www.nia.nih.gov/publication/why-population-aging-matters-global-perspective/trend-4-growing-burden-noncommunicable.

Adult non-communicable diseases are highly influenced by learned behaviors that occurred during adolescence. Throughout the world, adolescents regularly eat high-sugar, high-salt, and high-saturated-fat foods while avoiding regular exercise. More and more adolescents are becoming obese. It is estimated that less than one out of every four adolescents gets enough exercise, and that one in three is considered obese.

Cardiovascular disorders

Cardiovascular diseases (CVDs) include ischemic heart disease, hypertension, and stroke. Ischemic heart disease is a disturbance of heart function because of inadequate supply of oxygen to the heart muscle. Stroke is a sudden loss of function of the brain because of clotting or hemorrhaging. Ischemic heart disease caused the deaths of about 7.4 million people in 2014, and is the primary cause of death for all ages and both sexes. Globally, stroke was the second leading cause of death, and responsible for about six million fatalities. Combined, ischemic heart disease and stroke kill almost one in four people globally. Using data published by the *Journal of the American Medical Association*, Figure 10.6 illustrates the numbers of global deaths due to cardiovascular disease between 1990 and 2013. The countries with the top ten fastest rates of decline in CVD mortality during this period include Norway, Denmark, the United Kingdom, Portugal, Luxembourg, Israel, Bahrain, Qatar, South Korea, and Taiwan.

In low- and middle-income countries, stroke was the leading cause of death (10.5%), while ischemic heart disease was second (10%). Except for Eastern Asia and the Pacific, where stroke predominates, ischemic heart disease was the largest cause of death (except for sub-Saharan Africa, where communicable diseases cause more deaths). CVD occurs more commonly in Eastern Europe, especially in the former Soviet Union, than in Western Europe. While in high-income countries the majority of occurrences of CVD are in people over age 70, compared with low- and middle-income countries such as India, approximately half of all CVD-related deaths occur in people under 70. Worldwide, the three regions with the highest percentage of stroke-related deaths are Europe and Central Asia (20%), Eastern

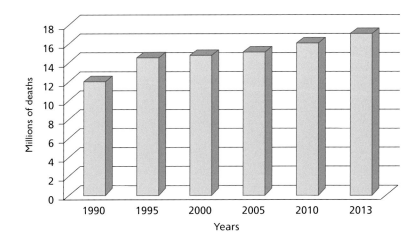

Figure 10.6 Global deaths due to cardiovascular disease, 1990–2013.

Source: O'Rourke et al., 2015.

Asia and the Pacific (19%), and the Middle East and North Africa (12%). Globally, stroke deaths average 11%.

In general, males have a higher risk of CVD than females, except for postmenopausal women, who have risks equivalent to those of men. Risks for stroke in both sexes are similar, and family history plays an important role. Both men and women have higher chances of developing heart disease if they had a male relative with the condition before 55 years of age, or if they had a female relative with it before 65 years of age. African and Asian ancestry also increases the risks. Aging plays an important part, since after the age of 55, your risk of stroke doubles every ten years. Modifiable risk factors for CVD include taking steps to lower hypertension, quitting smoking, lowering dietary cholesterol, increasing physical activity, and consuming alcohol only in moderation. Social-related risks for CVD include depression, poverty, stress, and social isolation.

The United Nations has suggested five priority areas that countries should concentrate on immediately: cardiovascular disease, tobacco use, obesity/poor diet/lack of exercise, harmful alcohol intake, and excessive dietary salt. To manage CVD, they recommend drug therapy to control hypertension, counseling for patients who have had a heart attack or stroke, and also counseling for people who have a risk that is greater than 30% for any type of cardiovascular event in the next ten years. They also recommend acetylsalicylic acid for acute myocardial infarction.

Most risks associated with CVD are linked to hypertension, high cholesterol, high body mass index, low amounts of fruits and vegetables in the diet, lack of exercise, and use of tobacco and alcohol. Foods high in salt, saturated fat, and trans fats must be decreased. Sugar intake must be limited, and refined grains must be replaced by whole grains.

You should remember

In the United States, approximately 70 million adults have hypertension, which is one out of every three adults. Hypertension is also known as the *silent killer* because it has no early significant symptoms.

Source: www.cdc.gov/bloodpressure/index.htm.

Cancer

Cancer is characterized by uncontrolled cellular growth and the ability to spread to other parts of the body. It affects people throughout the world, but is linked to more deaths in high-income countries (27%), Eastern Asia and the Pacific (22%), and Latin America as well as the Caribbean (16%) than elsewhere. Each type of cancer has different characteristics, affects different groups of people, has its own risk factors, and also has different methods of prevention and treatment. Cancer is the second leading cause of death worldwide, after cardiovascular disease.

As of 2012, 14.1 million new cancer cases occurred, and 8.2 million people had cancer-related deaths. Within the previous five years, 32.6 million people older than age 15 had been diagnosed with cancer. The most common types of cancer and prevalence of cancer deaths are listed in Table 10.5.

Recently, breast and cervical cancers have been increasing in prevalence. Breast cancer is the leading cause of cancer death for women globally and the leading cause of cancer death in low- and middle-income countries. It has increased by 20% in incidence since 2008. Cervical cancer is most prevalent in low-and middle-income countries.

Table 10.5 Most commonly diagnosed types of cancer and prevalence of cancer deaths

Most common types of cancer	Percentage
Lung	13
Breast	11.9
Colorectal	1.4

Most prevalent cancer deaths	Percentage
Lung	19.4
Liver	9.1
Stomach	8.8

You should remember

In the United States, the human papillomavirus vaccine is available to prevent cervical cancer. It is recommended for females between the ages of 9 and 26. The best time for them to receive this vaccine is between ages 10 and 11, prior to the onset of sexual activity.

Sources: www.wcrf.org/int/cancer-facts-figures/worldwide-data; http://journals.lww.com/ajnonline/abstract/2014/03000/ new_global_survey_shows_an_increasing_cancer.14.aspx.

Cancers have been documented to increase, in general, when populations in low- and middle-income countries begin to adopt lifestyles that are similar to those in high-income countries. For example, as women decide to have fewer children, have their first pregnancies later in life, and then breastfeed for shorter periods or not at all, breast cancer rates rise. Though more cases of cancer exist in wealthier countries, more people survive the disease because of earlier detection and more easily available treatments. While death rates from cancer are decreasing in the United States, they are increasing in many poorer countries.

There is a higher incidence for cancer in people older than age 65 since they have had more exposure to environmental risk factors and have accumulated changes in their genes. In general, tobacco is one of the most significant risk factors for cancer. Its use is directly linked to lung cancer, but it is also a risk for breast, prostate, and other types of cancer. Excessive alcohol use is linked to upper digestive tract, breast, liver, and colorectal cancers. Table 10.6 lists risk factors for various types of cancer.

Controlling tobacco use is the first priority in the prevention of cancer. Other factors include elimination or minimization of infectious agents by utilizing vaccines, antibiotics, and other drugs. Prevention of cancer is the most cost-effective way to reduce financial expenditures concerning the disease. Treatments for cancer are usually expensive and are seldom short-term. Unfortunately, in low- and middle-income countries, cancer is often detected much later in its development than in wealthier countries where better health care

Table 10.6 Risk factors for cancer

Risk factor	Related cancers
Tobacco use	Lung, breast, prostate
Alcohol use	Upper digestive tract, breast, liver, colorectal (men), pancreatic
Radiation exposure	Breast
Obesity	Breast (postmenopausal women), pancreatic, endometrial, kidney, esophageal
Human papillomavirus	Cervical
Diet high in red meat, low in fiber	Colorectal
Hepatitis B and C viruses	Liver
Schistosomiasis	Urinary bladder
Asbestos exposure	Lung
Air pollution	Lung
Sun exposure	Skin
Genetic predisposition	Breast
Lack of physical activity	Colon, breast, endometrial
Helicobacter pylori bacterium	Stomach

opportunities are available. In certain countries, up to 80% of cancers may be incurable by the time they are discovered.

Improved early detection is critical in reducing cancer throughout the world. Low-cost screening tests that are more effective are continually being developed, and are highly needed. Other methods of cancer screening such as **mammography, Pap smear**, and colorectal tests are becoming more available worldwide. There is, however, a worldwide shortage of radiation treatment centers and personnel. Adequate surgical facilities for cancer patients are also in great demand.

Focus on immunotherapy

Today, immunotherapy is being developed to fight cancer. It can stimulate the immune system to be more efficient and attack cancer cells. For example, in the United States, the poliovirus is being injected into brain tumors, causing the patient's immune system to attack the poliovirus and thereby destroy the tumors.

Diabetes mellitus

Diabetes mellitus is an illness caused by the inability to properly metabolize blood sugar. It is a major health problem for millions of people globally. In North America and the Caribbean, diabetes mellitus occurs most often, in 11.4% of the population. In the United States, more than 29 million people have diabetes. The difference is that diabetes in North America usually is not fatal. The regions with the highest percentages of death from diabetes are listed in Table 10.7.

The two most common types of diabetes are explained as follows:

- *Type 1 diabetes* – believed to be an autoimmune disorder, associated with family history, that destroys the cells in the pancreas that produce insulin, making the body unable to use *glucose* for energy; the patient must inject insulin, follow a strict diet, have daily exercise, and test blood sugar throughout each day. It usually begins before the age of 30, hence its former name, juvenile diabetes; it is also known as insulin-dependent diabetes mellitus. Other causes include environmental factors, increased maternal age at birth, and exposure to certain viruses
- *Type 2 diabetes* – the most common type, it is present in 90 to 95% of diabetics; the body either does not produce enough insulin, or cannot efficiently use the insulin that is made. It usually begins after the age of 30, hence its former name, *adult-onset diabetes*; it is associated with family history, diet, physical inactivity, obesity, insulin resistance, ethnicity, and increasing age.

It is estimated that diabetes affects 382 million people worldwide, with 8.3% of adults being diabetics. Overall, diabetes is the ninth leading global cause of death. Significantly, it is the eighth leading cause of death in high-income countries, but only the tenth leading cause of death in low- and middle-income countries. Even so, nearly 80% of all deaths from diabetes occur in low- and middle-income countries.

Complications of diabetes include blindness, kidney disease, nerve damage, coronary heart disease, and stroke. Approximately two-thirds of all diabetics have some related disability. Unfortunately, diabetes is rapidly becoming more prevalent everywhere in the world in relation to increasing obesity. While it is predicted to increase by 55% globally by the year 2035, some countries will see much larger percentages. For example, diabetes is expected to increase in prevalence by 109% in Africa, by 96% in the Middle East and North Africa, and by 71% in Southeast Asia by the year 2035.

Table 10.7 Deaths from diabetes

Area	Percentage of death
Latin America and the Caribbean	5
Eastern Asia and the Pacific	3
Middle East and North Africa	3

Sources: www.who.int/bulletin/Barcelo0103.pdf; http://care.diabetesjournals.org/content/39/3/472; www.ncbi.nlm.nih.gov/pubmed/24300017.

> ### You should remember
>
> The most common complications of diabetes are blindness, destruction of the kidneys, stroke, coronary heart disease, and amputation of the lower extremities. Approximately two-thirds of patients with diabetes are disabled.

Mental disorders

Mental disorders include a variety of different conditions. Anxiety disorders, bipolar disorder, schizophrenia, and depression are some examples. Another related area of health care concerns *behavioral disorders*, which include alcohol or drug use disorders and pervasive development disorders. There are four mental disorders that make up the majority of mental health cases globally, which include:

- Depression (or *unipolar depressive disorder*) – involves feelings of sadness, despair, loneliness, low self-esteem, and self-reproach
- Anxiety disorders – involving varying degrees of anxiety; one example is panic disorder, which is signified by attacks of acute, intense anxiety
- Schizophrenia – a mental illness signified by hallucinations, delusions, and changes affecting personality and outlook
- Bipolar disorder – a serious mood disorder signified by manic and depressive states.

The above four disorders make up a little more than 5% of health care cases in low- and middle-income countries. Of this percentage, up to 3% of cases are related to depression. Women suffer more disability in relation to these disorders (7.2%) than men (4.6%).

The ages between 15 and 49 are most affected by mental disorders. Major depressive disorder is this group's fourth leading cause of disability in low- and middle-income countries, while anxiety disorder ranks tenth. In high-income countries, major depressive disorders rank second in causes of disability. The subset of people most affected by mental disorders contains people between the ages of 15 and 19. Therefore, it is easy to see that mental disorders often begin in young age, continue for years, are often never cured, and result in widespread disability. They even result in death, such as when a disorder such as depression causes a person to commit suicide.

Southern Asia has the highest documented prevalence of depression in the world. Statistics for schizophrenia, bipolar disorder, and panic disorders vary widely between different areas of the world. It is projected that depression will see the greatest increase throughout the world up to the year 2030, reaching 8% in high-income countries and over 6% in low- and middle-income countries. Genetic and non-genetic risk factors influence mental disorders. These factors include childhood poverty, abuse, and violence.

Though adequate studies of mental health costs have been done only in high-income countries, in the United States, they are estimated to reach 2.5% of the gross national product (GNP). In Europe, these costs may reach 4% of the GNP. Indirect costs are substantial, and often related to mental illness-influenced accidents, injuries, and illnesses. Depressed workers in the United Kingdom were proven to have lost up to 45 days of work per year as a result of mental illnesses.

In many countries, there is a lack of understanding about mental disorders. There may also be inadequate funding for treatment, lack of health care professionals, and stigma among people concerning mental illness. Generally, there is lower-quality mental health care available in low- and middle-income countries than in high-income countries. WHO therefore recommends that countries establish mental health policies and appoint a part of their governments to focus on mental health. They advocate budgets for treatment programs, the training of health care workers, and the integration of mental health into primary health care.

Ideally, childhood mental disorders should be prevented as much as possible, depression should be medically treated along with adequate counseling, and psychotic disorders such as schizophrenia should be addressed appropriately. Steps that can be taken include reducing abuse of children and women, controlling bullying within schools, improving parenting skills, and treating people who have experienced wars, other conflicts, or significant emergencies.

Low- to middle-income countries should focus on community-based mental health care over the traditional psychiatric hospitalization methods. This will require changes in political and governmental organizations and how they view mental health. It is a crucial area of focus, since mental disorders contribute to 90% of the suicides that occur globally every year, which number between 800,000 and one million. Due to inadequate resources and attention, 80% of people with mental illnesses in low- and middle-income countries do not receive care.

You should remember

Throughout the world, mental health disorders contribute to more disability than any other category of health care, except for cardiovascular disorders.

Mental disorders in the United States include anxiety disorders, attention deficit hyperactivity disorder, bipolar and related disorders, depressive disorders, obsessive-compulsive disorders, schizophrenia, and post-traumatic stress disorder. The prevalence of these disorders is listed in Table 10.8.

Table 10.8 Prevalence of mental disorders in adults

Type of mental disorder	Prevalence (%)
Anxiety disorders	18
Post-traumatic stress disorder	8
Depressive disorders	6.6
Bipolar and related disorders	2.6
Attention deficit hyperactivity disorder	2.5
Obsessive-compulsive disorder	1.2
Schizophrenia	1

Source: www.cdc.gov/mmwr/preview/mmwrhtml/su6003a1.htm.

Effects of smoking

Tobacco use of any kind is the third leading attributable risk factor for death, in all economic situations, globally. Of the five million annual deaths from tobacco use, about 2.5 million are located in low-income countries. Approximately one in every five males over age 30 and one in every 20 females over age 30 die of a tobacco-related death, and this is a global fact. Cigarette smoking is increasing in many low- and middle-income countries, but decreasing in many high-income countries. Preference for smoking differs between males and females aged 13 to 15 in different countries (see Table 10.9). Smoking causes serious health problems and death – between 50 and 70% of smokers will die of related diseases. People between the ages of 35 and 69 constitute 50% of all tobacco-related deaths. Most male smokers live in Eastern Asia and the Pacific, while most female smokers live in Europe and Central Asia.

Focus on smoking

As many as 1.5 billion people smoke throughout the world, with Russia having the most smokers. The higher a person's socioeconomic status and level of education, the less likely he or she is to smoke.

Sources: www.washingtonpost.com/news/worldviews/wp/2012/10/19/who-smokes-most-a-surprising-map-of-smoking-rates-by-country/?utm_term=.c6edc44a20dd; www.tobaccofreemaine.org/channels/special_populations/.

The most common tobacco-related deaths are from respiratory disease, cardiovascular disease, and cancer. Tobacco is also linked to increased risks of becoming a diabetic. Though studies about the financial costs of smoking and related treatments focus on high-income countries, the general range is between 0.1 and 1.1% of gross domestic product (GDP). Another consideration is that although smoking is decreasing in the United States and many other countries, it is increasing in women in all countries and in men in low-income countries.

You should remember

Between 1950 and 2000, 70 million people died globally of smoking-related causes. Based on current trends and a larger population, another 150 million people will die between 2000 and 2025.

Source: www.ncbi.nlm.nih.gov/books/nbk11741/.

Table 10.9 Percentages of adolescents (aged 13 to 15) who smoke

Country	Male smokers	Female smokers
United States	21	15
Argentina	49	55
Russian Federation	30	24
Indonesia	41	6
Turkey	14	7

WHO created the *Mpower* program to control tobacco use, which consists of:

- The monitoring of tobacco use and ways to prevent it
- The protection of individuals from tobacco smoke
- The offer to help quit tobacco use
- Warnings about the dangers of tobacco use
- The enforcement of bans on the advertising, promotion, and sponsorship of tobacco products
- The raising of tobacco taxes.

Effects of alcohol use

The effects of alcohol use include significant disability related to normal living, including disruption of normal social, business, and personal relationships. It is more significant in high-income countries, where more than 1.5% of the population is negatively affected. In low- and middle-income countries, the percentage is lower, at 0.6%. Globally, alcohol use disorders are the ninth leading attributable risk factor for death, and the fifth leading risk factor for disability. Eastern Europe appears to be the worst in terms of alcohol use disorders in relation to disability, which is unusually high at 3.3%.

High-risk drinking is linked to hypertension, liver and pancreatic damage, heart disease, and hormonal abnormalities. Being intoxicated with alcohol is a proven risk factor for accidents, injuries, social problems, and death. Risky sexual behaviors and violence between individuals are both common effects of the overuse of alcohol. Dependence on alcohol may result in many negative physical and psychological consequences. In women who drink during pregnancy, fetal alcohol syndrome causes low birthweight and a variety of developmental disabilities.

The highest-risk drinkers are males in Europe and Central Asia between the ages of 45 and 59, with 21% of them being affected by high-risk drinking. More people participate in high-risk drinking below the age of 60. In high-income countries, studies have shown that risk factors for high-risk drinking include lower socioeconomic status and education. Table 10.10 lists percentages for alcohol consumption in adolescents in various areas of the world.

The costs of alcohol-related injury and death must incorporate not only those of the drinker, but also those of the people who are affected by his or her behavior. Alcoholics become less productive members of society, and may harm others because of driving while intoxicated, risky behaviors, and violence. Studies of the effects of alcohol use upon GDP show the highest costs have occurred in Italy (5.6%), New Zealand (4%), South Korea (3.3%), and the United States (2.7%).

Table 10.10 Alcohol consumption in adolescents (aged 15 to 19)

Area	Current drinkers (%)	Former drinkers (%)	Non-drinkers (%)
Europe	69.5	14.5	15.9
Southeast Asia	8.2	5.9	85.8
All continents	34.1	12	53.9

Source: http://apps.who.int/iris/bitstream/10665/66795/1/WHO_MSD_MSB_01.1.pdf.

Jim is a police officer who recently had to chase a suspect believed to have committed a burglary. After the chase and the man's arrest, Jim was sitting in his police car completing the incident report, and experienced shortness of breath, dizziness, discomfort in his chest, and tachycardia. Jim's father and brother had histories of cardiovascular disease, but Jim has never been diagnosed with the same condition, though he is overdue for his annual physical examination.

1 What conditions may Jim's symptoms signify?
2 Should Jim seek emergency medical care?
3 If Jim does have cardiovascular disease, what outcomes may be likely to occur?

Chapter highlights

This section answers the Objectives found at the beginning of the chapter.

1 **Describe various causes of communicable diseases.**

- Communicable diseases may be caused by bacteria, chlamydia, fungi, parasites, rickettsiae, and viruses.

2 **Describe the important link between tuberculosis and human immunodeficiency virus (HIV).**

- In a person's lifetime, the risk of developing active TB when you are not infected with HIV is only 10%. However, if HIV-positive, the *annual* risk of developing active TB is much higher – 30%. HIV is associated with a higher proportion of non-pulmonary TB compared to TB that is not related to HIV.

3 **List the five species of *Plasmodium* that cause malaria.**

- Plasmodium falciparum
- Plasmodium vivax
- Plasmodium ovale
- Plasmodium malariae
- Plasmodium knowlesi.

4 **Describe schistosomiasis and Chagas disease.**

- Schistosomiasis, or snail fever, is a parasitic infection caused by the genus *Schistosoma*. It is transmitted to humans by contact with water containing the infective stage of the parasite. *Schistosoma* may be found in the bladder, rectum, liver, lungs, spleen, intestines, and portal venous system. The disease causes abdominal pain, diarrhea, bloody stools, blood in the urine, liver damage, kidney failure, infertility, bladder cancer, poor growth, and learning difficulties. It affects more than 200 million people worldwide.
- Chagas disease is a protozoal infection caused by *Trypanosoma cruzi*, transmitted to humans by certain insects found mainly in poorer areas of Latin America. It may be acute or chronic, and can be asymptomatic or life-threatening. Acute infection,

more common in children, includes swelling of the eyelids on the side of the face nearest the bite, and a lesion at the site of the bite. Symptoms include fever, swollen lymph nodes, headache, enlargement of heart ventricles, heart failure, and enlarged esophagus or colon. Chagas disease affects more than seven million people worldwide. It is also referred to as *American trypanosomiasis* or *Brazilian trypanosomiasis*.

5 **Describe the symptoms of trypanosomiasis.**

- Symptoms of central nervous system involvement in trypanosomiasis include lethargy, sleepiness, headache, convulsions, and coma. The disease is fatal unless treated, though it may be years before the patient reaches the neurologic phase. It affects more than 30,000 people worldwide, and is also called sleeping sickness.

6 **Identify the risk factors for cardiovascular disorders.**

- The risk factors for cardiovascular disorders include family history, with a male relative being diagnosed before age 55, or a female relative being diagnosed before age 65. African or Asian ancestry also increases the risks, as well as being 55 years of age or older. Risk factors that can be modified include hypertension, smoking, high dietary cholesterol, insufficient physical activity, and overconsumption of alcohol. Depression, poverty, stress, and social isolation are also risk factors. Diets that are high in processed foods, refined grains, sugar, saturated fat, trans fat, and sodium, as well as low in fruits and vegetables, are definitively linked to increased risks for these disorders.

7 **List the risk factors for cancer.**

- Risk factors for cancer include tobacco use, alcohol use, radiation exposure, obesity, the human papillomavirus, diets high in red meat and low in fiber, the hepatitis B and C viruses, schistosomiasis, asbestos exposure, air pollution, sun exposure, genetic predisposition, lack of physical activity, and the Helicobacter pylori bacterium.

8 **Differentiate between the most common types of diabetes.**

- *Type 1 diabetes* – believed to be an autoimmune disorder, associated with family history, that destroys the cells in the pancreas that produce insulin, making the body unable to use glucose for energy; the patient must inject insulin, follow a strict diet, have daily exercise, and test blood sugar throughout each day. It usually begins before the age of 30, hence its former name, *juvenile diabetes*. Other causes include environmental factors, increased maternal age at birth, exposure to certain viruses, and increased weight and height development
- *Type 2 diabetes* – the most common type, it is present in 90 to 95% of diabetics; the body either does not produce enough insulin, or cannot efficiently use the insulin that is made. It usually begins after the age of 30, hence its former name, *adult-onset diabetes*. It is associated with family history, diet, physical inactivity, obesity, insulin resistance, ethnicity, and increasing age.

9 **Outline the four major mental health disorders throughout the world.**

- Depression (or *unipolar depressive disorder*) – sadness, despair, loneliness, low self-esteem, and self-reproach
- Anxiety disorders – degrees of anxiety; include panic disorder, which is signified by attacks of acute, intense anxiety

- Schizophrenia – hallucinations, delusions, and changes affecting personality and outlook
- Bipolar disorder – signified by manic and depressive states.

10 **Describe fetal alcohol syndrome.**

- Fetal alcohol syndrome is a set of congenital psychologic, behavioral, and physical abnormalities that tend to appear in infants whose mothers consumed alcohol during pregnancy.
- It causes low birthweight and a variety of developmental disabilities.

Summary

Communicable (infectious) diseases are those that may be transmitted via body discharges, other substances, inanimate objects, or by vectors such as insects. They may be caused by bacteria, chlamydia, fungi, parasites, rickettsiae, and viruses. Communicable diseases cause more disability than deaths in low- and middle-income countries. Many of these diseases can be prevented or treated by using vaccinations. The most fatal communicable diseases include lower respiratory conditions, AIDS, diarrheal diseases, tuberculosis, malaria, and measles. Other communicable diseases include influenza and neglected tropical diseases such as ascariasis, hookworm disease, trichuriasis, schistosomiasis, and filariasis.

Common non-communicable diseases include cardiovascular disease, cancer, diabetes mellitus, mental disorders, musculoskeletal disorders, and chronic respiratory disease. These types of disease are among the leading causes of death worldwide. Risk factors are highly related to lifestyle and health behaviors, such as the use of alcohol or tobacco, poor diet, and lack of sufficient exercise. Globally, the prevalence of non-communicable diseases is increasing. Therefore, there is still much work to be done to eradicate the causes of disease that are linked to lifestyle.

Review questions

1 Why may some communicable diseases be transmitted by vectors?
2 How many communicable diseases can be easily prevented or treated?
3 What is the cause of tuberculosis and how is it transmitted?
4 In what conditions is diarrhea an important symptom?
5 What are most common signs and symptoms of hookworm?
6 What are the risk factors associated with cardiovascular diseases?
7 Why is there a higher incidence of cancer in elderly people?
8 What is juvenile diabetes, and what are its complications?
9 What steps can be taken to reduce childhood mental disorders?
10 What are the most common tobacco-related deaths?

Bibliography

Adams, L.V., and Butterly, J.R. 2015. *Diseases of Poverty: Epidemiology, Infectious Diseases, and Modern Plagues.* Hanover: Dartmouth. Print.

Adeyi, O., and Smith, O. 2007. *Public Policy and the Challenge of Chronic Noncommunicable Diseases (Directions in Development).* Washington, D.C.: World Bank Publications. Print.

Baylor College of Medicine. 2016. Molecular Virology and Microbiology: Emerging Biodefense: Introduction to Infectious Diseases. Available at: www.bcm.edu/departments/molecular-virology-and-microbiology/emerging-infections-and-biodefense/introduction-to-infectious-diseases. Houston: Baylor College of Medicine.

Carter, D. 2014. New Global Survey Reveals Increasing Cancer. Available at: http://journals.lww.com/ajnonline/abstract/2014/03000/new_global_survey_shows_an_increasing_cancer.14.aspx. New York: Wolters Kluwer Health, Inc.

CDC. 2016. Diseases and Conditions – Popular Health Topics. Available at: www.cdc.gov/diseasesconditions/index.html. Atlanta: U.S. Centers for Disease Control and Prevention.

CDC. 2016. High Blood Pressure. Available at: www.cdc.gov/bloodpressure/index.htm. Atlanta: U.S. Centers for Disease Control and Prevention.

CDC. 2016. Mental Illness Surveillance. Available at: www.cdc.gov/mmwr/preview/mmwrhtml/su6003a1.htm. Atlanta: U.S. Centers for Disease Control and Prevention.

CDC. 2016. Non-communicable Diseases. Available at: www.cdc.gov/globalhealth/healthprotection/ncd/index.html. Atlanta: U.S. Centers for Disease Control and Prevention.

CDC. 2016. Zika Virus. Available at: www.cdc.gov/zika/index.html. Atlanta: U.S. Centers for Disease Control and Prevention.

Daniels, M.E., and Donilon, T.E. 2014. *The Emerging Global Health Crisis: Noncommunicable Diseases in Low- and Middle-Income Countries.* Washington, D.C.: Council on Foreign Relations Press. Print.

DeGraft-Adkins, A., and Agyemang, C. 2016. *Chronic Non-communicable Diseases in Low and Middle-Income Countries.* Wallingford, UK: CABI. Print.

Dowling, J., and Yap, C. 2014. *Communicable Diseases in Developing Countries: Stopping the Global Epidemics of HIV/AIDS, Tuberculosis, Malaria and Diarrhea.* New York: Palgrave Macmillan. Print.

Fisher, M. 2012. Who Smokes Most: A Surprising Map of Smoking Rates By Country. Available at: www.washingtonpost.com/news/worldviews/wp/2012/10/19/who-smokes-most-a-surprising-map-of-smoking-rates-by-country/?utm_term=.c6edc44a20dd. Washington, D.C.: The Washington Post.

Galambos, L., Sturchio, J.L. 2013. *Noncommunicable Diseases in the Developing World: Addressing Gaps in Global Policy and Research.* Baltimore: Johns Hopkins University Press. Print.

Hawker, J., Begg, N., Blair, I., et al. 2012. *Communicable Disease Control and Health Protection Handbook, 3rd Edition.* Hoboken: Wiley-Blackwell. Print.

Heymann, D.L. 2014. *Communicable Diseases Manual, 20th Edition.* Washington, D.C.: American Public Health Association. Print.

Just-Health.net. 2016. List of Non-communicable Diseases. Available at: www.just-health.net/non-communicable-diseases-list.html. New York: Just-Health.net.

Lewis, M.J., and MacPherson, K.L. 2012. *Health Transitions and the Double Diseases Burden in Asia and the Pacific: Histories of Responses to Non-Communicable Diseases.* London: Routledge. Print.

McQueen, D.V. 2013. *Global Handbook on Noncommunicable Diseases and Health Promotion.* New York: Springer. Print.

Merson, M.H., and Black, R.E. 2011. *Global Health: Diseases, Programs, Systems, and Policies, 3rd Edition.* Burlington: Jones & Bartlett Learning. Print.

Nanditha, A., Ma, R.C.W., Ramachandran, A., Snehalatha, C., Chan, J.C.N., Chia, K.S., Shaw, J.E. and Zimmet, P.Z. 2016. Diabetes in Asia and the Pacific: Implications for the

Global Epidemic. Available at: http://care.diabetesjournals.org/content/39/3/472. Crystal City: American Diabetes Association.

National Institute on Aging. 2016. Why Population Aging Matters: A Global Perspective. Available at: www.nia.nih.gov/publication/why-population-aging-matters-global-perspective/trend-4-growing-burden-noncommunicable. Washington, D.C.: U.S. Department of Health and Human Services.

NCBI. 2016. Tobacco Addiction. Available at: www.ncbi.nlm.nih.gov/books/nbk11741/. Bethesda: National Center for Biotechnology Information.

NCBI/PubMed.gov. 2014. Diabetes in the Middle-East and North Africa: An Update. Available at: www.ncbi.nlm.nih.gov/pubmed/24300017. Bethesda: National Center for Biotechnology Information.

New York State Department of Health. 2016. Communicable Disease Fact Sheets. Available at: www.health.ny.gov/diseases/communicable. Albany: New York State Department of Health.

O'Connell, J.K., et al. 2004. *The Health Care of Homeless Persons: A Manual of Communicable Diseases & Common Problems in Shelters & on the Streets*. Boston: The Boston Health Care for the Homeless Program. Print.

Partnership for a Tobacco-Free Maine. 2016. Special Populations: Tobacco's Targets. Available at: www.tobaccofreemaine.org/channels/special_populations/. Augusta: Maine Dept. of Health and Human Services.

Phaswana-Mafuya, N., and Tassiopoulos, D. 2011. *Non-Communicable Diseases (NCDs) in Developing Countries (Public Health in the 21st Century)*. New York: Nova Science Publishers, Inc. Print.

Piot, P., and Garey, L. 2015. *AIDS between Science and Politics*. New York: Columbia University Press. Print.

Project Hope. 2016. Noncomunicable Diseases. Available at: www.projecthope.org/what-we-do/noncommunicable-diseases. Millwood: Project Hope.

U.S. Department of Health and Human Services. 2016. Office of Global Affairs (OGA) – Communicable Diseases. Available at: www.globalhealth.gov/global-health-topics/communicable-diseases. Washington, D.C.: U.S. Department of Health and Human Services.

U.S. Department of Health and Human Services. 2016. Office of Global Affairs (OGA) – Non-Communicable Diseases. Available at: www.globalhealth.gov/global-healthtopics/non-communicable-diseases. Washington, D.C.: U.S. Department of Health and Human Services.

Webber, R. 2012. *Communicable Diseases: A Global Perspective, 4th Edition*. Wallingford, UK: CABI. Print.

World Cancer Research Fund International. 2012. Worldwide Data. Available at: www.wcrf.org/int/cancer-facts-figures/worldwide-data. London: World Cancer Research Fund International.

World Health Organization. 2012. *Prevention and Control of Noncommunicable Diseases: Guidelines for Primary Health Care in Low Resource Settings*. New York: World Health Organization. Print.

World Health Organization. 2016. Alcohol and Young People. Available at: http://apps.who.int/iris/bitstream/10665/66795/1/WHO_MSD_MSB_01.1.pdf. New York: World Health Organization.

World Health Organization. 2016. Diabetes in Latin America and the Caribbean. Available at: www.who.int/bulletin/Barcelo0103.pdf. New York: World Health Organization.

World Health Organization. 2016. Infectious Diseases. Available at: http://who.int/topics/infectious_diseases/en. New York: World Health Organization.

World Health Organization. 2016. Influenza. Available at: www.who.int/topics/influenza/en. New York: World Health Organization.

World Health Organization. 2016. Non-communicable Disease Fact Sheets. Available at: www.who.int/mediacentre/factsheets/fs355/en. New York: World Health Organization.

World Health Organization. 2016. Tuberculosis. Available at: www.who.int/mediacentre/factsheets/fs104/en/. New York: World Health Organization.

Emergencies

After study of the chapter, readers should be able to:

1. List the five levels of the emergency severity index and the time requirements of each level.
2. Give examples of man-made disasters.
3. Give examples of natural disasters.
4. List four items that should be included in a disaster preparedness plan.
5. Identify the people who are most vulnerable when a natural disaster occurs.
6. Explain when cardiopulmonary resuscitation should be performed.
7. Identify injuries and conditions that may require first aid.
8. List various types of fracture.
9. Discuss external and internal bleeding.
10. Compare hyperthermia with hypothermia.

Overview

Medical emergencies may involve acute illnesses or injuries of all types. Emergencies caused by natural disasters and terrorism are seemingly always in the news. Regardless of the type of medical emergency, it is important for health care professionals to remain as calm as possible and to think clearly. They must be trained and ready for any medical emergency. Immediate assistance can be given with more proficiency when the provider remains focused. Remember that efficient, prompt treatment can prevent serious disabilities and death.

Emergency and urgent care

Emergency care provides immediate services for patients with sudden and serious illnesses or injuries. However, it is sometimes used for uninsured or underinsured individuals who are not actually experiencing an emergency situation. An actual *medical emergency* is defined by the prudent layperson standard. This is defined in the *Social Security Act*, as follows:

> A condition with acute symptoms of sufficient severity, including severe pain, such that a *prudent layperson*, who possesses average knowledge of health and medicine, could reasonably expect the absence of immediate medical attention to result in:
>
> I   placing the health of the individual, or unborn child, in serious jeopardy,
> II serious impairment of bodily functions, or:
> III serious dysfunction of any bodily organ or part.

Trauma and other types of *emergent care* are classified by triage levels, using the emergency severity index *(ESI)*. Though there are other systems used for triage in the United States, ESI is the most widely used. There are five levels of ESI, classifying patients into groups based on the immediacy of their need for treatment. These are listed in Table 11.1.

As of the latest available (2011) CDC statistics, 2.2% of patients visiting an emergency department required no triage. According to the *Emergency Medical Treatment & Labor Act of 1986*, all patients presenting for treatment at an emergency department must be screened, evaluated, given the necessary stabilizing treatment, and admitted to the hospital when necessary – regardless of their ability to pay for services. According to the CDC, about 44 out of every 100 Americans visit an emergency department, with about 12 of these patients requiring hospitalization.

Urgent care focuses on illnesses, injuries, or other conditions that are serious enough for a reasonable person to seek care right away. It is a type of *ambulatory care*, in which the patient can walk into a medical facility for treatment, or may need assistance entering the facility. Urgent care usually involves physicians, nurse practitioners, or physician assistants providing care to walk-in patients, meaning that no previous appointment was made due to the immediacy of their conditions. Urgent care may be provided by *urgent care centers* or traditional physician practices.

Table 11.1 The five levels of the Emergency Severity Index (ESI)

Level	Time frame	Percentage of emergency patients
Immediate	Less than 1 minute	1.2
Emergent	1–14 minutes	10.7
Urgent	15–60 minutes	42.3
Semiurgent	61–120 minutes	35.5
Nonurgent	121 minutes–24 hours	8.0

Source: www.esitriage.org.

Note: These are the latest available statistics, from 2011.

> **Focus on urgent care**
>
> The first urgent care centers opened in the 1970s, and there are now more than 17,000 in the United States alone. Their advantages include shorter wait times than in emergency departments, lower co-payments, flexible hours, and the same quality of licensed health professionals.
>
> *Source:* www.medicaldoctormd.com/urgent-care/
> urgent-care-centers-on-the-rise/.

Triage

Triage is the process of determining which patients require treatment more urgently than others. It is best exemplified in an emergency situation such as a natural disaster, in which there may be many wounded people. It is important to follow these steps to perform triage in this type of situation:

- Wash your hands
- Put on examination gloves and any other applicable personal protective equipment
- Assess each wounded person quickly, based on the types of injuries and need for care
- Classify the wounded as *emergent*, *urgent*, *non-urgent*, or *deceased* – this helps to give the fastest treatment, based on need
- Label patients using *disaster tags* and pens as follows:

  - Emergent patients are labeled as number one, and must be sent for treatment immediately – these include those who are hemorrhaging, in shock, or otherwise need immediate care
  - Urgent patients are labeled as number two, and are sent for basic first aid, requiring care within a few hours – these include lacerations that can be dressed to stop bleeding, but sutured at a later time
  - Non-urgent patients are labeled as number three, and are sent to volunteer helpers providing empathy and refreshments while they wait – they are not in a critical situation, and include people who may only be emotionally upset and not physically injured
  - Deceased patients are labeled as number four, and are moved to a separate area where they will be safe from being disturbed – they will then be identified so that proper action can occur.

Natural and man-made disasters

A disaster is any occurrence causing damage, loss of life, deterioration of health and health services, and ecological destruction that is serious enough to require a significant response from people outside the affected area. Disasters may be natural or man-made, and, regardless of their cause, result in human suffering and the need for other people to assist. Examples of man-made disasters include injuries resulting from the use of chemical weapons by terrorists, or when industrial accidents cause environmental toxins to enter the air, water, and soil.

The use of bioterror is one of the greatest threats of today, in which germs or other biological substances are deliberately released to harm the population. In 2001, several cases of anthrax occurred due to terrorists deliberately putting infectious anthrax into letters sent through the mail, resulting in five deaths. Substances considered "high-risk" that are used in bioterrorism include tularemia, anthrax, smallpox, botulinum toxin, bubonic plague, and viral hemorrhagic fevers such as Ebola.

You should remember

The events of September 11, 2001 resulted in the deaths of more than 3,000 Americans in New York. It resulted in billions of dollars in costs for health care, the military (which invaded Afghanistan), and rebuilding.
Sources: www.digitalhistory.uh.edu/disp_textbook.cfm?smtid=2&psid=3379; www.crainsnewyork.com/article/20150910/health_care/150919993/two-federal-programs-covering-medical-care-for-9-11-first-responders-of-the-sept-11-attacks-expire-next-year-and-with-uncertainty-over-their-future-survivors-could-be-left-with-hefty-bills; www.nationalpriorities.org/campaigns/how-military-spending-has-changed/; www.iags.org/costof911.html.

Focus on health effects of 9/11

Thousands of tons of toxic debris resulted from the collapse of the Twin Towers in New York City, exposing many rescuers, recovery workers, and residents to carcinogens and other toxins. It is estimated that 18,000 people have developed illnesses as a result of the toxic dust caused by this man-made disaster.
Sources: www.medicalnewstoday.com/articles/234030.php; www.bbc.com/news/world-us-canada-14738140.

Because of civil wars and other man-made disaster situations, the term *complex humanitarian emergency (CHE)* has been created. This is defined as a complex, multi-party, intra-state conflict that results in a humanitarian disaster that could risk or threaten regional and international security. These emergencies, like natural disasters, have the potential to cause the deaths of many people, or to displace people and cause many to become political refugees, such as the thousands of refugees fleeing the war in Syria and entering Europe. Examples of man-made and natural disasters are listed in Table 11.2.

Natural disasters occur all over the world, but may be easier to predict in areas that are more prone to phenomena such as earthquakes, hurricanes, typhoons, flooding, or volcanic eruptions. Because of the repeated occurrences of earthquakes throughout the West Coast of the United States, trained disaster preparedness teams are maintained and ready to act quickly when needed.

Disaster preparedness helps people to prepare for natural disasters, reducing their impact upon health. When creating a *disaster preparedness plan*, it is important to include the following:

- An identification of the area's vulnerabilities
- Scenarios of what might occur and how likely these situations are

Table 11.2 Examples of man-made and natural disasters

Man-made disasters	Natural disasters
1990 to 2004 – Liberia – civil war caused 500,000 people to be internally displaced and created more than 125,000 refugees	1989 – San Francisco, California – a powerful earthquake injured hundreds of people, killed 9, and seriously damaged bridges, roads, and buildings
1996 to 2006 – Nepal – conflict between the government and rebels caused up to 200,000 internally displaced people	2005 – New Orleans, Louisiana – Hurricane Katrina killed more than 1,200 people because of its intensity and the flooding that followed
2001 – New York City – Islamic terrorists attacked by using commercial jet airliners, killing more than 3,000; they also targeted Washington, D.C. and other areas	2010 – Pakistan flooding, leaving millions of people homeless and killing more than 1,600; Mexico landslide following rain that buried hundreds of houses and killed 11 people
2010 – Gulf of Mexico oil spill, poisoning the water and killing 11 people	2011 – Japan – earthquake and **tsunami** that caused a nuclear power plant explosion, and the release of radioactivity into the atmosphere; United States – Hurricane Irene caused billions of dollars in damage and killed 56 people; the Philippines – Tropical Storm Washi caused flooding and killed 1,268 people
2011 – Syria – civil war, still ongoing, has caused 6.5 million internally displaced people and more than 2.8 million refugees	2012 – Pakistan – an avalanche hit a military base and killed 140 people; Russia – flooding resulted in the deaths of 172 people; United States – Hurricane Sandy caused billions of dollars in damages and killed more than 100 people
2011 – Libya – still ongoing conflict between various government forces has led to more than 80,000 internally displaced people	2013 – United States – flash flooding damaged many homes and the infrastructure in Colorado, killing at least 6 people; the Philippines – an earthquake injured 300 people and killed 144; the Philippines – Typhoon Haiyan destroyed many islands, with 4,011 people dead and 1,602 missing
2015 – Paris, France – terrorists from the group known as "ISIS" used suicide bombers and gunmen to attack citizens, killing 129 and injuring more than 350	2014 – Solomon Islands – flooding due to Tropical Cyclone Ita affected more than 50,000 people and killed at least 22; India and Pakistan – flooding killed more than 557 people; China – earthquakes damaged or destroyed more than 42,000 houses and killed at least 617 people

Source: www.disasterium.com.

- An explanation of the roles different people will have if a disaster occurs
- A training program for first responders and disaster management teams.

A good strategy for long-term disaster preparedness is to improve the construction of hospitals, water systems, and other supportive factors so that they are better able to withstand the effects of a disaster. It is also important to determine the best, most cost-effective methods by which assistance can be brought in once a disaster occurs. It is advisable, in areas of the world that are more prone to natural disasters, to build temporary buildings that are strongly constructed, which can be left in place to serve as hospitals should another disaster occur. Disaster-prone communities should create lists of most-needed items, based on previous natural disasters.

Most natural disasters cause extreme devastation along with injuries and deaths. They often impact the environment, resulting in long-term effects that harm people slowly due to toxins, unsanitary conditions, and infectious microorganisms. Fortunately, with improved disaster preparedness techniques, fewer people are dying as a result of natural disasters in more developed countries, even though there are more disasters occurring than ever before. Low- and middle-income countries are more severely affected by natural disasters than higher-income countries. More than 90% of natural disaster-related deaths occur in low- and middle-income countries. This is probably linked to the fact that houses and other structures are often of lower-quality construction in these countries, and are therefore unable to withstand many disaster conditions.

Perhaps the best overall suggestion regarding disaster preparedness is for various disaster relief teams to work together and coordinate their efforts. The collective knowledge of these individuals, when shared, improves future relief efforts for everyone. In this way, standards that focus on the most important disaster relief priorities can be established and followed, ensuring a better overall outcome.

> ## You should remember
>
> In the years 2000–2009, the countries most affected by natural disasters included China, the United States, Indonesia, the Philippines, and India. These countries account for about 34% of total disaster occurrences worldwide.
>
> *Source:* www.worldatlas.com/articles/the-countries-with-the-most-natural-disasters-worldwide.html.

Health care during natural disasters

Health care differs between types of natural disasters due to the resulting injuries and conditions that are caused. An earthquake, for example, kills many people very quickly, but can also result in permanent orthopedic, mental, and cardiovascular diseases. The effects of an earthquake are related to how much infrastructure damage is caused, and how many people lose their homes as a result. Another example is when a volcano erupts, resulting in ash, mud, and potential flooding due to effects upon natural structures such as water reservoirs. People are displaced from their homes, water supplies become unsafe, and many people experience mental health problems due to the shock of a volcanic eruption.

Tsunamis usually kill many more people than they injure, due to drownings, trauma, and heavy objects being blown about. Survivors experience gastrointestinal infections, respiratory infections, and skin diseases. Many natural disasters result in widespread famine and, sometimes, various epidemics. People who are very young, very old, or chronically ill are most vulnerable when a natural disaster occurs.

Immediately after a natural disaster, it is critical that the health of the affected people is assessed, in order for the relief effort to be successful. Those who are injured must receive care, based on the levels of triage. Urgent psychological problems must be addressed. Disease surveillance must be organized, which will continue throughout the time it takes to restore the people of the affected area to normal conditions, or at least as close as possible to normal conditions. Safe water and food are essential, as is adequate shelter. Many countries require the help of other countries when they experience a natural disaster. Assistance must be coordinated so that it matches the conditions of the disaster survivors. External assistance must include all needed participants, be cooperative, work to complement the skills and talents of the participants, be based on evidence, be transparent so that all activities can be assessed, and involve the affected communities.

Focus on natural disasters

According to the World Health Organization, natural disasters kill about 90,000 people globally every year, and affect nearly 160 million people. They have an immediate impact on human life and often cause destruction of physical, biological, and social environments. This results in longer-term impacts on health, well-being, and survival.

Source: www.who.int/environmental_health_emergencies/natural_events/en/.

The general impact of natural disasters upon health systems affects the health workforce, health information management, medical products and technologies, financing, leadership, governance, and health service delivery. Hospital-acquired infections, injuries, and even violence may cause illness, disability, and death. Health care providers may also be displaced because of insecurity or destruction of housing. They may have psychological trauma because of displacement and the illnesses, deaths, or disabilities of their colleagues. Health information management systems may collapse, or be unable to effectively monitor the status of health performance. Medical supplies and equipment may be stolen. Insecurity and poor access may cause a breakdown of supply chain management systems, resulting in a lack of adequate drug supplies.

With natural disasters, health resources may be diverted to other areas, resulting in reduced spending on needed health services. The cost of delivering health care is often increased. Strategic policy frameworks for health care often break down, and there may be a lack of supervision, monitoring, and evaluation of services. Health regulations and accountability are often unenforceable. As a result of breakdowns in health financing, leadership, and governance, there may be reduced access to health care, reduced immunizations, lower quality of the health care services that remain available, and even unsafe health care services.

Natural or man-made disasters usually impact the health of affected areas. Usually, addressing the social factors of health soon after a disaster will reduce the impact of the disaster. Risk and vulnerability reduction measures should be implemented before, during, and after disasters. Morbidity and mortality during a disaster can be reduced by developing and implementing emergency preparedness and response programs. Finally, the use of a health system-based approach to emergency response can ensure better recovery of affected areas after a disaster occurs.

Emergency procedures

Emergency procedures focus on giving needed care to a person prior to fully trained medical personnel arriving on the scene. There are various steps involved in giving emergency care, all of which are designed to protect rescuers and victims. The steps for emergency procedures include:

- Assessing the environment – You must first determine whether you can safely approach the victim, and whether calling for additional help is a better choice than approaching a hazardous area alone. For a conscious victim, tell him or her you are calling for help and will return quickly. When you call 9-1-1 for Emergency Medical Services (EMS), listen carefully to the trained operator and answer all questions as accurately as possible. He or she will ask the victim's name and location, the type of emergency, and if any treatment has been given. The proper emergency services personnel will then be dispatched. Often, the operator will advise you on what steps to take until they arrive. You must remain safe so that you can continue to assist the victim, so continual monitoring of the safety of the emergency scene must occur.
- Obtaining consent – If the victim is conscious, identify yourself, and state that you intend to give assistance. Obtain permission before administering any care. If the victim is a child, determine whether a parent or a guardian is nearby in order to obtain consent for care. You should not administer care to any conscious victim who does not want you to help – each person has the right to refuse care. If care is obviously needed but the victim refuses help, call EMS immediately. When a victim is unconscious, you may administer care without consent.
- Determining what has occurred – Ask the victim what happened if he or she is conscious, or look for clues as to what might have happened if the victim is unconscious. Clues include medication bottles, substances that might have been used as poisons, and medical alert bracelets or other identifiers. Also search for any other potential victims. Whatever you find, inform EMS.
- Following standard precautions – This must occur if you come into contact with body fluids. It is suggested that you carry disposable gloves and barrier devices used for mouth-to-mouth resuscitation. Another suggestion is to carry a first aid kit.
- Getting help from others – If other people are in the area, ask them for help. The most experienced person should be the one who assists the victim. Less experienced people can be sent to call for help. Other people can help direct traffic away from the scene, keep onlookers out of the way, search for additional clues, and assist other victims.
- Keeping the victim in one place – A victim with a neck or back injury can be permanently paralyzed if moved, so this should never occur. The only time you should move a victim is if he or she is in imminent danger and must be moved somewhere safer. The victim's spine must be kept in straight alignment if moving is necessary. If you must turn a victim who has a neck or back injury, turn the body as one unit to prevent injury to the spinal cord. If you must move an injured arm or leg, support it well while moving to prevent further damage to blood vessels or nerves.

- Remaining calm – You must remain calm at all times, and reassure the victim if he or she is conscious, as well as any other people assisting. It is vital to think and act clearly and carefully. It is usually best to call EMS immediately since they are specially trained in handling emergencies.

The Good Samaritan Act protects caregivers and rescuers when they try to help someone in an emergency, as long as no gross negligence occurs and nothing is willfully done to harm the victim. Each state has its own variation of Good Samaritan laws. They generally prevent the caregiver or rescuer from liability while trying to give aid. Civil or other damages cannot be brought against the caregiver or rescuer unless gross negligence occurs. Unfortunately, many emergency situations involve extreme injuries that cannot be treated, and often victims die before sufficient medical help can arrive. A caregiver or rescuer can only try his or her best to help a victim, and must understand that efforts to help are better than not attempting to assist a victim, regardless of the outcome.

Cardiopulmonary resuscitation

Cardiopulmonary resuscitation (CPR) is administered when a person is not breathing and does not have a pulse. When sufficient oxygen is not received, the heart stops and the brain will not receive necessary blood flow. Therefore, the victim is at high risk of brain damage and death. Immediate CPR is required to save the victim's life, which involves *chest compressions*, with or without *rescue breathing*, based on whether the rescuer is trained in CPR. Chest compressions circulate oxygenated blood throughout the body until the heartbeat and independent breathing are restored. Rescue breathing provides oxygen to the lungs. Situations in which CPR is commonly performed include choking victims who are unconscious, drownings, heart attacks, and electric shocks.

The American Red Cross and American Heart Association recommend that all citizens receive training in CPR, since this training increases the likelihood that many more lives could be saved. An injured person has a better chance of survival when care is administered immediately prior to the arrival of medical help, rather than not receiving any care until medical help arrives.

The steps of CPR are as follows:

- Check to see if the victim is breathing – if not, begin CPR chest compressions immediately.
- Only check for a pulse if you have been trained to perform CPR.
- A person who is untrained in CPR should only provide chest compressions and not attempt to perform rescue breathing.
- Chest compressions are performed by placing the heel of one hand on the victim's breastbone, and the other hand directly on top of the first hand; position your body above the victim's chest and administer 30 rapid, hard chest compressions (at a rate of 100 or more per minute); the chest should be depressed at least two inches with each compression, and you must allow the chest to rise between each compression.
- If the rescuer is trained in CPR, after 30 chest compressions, the victim's head should be tilted back and the chin should be lifted (see Figure 11.1); two rescue breaths should then be administered, ideally using a barrier device; if such a device is not available, the rescuer should cover the victim's mouth tightly with his or her mouth, pinch the victim's nose closed, and give two breaths lasting one second each – the chest should rise with each breath.
- Cycles of 30 chest compressions (and two breaths, if these are being performed) should continue until the victim starts breathing or EMS personnel arrive.

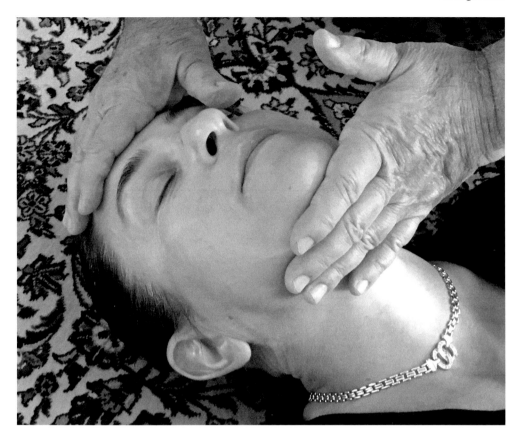

Figure 11.1 The head-tilt chin-lift technique used in CPR.

Automatic external defibrillator

For any victim who is not breathing normally and is unresponsive, an **automatic external defibrillator** (AED) should be used as well as CPR. An AED is a portable machine that monitors heart rhythm and can introduce an electric shock to the heart to restore normal rhythm (see Figure 11.2). Generally, AEDs are found in schools, airports, shopping malls, golf courses, and other large gathering places. They are simple to use without training, and have lights, text messages, and voice prompts that tell the rescuer each step needed to use them.

The steps required to use an AED are as follows:

- Determine if the victim is responsive by shaking him or her, and shouting "Are you okay?"
- If he or she is not breathing, begin CPR immediately. This should occur while the AED is being brought to the location of the victim. If possible, ask another person to help you and provide instructions as needed, or have the person call 9-1-1 and obtain the AED.
- Turn on the AED and follow the step-by-step instructions. The other person or yourself should continue CPR while the AED is being operated.
- The victim's shirt should be removed and the chest prepared for the placement of the AED's electrodes. The skin must be dried if it is wet, and any transdermal medication patches should be removed and the areas cleaned. If the victim has excessive chest hair,

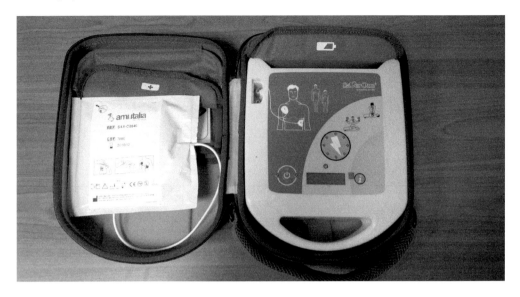

Figure 11.2 Automatic external defibrillator.

scissors or a razor should be used, if available, to quickly trim it – these are often included in the AED's equipment. Metal necklaces or underwire bras must be removed since they may conduct electricity and burn the patient.

- Verify that the victim does not have an implanted pacemaker or similar device – their outlines are visible under the chest or abdominal skin; also check for medical alert bracelets and body piercings.
- Remove the AED electrode pad paper backings and place the pads as instructed. You may need to move the pads at least one inch away from implanted devices or piercings so that electrical current can flow between the pads.
- You may need to connect the wires from the pads to the AED.
- As the AED analyzes heart rhythm, follow instructions and do not touch the victim at all, including avoiding CPR at this time. The AED will indicate if no electric shock is necessary and instruct you to resume CPR.
- If a shock is necessary, make sure no one is touching the victim or anything that the victim is lying on, besides the floor or ground. Some AEDs will deliver the shock automatically; for others, you must press a button do deliver the shock. The AED will analyze the victim's heart rhythm again, and no one should touch the patient during this time.
- Continue to follow all instructions given by the AED until EMS arrives.

It is advised that all health care professionals receive training in the proper use of an AED. This is provided through the American Heart Association and the American Red Cross.

First aid

First aid involves providing emergency care following an accident or sudden illness. Its goal is to minimize the effects of injury or illness until a physician can treat the patient. According to the American Red Cross, all people should take a first aid and safety course so that they know what to do in emergencies, how to give first aid, and how to prevent harm to others. The *golden rule* in first aid is to do no further harm. Caregivers should not attempt anything that they do not have the skills to perform. Instead, they should seek help immediately, increasing the chances that the victim's life will be saved.

Seizures

Seizures involve uncontrolled muscle movements, abnormal sensations, and a partial or complete loss of consciousness. They are caused by abnormal discharges of electrical signals within the brain. A seizure signifies an underlying disorder and is not actually a disease itself. Underlying disorders that may result in seizures include epilepsy, drug toxicity, head injuries, and other conditions. Seizure symptoms often develop quickly, and last from one second to several minutes. Common symptoms that may occur before a seizure include:

- Bitter or metallic taste in the mouth
- Visual abnormalities, including the appearance of flashing lights, blurred vision, or the perception of hallucinations.

During a seizure, symptoms may include:

- Muscle twitching or tightening
- Sudden loss of muscular control.

After a seizure, the victim often has no memory of a specific period of time.

To treat a seizure victim, the most important factor is protecting him or her from injury by moving any potentially harmful objects away. If the victim has fallen and has lost consciousness, attempts should be made to protect the neck and spine until EMS arrives. It is important to check the victim's responsiveness, airway, and breathing. It is important to make sure that the airway stays clear and open, while not causing injury or becoming injured, since seizure victims often vomit. You should help the victim roll onto one side, which helps vomit, blood, and other secretions drain from the mouth. Also, secretions can be removed from the victim's mouth by using suction devices if they are available.

Shock

Shock is a condition in which there is a sudden reduction in blood flow, depriving the vital organs of oxygen. It is related to heart disease, hemorrhage, infections, and other conditions. As shock develops, the body increases the strength of heart contractions and the heart rate as it constricts blood vessels. Progression of shock makes it harder for the body to adjust, and tissue and organ damage eventually becomes severe. At this point, shock is irreversible and the victim will die.

Signs and symptoms of shock include:

- Low blood pressure
- Weak, rapid pulse
- Restless or signs of fever
- Nausea
- Thirst
- Skin that is cool and clammy, which may become pale, with lips and earlobes appearing bluish in color.

Since shock may develop from so many different factors, health care professionals must be prepared to treat it in any type of emergency. The steps for treating shock include:

- Calling EMS immediately
- Monitoring the victim's airway and keeping it open
- Controlling bleeding
- Administering oxygen if directed by a physician
- Immobilizing the victim to protect against spinal injuries
- Splinting fractured bones
- Preventing loss of body heat by covering the victim with a blanket, especially if he or she is cold
- Elevating the victim's legs and feet to help blood circulate to the vital organs.

Diabetic emergencies

People who have diabetes mellitus either do not produce insulin, do not produce enough insulin, or cannot effectively use insulin in their body cells. Some diabetics need medication to regulate blood sugar levels and must monitor dietary intake. Inadequate regulation of blood sugar results in either *hypoglycemia* or *hyperglycemia*. Hypoglycemia (low blood sugar) and hyperglycemia (high blood sugar) can both cause coma and death if they are untreated. These diabetic emergencies can result from the following factors:

- Incorrect amount of synthetic insulin being administered
- Excessive or inadequate food or exercise
- Physical stress caused by a cold, flu, or other illness
- Mental or emotional stress.

Hypoglycemia occurs more quickly than hyperglycemia, and is signified by hunger, sweating, confusion, pale skin, and lack of coordination. A person with hypoglycemia should be given a sweetened drink or snack to help raise blood sugar levels. This usually occurs within five to 15 minutes. If the person becomes unconscious, immediate treatment is required. This means an injection of glucagon or emergency treatment in a hospital.

Hyperglycemia develops slowly, and is signified by a "fruity" smell to the breath, extreme thirst or hunger, extreme urination, vomiting, flushed skin, confusion, and rapid pulse. To treat a hyperglycemic person, find out if he or she is a diabetic and is due for an insulin injection. If insulin is needed, help the person in administering the insulin. Ask another person to call EMS and remain with the diabetic person as you monitor vital signs.

Fainting

Fainting is a brief loss of consciousness that is not caused by trauma. It usually occurs suddenly, and is often linked to low blood sugar or excessive standing for a long period of time. Sometimes, fainting occurs when a person has been sitting and then stands too quickly, which may produce a reduction in blood pressure. This is referred to as *orthostatic hypotension*. It is important to note that loss of consciousness may also occur after a head injury such as a *concussion*.

Signs that occur prior to a person fainting include dizziness, nausea, weakness, and blurred vision. If you are present when a person faints, help him or her to lie down on the floor, face up, with the legs elevated above the heart. Do not put a pillow under the victim's head. Loosen the clothing so that breathing is not restricted. If the victim vomits before regaining consciousness, turn the head to one side to help keep his or her airway clear. You may roll the victim onto one side if there is no neck or spinal cord injury. A fainting victim should regain consciousness in less than five minutes. If not, or if there are additional signs and symptoms, call EMS immediately.

Fractures

Fractures are broken bones, which usually occur due to an external injury to the body. However, fractures can also occur in thin or brittle bones because of diseases such as osteoporosis, which is a weakening of bones due to loss of calcium, often seen in older people. Fractures may be closed, in which the skin is not broken, or open, in which the bone breaks through the skin. Fractures are signified by pain, swelling, and loss of function. Fractures can also cause the affected area of the body to appear deformed. Prevention of fractures includes weight-bearing exercises, avoiding overextension of joints, proper diet with enough calcium and vitamin C, stretching, good posture, proper body position when working, proper lifting techniques, and the use of protective equipment such as seat belts or helmets.

When treating a fracture, it is important to immobilize the broken bone using a splint (see Figure 11.3). You should not move the victim until the affected limb is immobilized unless safety is compromised. Do not give the victim anything by mouth. If no medical supplies are available, splints may be made out of thick twigs from trees, or from wooden boards. Strips of cloth can be used to attach splints. Check for circulation to make sure the splint is not too tight, so that no further tissue damage occurs. You should never test a fractured area for function, nor attempt to realign a bone, since there is the possibility of causing further tissue damage, hemorrhaging, nerve damage, or a blood clot. Open fractures should be covered with a dressing before being immobilized, which helps to prevent additional contamination. The wound should not be washed, and you should not remove anything from the wound. Various types of fracture are explained in Table 11.3.

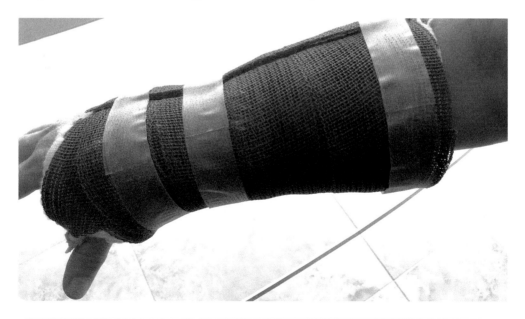

Figure 11.3 Immobilizing a broken bone with a cast.

Table 11.3 Types of fractures

Type	Explanation
Simple (closed)	A break in a bone's continuity, with no breaking through of the skin or overlying soft tissue
Compound (open)	A break in a bone's continuity in which the bone extends through adjacent or overlying soft tissue or the skin; it is a surgical emergency; another example is when a bullet wound causes a bone fracture
Incomplete (greenstick)	The bone is bent, and the complete cross-section of the bone is not involved; most common in children
Comminuted	The bone has been splintered or crushed into three or more pieces
Spiral (torsion)	Caused by a twisting motion, in which a bone is twisted apart; the fracture line resembles a spiral
Transverse	The broken piece of bone is at a right angle to the bone's axis
Oblique	The break has a curved or sloped pattern, known as an oblique direction
Buckled (impacted)	One bone fragment is firmly driven into the other, commonly seen in arm fractures in children
Pathologic	Caused by a disease that weakens the bones, such as osteoporosis, osteomalacia, or neoplasia
Stress	A hairline crack in a bone
Longitudinal	A fracture extending along the length of a bone

Sprains

Sprains are torn ligament fibers. They cause a joint to become loose, as well as pain and swelling. A sprained joint will still function unless there has been a complete tear. To treat a sprain, remove any constricting clothing or jewelry. Apply cold compresses as quickly as possible, repeating every 3–4 hours, for 15–20 minutes each time. Never place ice directly on the skin. If the injury occurred in a limb, elevate it. If pain is severe, contact a physician. A physician should also be contacted if there is loss of function, impairment of circulation below the injured area, or if the area is misshapen. The injured area should be rested for at least 24 hours, and should not be used if pain occurs with movement. If the injury does not improve, contact a physician.

Strains

Strains occur when muscle fibers are suddenly torn during exertion. They are also known as *pulled muscles*. When a strain occurs, the victim will feel a sudden tearing sensation. This will be followed by pain and swelling. The same treatment measures should be used for a strain as for a sprain.

Wounds

A *wound* is damage to the body's soft tissues because of violence or trauma. When giving first aid for wounds, the area should be cleaned and protected from further damage. Wounds include tears or open areas anywhere on the body. You should not attempt to clear large wounds or remove any embedded objects. However, you may remove any obvious loose debris. A *sucking wound* involves bubbling from the neck or chest, and difficulty breathing. This type of wound needs to be sealed as quickly as possible. If possible, apply an airtight dressing over the site, such as plastic wrap or a plastic bag, tin foil, or other non-porous material. If this is not available, use a regular gauze pad or clean cloth coated with petroleum jelly. Leave one edge of the airtight dressing untapped or unsealed. Do not move the patient unless necessary, and do not give anything by mouth.

An *amputation* is when part of the body has been severed. You should save the severed part since there is a possibility it can be reattached. Give the victim appropriate first aid. If the missing body part is not visible, try to locate it. If found, rinse the body part, wrap it in a moistened cloth, and place it inside a plastic bag or other container. If available, place the container inside another containing ice and water. Do not place ice directly on the severed body part. Write the patient's name and time of the accident on the container, and make sure the amputated body part remains with the victim during transport to the hospital.

Burns

Burns may be caused by fire, heat, chemicals, electrical current, or radiation. A burn's severity is determined by its size, depth, and location on the body. The three types of burns are described as follows:

- First-degree (superficial) burns – only the top layer of skin (epidermis) is involved; the skin is red and dry (see Figure 11.4a)
- Second-degree (partial-thickness) burns – the burned area continues and extends beyond the epidermis to the dermis; the skin is reddened, wet, painful, swollen, and blistered (Figure 11.4b)
- Third-degree (full-thickness) burns – the burned area continues into deeper tissues beyond the dermis; all skin layers are destroyed, as well as fat, muscles, bones, and nerve tissues; the skin will appear red, brown, black, or charred (Figure 11.4c)

The amount of pain the victim feels does not determine the severity of the burn. This is because deeper burns can be painless due to destruction of nerve endings.

Treating burns involves methods to stop the cause of the burns, cooling the burned area, and covering it loosely with clean, dry dressings.

If the victim's clothing is on fire, it must be extinguished as quickly as possible. If smoke is present, move the victim to a well-ventilated area. However, only move accident victims if

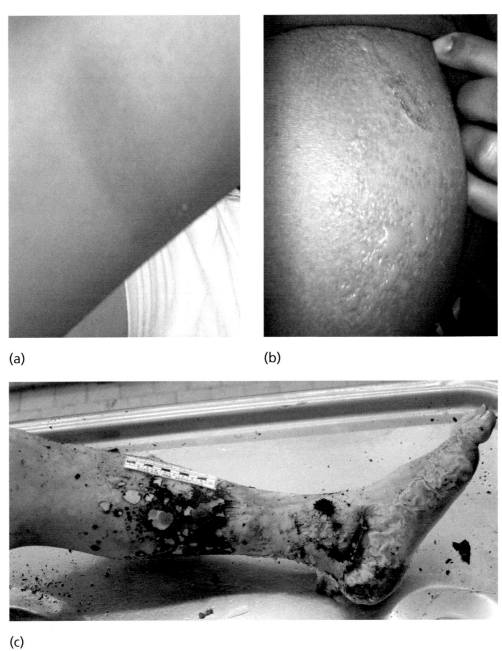

(a)

(b)

(c)

Figure 11.4 Types of burns: (a) first-degree; (b) second-degree; (c) third-degree.

this is necessary for their protection. Always maintain body alignment when moving a victim. Cool water should be run over the burned area for several minutes, or the area should be immersed in cool water. Also, a cool and wet cloth can be used on areas that cannot be immersed, and additional cool water can be poured onto the cloth as needed. Ice should not be applied except for a minor first-degree burn. If clothing is stuck to a burn, do not use force to remove it. Do not break blisters. Cover burned areas with sterile, non-adhesive dressings if available, or if not, clean clothes. For severe burns, do not apply ointments. Always apply any bandages loosely, and never use cotton as a dressing. Prevent the victim from becoming chilled.

Every burn victim must be assessed for possible respiratory damage because of the inhalation of smoke or chemical fumes. Respiratory system damage can cause swelling that may impair normal breathing. Discolored areas around the nose or mouth may indicate respiratory system damage. Even if the victim does not have difficulty breathing, if he or she has been exposed to smoke or chemical fumes, or has discolored areas on the face, consider that respiratory system damage is likely. Effects of this damage may not manifest until 24 hours later.

A *radiation burn* is most often seen in the form of a sunburn, caused by the ultraviolet radiation in the sun's rays. It may also be linked to thermal (electromagnetic) radiation, radio frequency energy, ultraviolet light, and ionizing (subatomic particle) radiation. If a victim has been burned by a form of radiation, move him or her away from the source of the radiation. Follow the previous steps to cool the burn, apply a dressing, and prevent chilling.

For chemical burns, prevent any further contact with the chemical that cause the burn. Move the victim to a well-ventilated area if there are chemical fumes. Use cool water to flush the burn area until EMS arrives, remembering to flush the burn *away from the body* so that no more of the chemical will contact the body and cause additional burns. If the eyes are burned, flush them continuously with cool water. If only one eye is burned, flush it from its inner aspect toward its outer aspect so that the other eye will not be harmed. For burns by electrical current, never touch the victim if he or she is still in contact with a live electrical wire. Have electrical power turned off before touching the patient. Do not cool the burn, but apply a clean, dry dressing. Prevent chilling, and do not move the victim if possible since other injuries may be present.

Bleeding

Bleeding occurs when there is damage to a blood vessel. Heavy bleeding is known as *hemorrhaging*. *External bleeding* occurs when blood drains out of the body through a break in the skin. It indicates damage to tendons or muscles, and loss of sensation distal to the wound indicates nerve damage. If external bleeding does not stop on its own, first aid is needed to stop the bleeding so that excessive blood loss does not occur. A leg or an arm that is bleeding should be elevated above heart level unless prohibited by discomfort or a neck or back injury.

To stop external bleeding, apply direct pressure with a clean piece of cloth or a sterile dressing. Pressure dressings can be used if the rescuer must use his or her hands to perform additional first aid. Once soaked with blood, a dressing should be left in place and covered with another dressing. You should not look under a dressing to see if bleeding has stopped. If bleeding from an arm or a leg wound does not stop after 15 minutes of direct pressure, use pressure-point bleeding control. For an arm wound, the pressure point is on the brachial artery, located between the large muscles on the inside of the arm. Press firmly with your fingers until you no longer feel a pulse. For a leg wound, the pressure point is on the femoral artery, in the groin, at the bend of the leg. Press firmly with your palm or with both palms, against the pelvic bone, until you no longer feel a pulse.

> ### You should remember
>
> Never apply pressure over an embedded object, the eyes, or on a head injury if you suspect that the patient has a skull fracture.

Arterial bleeding is bright red and "spurts" out with every heartbeat. This is potentially life-threatening and must be stopped as quickly as possible. *Venous bleeding* is darker in color and flows evenly, yet can still result in significant blood loss. For all types of external bleeding, universal precautions must be followed. The victim may be weak, confused, and have varying levels of consciousness. You should call EMS in cases of heavy external bleeding or if other injuries are suspected. **Tourniquets** are rarely used in emergencies due to the potential for additional harm. They should be reserved as last resorts to save the life of the patient. A tourniquet is a tight band that is placed around an arm or a leg to stop bleeding from an injury below.

Internal bleeding occurs inside the body, and is more difficult to detect. It may signify abdominal or other serious injuries. Therefore, EMS should be called as soon as possible. It should be suspected if the victim has a broken bone, has been in a car accident, has been struck by an object, or has had other types of trauma. Any victim with suspected internal bleeding must be evaluated by a medical professional. It may be signified by blood in the stool, urine, vomit, or from the vagina. Other signs include abdominal distention or tenderness, nausea, confusion, weakness, or decreased level of consciousness. The patient should not be given anything to eat or drink since this can cause vomiting, and should be placed on his or her back with the knees elevated and a pillow under the head (see Figure 11.5).

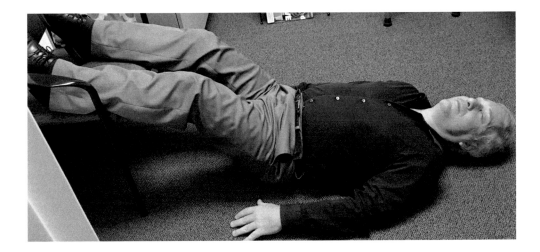

Figure 11.5 Place emergency patients in the shock position, unless they have spinal injury.

A blanket should be used if there is abdominal discomfort. For bruised areas, which are caused by bleeding within the skin and soft tissues, cold compresses should be applied. Overall, the victim should be kept still and treated for shock. You should stay with the victim until medical assistance arrives. Apply chest compressions, with or without rescue breathing, if needed.

Hypothermia

Exposure to excessively cold temperatures can cause **hypothermia**, in which the body temperature drops below normal. Other conditions that cause hypothermia include wet clothing and immersion into cold water. In a cold room, hypothermia can develop in the elderly, newborns, and people who are in poor health. When mild, hypothermia causes the skin to feel cold, shivering, and the victim to experience confusion and lack of coordination. Once it becomes severe, shivering stops, coordination problems worsen, the speech becomes slurred, it becomes difficult to see, and the heart rate slows. The victim feels drowsy and wants to be left alone, often becoming irrational and uncooperative. Untreated severe hypothermia will result in coma and death.

To treat hypothermia, when respirations are less than six per minute, rescue breathing is required. The victim should be moved inside some form of shelter if possible. Wet clothes should be removed and replaced with dry clothes. No constricting clothes or jewelry should be left on the victim, however. Direct heat must be avoided, though warm towels or linens may be applied to the neck, chest, and groin. If the victim is able to drink liquids, administer warm and sweet fluids. The victim should be wrapped in an insulated blanket or aluminum foil, including the neck and head. You can also lie beside the victim to help raise the body temperature.

Hyperthermia

Exposure to excessively warm temperatures and high humidity can cause **hyperthermia**, in which the body temperature rises above normal. Hyperthermia results in loss of body fluids due to excessive perspiration, loss of salt from the body, and dehydration. Hyperthermia may be aggravated by certain medical conditions and even medications. In a room that is overheated and poorly ventilated, the elderly, newborns, and people in poor health may develop hyperthermia. Excessive exercise, obesity, and drinking alcohol can also cause hyperthermia. The most severe heat-related illnesses include heat stroke, heat exhaustion, and heat cramps.

Heat stroke is the most severe hyperthermic condition, and is life-threatening. The skin is dry, hot, and reddened. The victim may be confused, weak, and even experience seizures. The pupils of the eyes will be constricted, the pulse will be weak and rapid, and the breathing will be shallow and rapid. Body temperature will be above 102 °F (38.9 °C), and the victim may be unconscious. It is crucial to call EMS immediately and avoid administering any liquids. If EMS is not available immediately, the victim should be immersed in cold water, but requires constant monitoring of alertness, pulse, and respirations.

CASE STUDY

You are working in the emergency department when three unrelated patients enter. The first is a 41-year-old male who has been involved in a bicycle accident. His right arm is in a sling, and he states that he fell off his bike, landing on that arm. He has pain in his wrist and a laceration on his left elbow. He also states he was wearing a helmet at the time of the accident. The second is a 7-year-old boy, accompanied by his father. The boy has abdominal pain, and did not want to play with his friends or eat previously in the day. During triage, the boy vomits. He has a slight temperature, and continues to complain about his "sore tummy." The last patient is a 33-year-old female who complains of vomiting through the previous night, and of having diarrhea. She states that she has abdominal cramps, but has no fever or chills.

1 Of these patients, which do you believe should be treated first?
2 Would food poisoning be a consideration for the female patient?
3 Which ESI level do you think applies to each patient?

Chapter highlights

This section answers the Objectives found at the beginning of the chapter.

1 **List the five levels of the emergency severity index and the time requirements of each level.**

- Immediate – less than one minute
- Emergent – within one to 14 minutes
- Urgent – within 15 to 60 minutes
- Semiurgent – within 61 to 120 minutes
- Nonurgent – within 121 minutes to 24 hours.

2 **Give examples of man-made disasters.**

- Wars and other human conflicts
- Injuries resulting from the use of chemical weapons, such as in terrorist attacks
- Oil spills and other industrial accidents that cause environmental toxins to enter the air, water, and soil.

3 **Give examples of natural disasters.**

- Earthquakes, hurricanes, typhoons, other severe storms, flooding, landslides, tsunamis, avalanches, volcanoes.

4 **List four items that should be included in a disaster preparedness plan.**

- An identification of the area's vulnerabilities
- Scenarios of what might occur and how likely these situations are
- An explanation of the roles different people will have if a disaster occurs
- A training program for first responders and disaster management teams.

5 **Identify the people who are most vulnerable when a natural disaster occurs.**

- People who are very young, very old, or chronically ill are most vulnerable when a natural disaster occurs.

6 **Explain when cardiopulmonary resuscitation should be performed.**

- Cardiopulmonary resuscitation (CPR) is administered when a person is not breathing and does not have a pulse. Training in CPR increases the likelihood that many more lives could be saved. An injured person has a better chance of survival when care is administered immediately prior to the arrival of medical help, rather than not receiving any care until medical help arrives.

7 **Identify injuries and conditions that may require first aid.**

- First aid involves providing emergency care following an accident or sudden illness. Examples of injuries that may require first aid include fractures, sprains, strains, wounds, burns, and bleeding. Conditions that may require first aid include hypothermia and hyperthermia.

8 **List various types of fractures.**

- Types of fractures include simple (closed), compound (open), incomplete (greenstick), comminuted, spiral (torsion), transverse, oblique, buckled (impacted), pathologic, stress, and longitudinal.

9 **Discuss external and internal bleeding.**

- External bleeding occurs when blood drains out of the body through a break in the skin. It indicates damage to tendons or muscles, and loss sensation distal to the wound indicates nerve damage. If external bleeding does not stop on its own, first aid is needed to stop the bleeding so that excessive blood loss does not occur. For all types of external bleeding, universal precautions must be followed. You should call EMS in cases of heavy external bleeding or if other injuries are suspected.
- Internal bleeding occurs inside the body, and is more difficult to detect. It may signify abdominal or other serious injuries. Therefore, EMS should be called as soon as possible. It should be suspected if the victim has a broken bone, has been in a car accident, has been struck by an object, or has had other types of trauma. Any victim with suspected internal bleeding must be evaluated by a medical professional. It may be signified by blood in the stool, urine, vomit, or from the vagina. Other signs include abdominal distention or tenderness, nausea, confusion, weakness, or decreased level of consciousness.

10 **Compare hyperthermia with hypothermia.**

- Hypothermia is caused by exposure to excessively cold temperatures, resulting in the body temperature dropping below normal. It may also be caused by wet clothing and immersion into cold water. Hypothermia (or hyperthermia) may more commonly affect the elderly, newborns, and people who are in poor health. Mild hypothermia causes cold skin, shivering, confusion, and lack of coordination. Severe hypothermia causes shivering to stop, coordination problems to worsen, slurred speech, vision difficulties, slowed heart rate, drowsiness, irrational and uncooperative behavior, and eventually coma and death.

- Hyperthermia is caused by exposure to excessive warm temperatures and high humidity, resulting in the body temperature rising above normal. Body fluids are lost due to excessive perspiration, salt is lost, and dehydration develops. Hyperthermia may be aggravated by certain medical conditions and even medications. It can also be caused by excessive exercise, obesity, and drinking alcohol. The most severe heat-related illnesses include heat stroke, heat exhaustion, and heat cramps.

Summary

Emergency and urgent care generally focuses on patients with more immediate health care needs. These people often need medical attention in order to avoid jeopardizing health, causing impairment of bodily functions, or causing serious dysfunction of bodily organs or parts. The determination of patients needing immediate care is based on levels of triage, which include immediate, emergent, urgent, semiurgent, and non-urgent. Triage is a common part of health care for people involved in natural or man-made disasters. Disaster preparedness helps protect against natural disasters and reduce their impact upon health. Good disaster preparedness requires teams of people working together with coordinated efforts. Health care workers, at all levels, must cooperate in order to combat the severe damage that disasters often cause, which affect all levels of the health care system and its potential effectiveness.

Review questions

1 What is urgent care?
2 When is cardiopulmonary resuscitation indicated?
3 What is triage?
4 What is the Good Samaritan Act?
5 When is an automatic external defibrillator used?
6 What are the signs and symptoms of shock?
7 What factors may cause diabetic emergencies?
8 What are the three types of burns?
9 What are the signs and symptoms of hypothermia?
10 What is heat stroke?

Bibliography

Abbott, P.L. 2013. *Natural Disasters, 9th Edition.* New York: McGraw-Hill Education. Print.
Advanced Life Support Group. 2014. *Emergency Triage, 3rd Edition.* London: BMJ Books. Print.
Agency for Healthcare Research and Quality. 2016. Agency for Healthcare Research and Quality. Available at: www.ahrq.gov/professionals/systems/hospital/esi/esi1.html. Rockville: Agency for Healthcare Research and Quality.

American Academy of Orthopedic Surgeons (AAOS). 2013. *Emergency Care and Transportation of the Sick and Injured, 10th Edition*. Burlington: Jones & Bartlett Learning. Print.

American Red Cross. 2016. Disaster Preparedness. Available at: www.redcross.org/what-we-do/international-services/disaster-preparedness. Washington, D.C.: The National American Red Cross.

Angelini, D.J., and LaFontaine, D. 2012. *Obstetric Triage and Emergency Care Protocols*. New York: Springer Publishing Company. Print.

Booth, K.A., Whicker, L.G., and Wyman, T.D. 2013. *Medical Assisting: Administrative and Clinical Procedures with Anatomy and Physiology, 5th Edition*. New York: McGraw-Hill. Print.

Bradley, A.T. 2013. *The Disaster Preparedness Handbook: A Guide for Families, 2nd Edition*. New York: Castle Books. Print.

Buttaravoli, P., and Leffler, S.M. 2012. *Minor Emergencies: Expert Consult, 3rd Edition*. Philadelphia: Saunders. Print.

Campo, T.M., and Lafferty, K. 2010. *Essential Procedures for Practitioners in Emergency, Urgent, and Primary Care Settings: A Clinical Companion*. New York: Springer Publishing Company. Print.

CDC. 2016. Disasters – Hurricanes. Available at: http://emergency.cdc.gov/disasters/hurricanes/hcp.asp. Atlanta: U.S. Centers for Disease Control and Prevention.

CDC. 2016. Emergency Department Visits. Available at: www.cdc.gov/nchs/fastats/emergency-department.htm. Atlanta: U.S. Centers for Disease Control and Prevention.

Crain's New York Business. 2015. 9/11 First Responders May Get Left Holding the Bill. Available at: www.crainsnewyork.com/article/20150910/health_care/150919993/two-federal-programs-covering-medical-care-for-9-11-first-responders-of-the-sept-11-attacks-expire-next-year-and-with-uncertainty-over-their-future-survivors-could-be-left-with-hefty-bills. New York: Crain's New York Business.

Digital History. 2001. Osama Bin Laden. Available at: www.digitalhistory.uh.edu/disp_textbook.cfm?smtid=2&psid=3379. Houston: University of Houston / Digital History.

Disasterium – Natural and Man Made Disasters. 2016. Information About Disasters. Available at: www.disasterium.com. New York: Disasterium.

Emergency Severity Index (ESI). 2016. Emergency Severity Index Home Page. Available at: www.esitriage.org. Boston: Emergency Severity Index (ESI).

FEMA / Ready.gov. 2016. FEMA / Ready.gov Home Page. Available at: www.ready.gov. Washington, D.C.: FEMA / Ready.gov.

Goodwin-Veenema, T. 2012. *Disaster Nursing and Emergency Preparedness for Chemical, Biological, and Radiological Terrorism and Other Hazards, 3rd Edition*. New York: Springer Publishing Company. Print.

Goyal, D.G., and Mattu, A. 2012. *Urgent Care Emergencies: Avoiding the Pitfalls and Improving the Outcomes*. Hoboken: Wiley-Blackwell. Print.

Guiberson, B.Z. 2014. *Disasters: Natural and Man-Made Catastrophes Through the Centuries*. New York: Square Fish. Print.

HealthITBuzz. 2014. HIE Supports Disaster Preparedness and Emergency Services. Available at: www.healthit.gov/buzz-blog/ehr-case-studies/disaster-preparedness-health-information-exchange. Washington, D.C.: HealthIT.gov.

Informed, Derr, P., Tardiff, J., and McEvoy, M. 2013. *Emergency & Critical Care Pocket Guide, 8th Edition*. Burlington: Jones & Bartlett Learning. Print.

Institute for the Analysis of Global Security. 2003. How Much Did the September 11 Terror Attacks Cost America? Available at: www.iags.org/costof911.html. Potomac: Institute for the Analysis of Global Security.

Knickman, J.R., and Kovner, A.R. 2015. *Jonas and Kovner's Health Care Delivery in the United States, 11th Edition*. New York: Springer Publishing Company. Print.

McEntire, D.A. 2006. *Disaster Response and Recovery*. New York: Wiley. Print.

Medical Doctor MD – Updates on Medicine. 2011. Urgent Care Centers on the Rise. Available at: www.medicaldoctormd.com/urgent-care/urgent-care-centers-on-the-rise/. Trenton: MedicalDoctorMD.com.

MedlinePlus. 2016. Recognizing Medical Emergencies. Available at: www.nlm.nih.gov/medlineplus/ency/article/001927.htm. Bethesda: U.S. National Library of Medicine.

Mitchell, D., and Haroun, L. 2011. *Introduction to Health Care, 3rd Edition*. Boston: Delmar Cengage Learning. Print.

National Institutes of Health. 2016. Work-Related Medical Emergencies. Available at: www.ors.od.nih.gov/sr/dohs/occupationalmedical/pages/med_emergencies/aspx. Bethesda: National Institutes of Health.

National Priorities Project. 2016. How Military Spending Has Changed Since 9/11. Available at: www.nationalpriorities.org/campaigns/how-military-spending-has-changed/. Northampton: National Priorities Project.

Nordqvist, C. 2011. 911 Ten Years On – The Health Effects on Rescue Workers. Available at: www.medicalnewstoday.com/articles/234030.php. Brighton: Medical News Today.

Preparedness.com. 2015. Preparedness.com Home Page. Available at: http://preparedness.com. Gradenville: Preparedness.com.

PreventionWeb. 2016. The Economic Cost of the Social Impact of Natural Disasters. Available at: www.preventionweb.net/files/11214_WHOpresentationontheimpactofnatural.pdf. Geneva: PreventionWeb.

Questcare Urgent Care. 2016. Urgent Care Centers See Continued Growth. Available at: http://questcareurgent.com/immediate-care-urgent-care-centers-see-continued-growth. Dallas: Questcare Urgent Care.

Reliefweb.int. 2013. Statistical Review of Natural Disasters. Available at: http://reliefweb.int/report/world/annual-disasterstatistical-review-2013-numbers-and-trends. Chicago: Reliefweb.int.

Shea, S.S., and Hoyt, K.S. 2014. *Pocket Reference Guide for Health Providers, NPs, PAs & Other Medical Professionals: A Useful Approach to Emergent/Urgent & Ambulatory Care, 2nd Edition*. Seattle: CreateSpace Independent Publishing Platform. Print.

Shukman, D. 2011. Toxic Dust Legacy of 9/11 Plagues Thousands of People. Available at: www.bbc.com/news/world-us-canada-14738140. London: BBC.

Skolnik, R. 2015. *Global Health 101 (Essential Public Health), 3rd Edition*. Burlington: Jones & Bartlett Learning. Print.

University Hospitals EMS Training and Disaster Preparedness Institute. 2016. Simple Triage and Rapid Treatment. Available at: www.emsconedonline.com/pdfs/starttriage.pdf. Cleveland: University Hospitals.

Urgent Care Association of America. 2016. Industry News. Available at: www.ucaoa.org/?industrynews. Chicago: Urgent Care Association of America.

Visser, L.S., Montejano, A.S., and Aarne-Grossman, V. 2015. *Fast Facts for the Triage Nurse: An Orientation and Care Guide in a Nutshell*. New York: Springer Publishing Company. Print.

World Health Organization. 2011. Disaster Risk Management for Health OVERVIEW. Available at: www.who.int/hac/events/drm_fact_sheet_overview.pdf. New York: World Health Organization.

World Health Organization. 2016. Environmental Health in Emergencies. Available at: www.who.int/environmental_health_emergencies/natural_events/en. New York: World Health Organization.

World Health Organization. 2016. Environmental Health in Emergencies – Natural Events. Available at: www.who.int/environmental_health_emergencies/natural_events/en/. New York: World Health Organization.

WorldAtlas. 2014. Countries with Natural Disasters. Available at: www.worldatlas.com/articles/the-countries-with-the-most-natural-disasters-worldwide.html. St. Laurent: WorldAtlas.

Young, T. 2015. *Start Prepping! Get Prepared – For Life: A 10-Step Path to Emergency Preparedness So You Can Survive Any Disaster*. Seattle: CreateSpace Independent Publishing Platform. Print.

Unit V

Safety in the workplace

Contents

12 Infection control 283

Overview 283
Classification of microorganisms 285
Infectious disease process 288
Chain of infection 288
Hand hygiene 293
Microorganism control 294
Personal protective equipment 295
Antiseptics, disinfectants, and sterilization 296
Surgical asepsis 299
Case study 299
Chapter highlights 299
Summary 301
Review questions 301
Bibliography 302

13 Occupational Safety and Health Administration (OSHA) standards 303

Overview 303
OSHA Bloodborne Pathogens Standard 304
Components of the OSHA Standard 311
OSHA Hazard Communication 315
Fire safety and emergency plan 318
Chemical hazards and safety 322
Physical safety 324
Latex allergy 325
Ergonomics 325
Radiation hazards 328
Workplace violence 328

Employee responsibilities 328
Case study 329
Chapter highlights 329
Summary 331
Review questions 332
Bibliography 333

Chapter 12

Infection control

Objectives

After study of the chapter, readers should be able to:

1 Differentiate between the structures of bacteria and viruses.
2 Give examples of diseases caused by bacteria and viruses.
3 Explain how fungi grow, and in which individuals they primarily cause disease.
4 List the ways that protozoal infections spread, and give examples of common protozoal infections.
5 Identify the six essential links in the chain of infection.
6 List examples of diseases transmitted by direct contact, and diseases caused by airborne particles.
7 List some factors that influence a host's susceptibility to disease.
8 List examples of personal protective equipment.
9 Identify the type of infection control procedure that is the most effective against microorganisms, and examples of how it is utilized.
10 Differentiate between surgical asepsis and medical asepsis.

Overview

One of the most important programs of disease surveillance within health care facilities concerns the investigation, prevention, and control of infections and their causative microorganisms. Infection control can include the policies and procedures of a hospital or other health care facility to minimize the risk of spreading *nosocomial* or *community-acquired* infections to patients or staff members. The majority of microorganisms are beneficial to humans. However, harmful microorganisms called **pathogens** are linked to infections of different organs or body systems. Infection control includes the concepts of how disease is transmitted, along with how the body responds. Health care professionals understand the methods used to minimize the chances of disease transmission. This begins with proper hand hygiene. This chapter focuses on microorganisms, the chain of infection, and how to control pathogenic activity. These concepts may reduce transmission of diseases, with potentially life-saving outcomes.

Classification of microorganisms

Common infectious agents are microorganisms that are classified as bacteria, viruses, fungi, protozoa, and rickettsia. Infection control practices such as sanitization, disinfection, and sterilization are methods to break these links in the chain of infection, and are discussed later in this chapter.

Bacteria

Bacteria are small unicellular microorganisms lacking a true nucleus or cellular metabolism. More types of bacteria exist than any other microorganism. They are able, under the right conditions, to multiply extremely quickly. Bacteria are classified according to their shapes, examples of which include cocci, bacilli, and spirilla (see Figure 12.1). Cocci are spherical in shape. **Diplococci** are spherical or coffee bean-shaped and usually appear in pairs. **Streptococci** have spherical or oval shapes and occur in chains, while **staphylococci** are spherical and occur in grape-like clusters. **Bacilli** are rod-shaped, and are divided into **coccobacilli** and streptobacilli. Another type is the spiral-shaped **spirilla**.

Bacteria are also classified by their ability to grow in the presence or lack of oxygen. They are called *aerobic* when growing faster in the presence of oxygen, and are called **anaerobic** when growing faster in the absence of oxygen. When they can grow in either condition, they are called *facultative*. Most bacteria are aerobic, while most normal flora are anaerobic. Bacteria can also be differentiated by certain biochemical reactions occurring inside their cell walls.

Bacteria require food in order to survive. Most of them multiply using simple cell division, but some forms of bacteria produce **spores**, which are a resistant stage that is able to withstand unfavorable environments. When conditions become favorable once again, spores germinate, forming new cells. They are resistant to disinfectants, drying, and heat. A wide range of illnesses is caused by pathogenic bacteria. Examples include diarrhea, gonorrhea, pneumonia, sinusitis, and urinary tract infections.

Viruses

Viruses are microorganisms that can only live inside cells, and are the smallest of all microorganisms, only able to be viewed by using an electron microscope. They are unable to get nourishment or reproduce outside cells. Viruses are much simpler than bacteria, and are not usually considered cellular. Their core consists of DNA or RNA that is surrounded by a protein coating. Certain viruses can create an additional coating, or *envelope*, that protects against attack by the immune system. Viruses damage cells they inhabit by blocking normal protein synthesis. They also cause damage by using their host cell's mechanism for metabolism to reproduce. An example of the hepatitis B virus is shown in Figure 12.2.

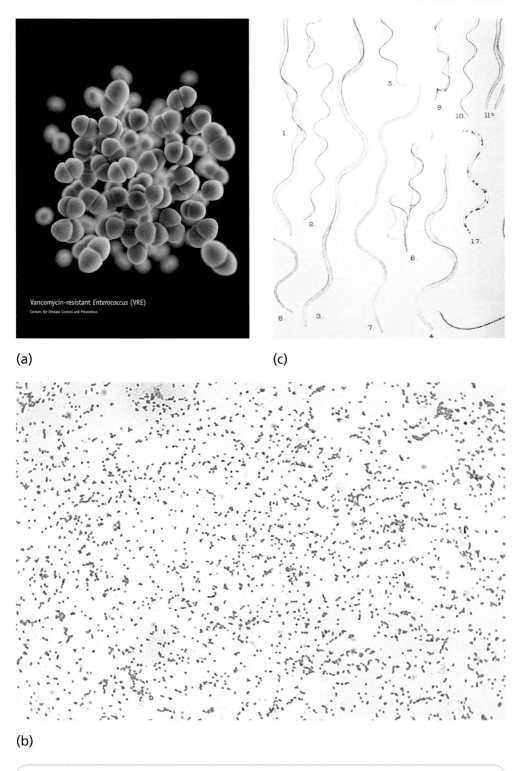

(a)

Vancomycin-resistant *Enterococcus* (VRE)
Centers for Disease Control and Prevention

(c)

(b)

Figure 12.1 Types of bacteria: (a) cocci; (b) bacilli; (c) spirilla.

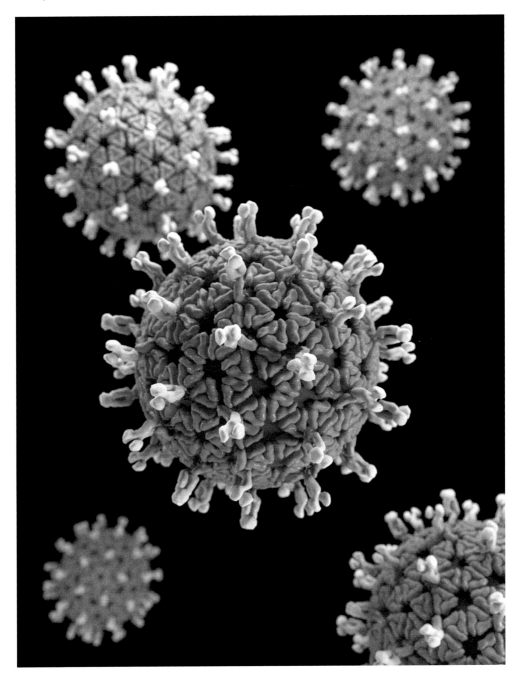

Figure 12.2 Example of a virus.

Viruses are classified by the physiochemical characteristics of their virions, along with their mode of transmission, host range, symptomatology, and various other factors. A specific viral infection may cause different symptoms between individual people. Some viruses immediately trigger a disease response, while others remain latent for years. Examples of viral infections include the common cold, genital herpes, hepatitis, influenza, measles, the infections caused by HIV, and the West Nile virus.

Fungi

Fungi are simple parasitic plants that depend on other life forms for a nutritional source. *Molds* are multi-celled fungi that can be found indoors as well as outdoors. They grow best when conditions are warm, damp, and humid. Molds form *spores* in order to reproduce and spread. This is a mode of reproduction in which the organism breaks up into many pieces. Mold spores can survive extreme environmental conditions, such as dry conditions that would not support normal mold growth.

Yeasts are single-celled fungi made up of oval or round cells. They are found in soils and on plant surfaces, in sugary mediums such as fruits and flower nectar, and as mild to potentially dangerous pathogens in humans. The multiplication of yeast cells occurs by a *budding* process, via the formation of cross walls or *fission*, and sometimes by a combination of these processes. There are approximately 100 types of fungi common in humans. Only about ten of these are pathogenic. Examples of pathogenic fungal conditions include histoplasmosis, *candida albicans* (a yeast infection), and *tinea pedis* (athlete's foot).

Like bacteria, fungi break down complex organic substances. They are also essential in the recycling of carbon and various elements. Fungi are used as foods, and in fermentation to develop medical and industrial substances. These substances include antibiotics and other drugs, antitoxins, and alcohol.

Protozoa

Protozoa are the lowest forms of animal life, and are much larger than bacteria. They are single-celled eukaryotic parasites that are capable of movement, and are found in soil and water (see Figure 12.3). Most protozoa feed off dead or decaying organic matter. Protozoal infections spread through ingestion of food or water that is contaminated, or through insect bites. Common protozoal infections include amebic dysentery, gastroenteritis, malaria, and vaginal infections such as Trichomonas vaginitis. Protozoal infections are leading causes of death in developing countries because of poor sanitation conditions. They are also common in immunocompromised patients.

Rickettsia

Rickettsia is a genius of *Rickettsiae*, known as *obligate* parasites because they depend completely on their host in order to survive. *Rickettsiae* are larger than viruses, and can be seen under conventional microscopes after staining procedures. These intracellular parasites must enter living cells in order to reproduce. Rickettsial infections are spread through flea, tick, mite, and lice bites. Common examples of these infections include typhus and Rocky Mountain spotted fever. Different rickettsial infections cause similar symptoms, including fever, a characteristic rash, malaise, and severe headache.

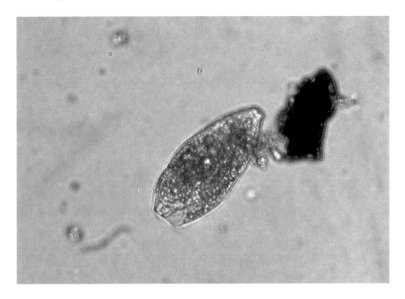

Figure 12.3 Protozoa.

Infectious disease process

There are five unique stages of the infectious disease process, which begin once an individual has been exposed to a pathogen. These stages are as follows:

- *Incubation or "silent" stage* – Often, the actual time when a pathogen gains entry and begins replicating is not known. This stage can be of widely varying lengths. It ends once disease signs and symptoms begin.
- *Prodromal stage* – Starts with signs and symptoms of disease, and usually lasts one to two days. At this time, the disease process is occurring.
- *Acute stage* – The disease process reaches its most severe peak, with the symptoms helping in the determination of which disease has developed.
- *Declining stage* – The symptoms begin to lessen and health begins to return to normal. However, the infection is still present during this stage.
- *Convalescent stage* – Symptoms are nearly gone, health status is nearly normal, and the pathogen has been almost entirely eliminated.

Chain of infection

The elements of an infectious process constitute the chain of infection. It is interactive, involving an agent, the environment, and a host. There are several essential links in the chain of infection that allow transmission of microorganisms to occur. Figure 12.4 identifies the six essential links. The infectious process cannot occur without transmission of microorganisms. By understanding the chain of infection, disease can be prevented or controlled by breaking the links in the chain. This occurs when one or more interactive links of the agent, host, or environment are interrupted.

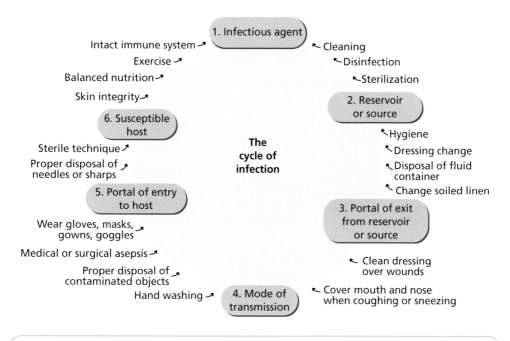

Figure 12.4 Chain (cycle) of infection.

Causative agent

A causative agent is any entity that may cause disease, and includes:

● *Biological agents*: Live organisms that invade a host, including bacteria, viruses, fungi, protozoa, and rickettsia
● *Chemical agents*: Substances that interact with body cells and tissues, including food additives, industrial chemicals, medications, and pesticides
● *Physical agents*: Environmental factors applied to tissues systemically, which alter physiologic processes, including: heat, light, noise, and radiation.

The primary concern regarding the chain of infection is how biological (infectious) agents affect the host.

Reservoir

The reservoir is the place where an agent is able to survive. An agent that is present in a reservoir is able to colonize and reproduce. For growth of pathogens, the reservoir must contain nutrients such as oxygen or organic matter, a certain temperature range, moisture, a compatible pH level, and the proper amount of light exposure. Common reservoirs include animals, the environment, fomites, and humans. Fomites can be surgical dressings or instruments that are contaminated with infectious agents. Infected animals or humans can either have symptoms or be asymptomatic (symptom-free) carriers of the infectious agent. In both examples, the agent can be transmitted to others.

Portal of exit

The portal of exit is the route used by an infectious agent to leave the reservoir so that it can be transferred to a susceptible host. The agent may leave the reservoir through blood, wounds that are draining, feces, saliva, semen, sputum, urine, and vaginal secretions.

Mode of transmission

The mode of transmission occurs between the portal of exit from the reservoir and the portal of entry into a susceptible host. Infectious agents usually have a specific mode of transmission, though some pathogens may be transmitted by more than one (see Table 12.1).

Contact transmission involves an agent being physically transferred from an infected person to an uninfected person. This can occur several ways: direct contact by physically touching the infected person, or indirect contact with the infected person's secretions (see Figure 12.5).

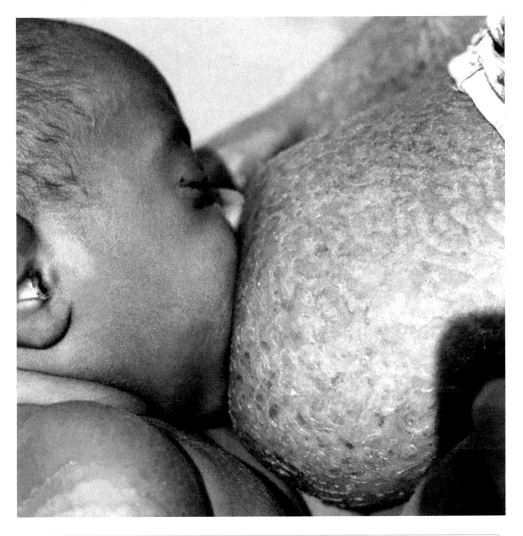

Figure 12.5 How contact transmission occurs.

Table 12.1 Modes of transmission

Mode	Examples
Contact	Bathing
	Bed linens
	Clothing
	Diagnostic equipment
	Direct, with infected person
	Dressings
	Healthcare equipment
	Indirect contact (with fomites)
	Instruments used for treatments
	Laboratory analysis specimen containers
	Personal belongings
	Personal care equipment
	Rubbing
	Secretions from client
	Toileting (feces and urine)
	Touching
Airborne	Coughing
	Inhaling microorganisms in moisture or dust particles
	Sneezing
	Talking
Vehicle	Blood
	Contact with contaminated inanimate objects
	Drugs
	Food
	Urine
	Water
Vector-borne	Animals
	Contact with contaminated animate hosts
	Insects

Diseases caused by direct contact include colds, influenza, and sexually transmitted diseases. Transmission by touching is the most common way that pathogens are transmitted.

Airborne transmission occurs when a susceptible person is infected because of contact with contaminated droplets or dust particles suspended in the air, such as from sneezing. The longer particles are suspended, the higher the chance they will find an available port of entry. Measles is an organism that relies on airborne transmission. Anthrax spores are also transmitted in an airborne powder form.

> **You should remember**
>
> When a person sneezes, more than 100,000 droplets emerge from the respiratory tract at more than 100 miles per hour. The droplets quickly spread in the air, potentially causing another person to breathe them in. Therefore, covering the mouth and nose when sneezing is always suggested.

Vehicle transmission occurs when agents are transferred to susceptible hosts via contaminated inanimate objects. These include blood, drugs, foods, and water. Salmonellosis is an example of a disease that is transmitted through contaminated food.

Vector-borne transmission occurs when agents are transferred to susceptible hosts by creatures such as fleas, lice, mosquitoes, and ticks (see Figure 12.6). Lyme disease is an example of vector-borne transmission, and is transmitted by the bites of ticks.

Portal of entry

A **portal of entry** is the route through which an infectious agent enters a host. They include the following:

- Circulatory system – bites of insects or rodents
- Gastrointestinal system – ingestion of contaminated food or water
- Genito-urinary tract – contamination with infected semen or vaginal secretions

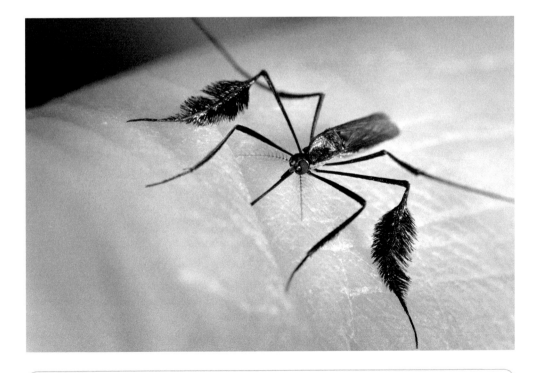

Figure 12.6 How vector-borne transmission occurs.

- Integumentary system – breaks in skin or mucous membranes
- Respiratory tract – inhalation of contaminated droplets
- Transplacental – via transfer from mother to fetus through the placenta and umbilical cord.

A microorganism must overcome surface barriers such as the skin, various enzymes, and mucus. Each of these may have direct antimicrobial activity, or inhibit the ability of the microorganism to attach to the host. Neither the skin's surface nor the mucous membranes of body cavities are supportive environments for most microorganisms. Therefore, the majority of pathogens must cross these barriers to reach tissues below. Any microorganism that penetrates will encounter two types of resistance: non-specific resistance mechanisms and the specific immune response.

Susceptible host

A host is any organism that can be affected by an agent. It may also be described as an individual who is at risk of contracting an infectious disease. A susceptible host is a person lacking resistance to an agent, meaning he or she is vulnerable to a disease. A compromised host has impaired defense mechanisms, and therefore is more susceptible to infection. A host's susceptibility to infections involves the following factors:

- *Age* – immunity declines with advancing age
- *Concurrent disease* – other present diseases increase susceptibility
- *Heredity* – causes some people to be more susceptible to infection than others
- *Immunization/vaccination status* – some people are not fully immunized
- *Lifestyle* – defenses can be altered by behaviors such as drug use (including sharing needles), tobacco use, and having multiple sexual partners
- *Nutritional status* – being overweight or obese makes a person more prone to illness
- *Occupation* – certain jobs involve more exposure to pathogens such as chemical agents
- *Stress* – a compromised emotional state lowers a person's defense mechanisms.

Focus on hospital-acquired infections

Hospital-acquired infections are also called *nosocomial infections* or *health care-associated infections.* These types of infections usually fall into four categories: urinary tract infections, surgical wound infections, pneumonia, and septicemia.

Hand hygiene

The most important means of preventing spread of infection is frequent, effective hand hygiene. This is true for all health care workers as well as patients, family members, and others. Hands must be washed with the correct technique. Extended scrubbing is not needed every time, unless the hands are excessively contaminated. Antimicrobial soap containing chlorhexidine (such as Hibiclens®, which has antiseptic residual action that lasts for several hours) should be used. However, even washing the hands with this substance does not sterilize them, because skin cannot be completely sterilized. Though most pathogens will be removed, normal non-pathogenic flora will remain. Proper hand washing requires both running water and friction. The water should be warm, since water that is too cold or too hot will cause the skin to become chapped. Friction is created by firm rubbing of all surfaces of the hands and wrists (see Figure 12.7).

Hand washing performed before gloving for a surgical procedure is known as a *surgical scrub*. This includes a two- to six-minute scrub, or the length of time that is recommended by the antimicrobial soap manufacturer.

When a sink is not available for hand washing, or if the hands are not visibly soiled between patients, a practical way to cleanse the hands is by using an alcohol-based hand-rub preparation, in the form of a gel or foam. It must be applied and spread over the hands in the same way that soap would be used.

You should remember

Hand hygiene is the first line of defense against infection, and is the single most important practice in preventing the spread of infection.

Microorganism control

Though microorganisms are beneficial, some of their effects are undesirable, such as infectious disease and spoiling of food. It is vital to be able to kill a large variety of microorganisms, or inhibit their growth, in order to minimize their destructive effects. Goals for controlling growth of microorganisms include:

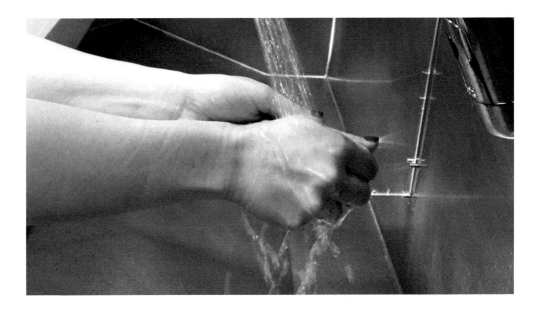

Figure 12.7 Hand washing.

1   Destruction of pathogens
2   Prevention of pathogen transmission
3   Reduction or elimination of microorganisms that may contaminate food, water, or other substances.

Control of microorganisms requires physical, chemical, and biological agents. Terms such as *antiseptic* and *disinfectant* must be thoroughly understood. Confusion exists about which treatments inhibit growth of microorganisms or actually kill them. The types of agents used to control microorganisms are listed in Table 12.2.

> ### Focus on emerging infectious diseases
>
> Emerging infectious diseases are important, particularly since their incidence has not been stabilized. This relates to people traveling more frequently today, for farther distances than ever before. The possibility of transferring an emerging disease from its country of origin to a new area is much greater now.

Personal protective equipment

All types of clothing and equipment worn to protect against physical hazards may be called *personal protective equipment (PPE)*. In health care, this includes gloves, eyewear such as goggles, face shields, masks, gowns, aprons, laboratory coats, hair covers, and shoe covers. The amount of PPE required for certain procedures is directly linked to the chance of exposure to blood and other potentially contaminated substances.

Table 12.2 Control of microorganisms

Physical agents	Chemical agents	Mechanical controls	Biological agents
Dry heat: incineration and dry ovens (sterilization)	**Gases:** (sterilization and disinfection)	**Air filtration:** (sterilization)	**Predators:** (antisepsis)
Moist heat: steam under pressure (sterilization); boiling or hot water/pasteurization (disinfection)	**Animate liquids:** (chemotherapy and antisepsis)	**Liquid filtration:** (sterilization)	**Viruses:** (antisepsis)
Ionizing radiation: X-ray/cathode/gamma (sterilization)	**Inanimate liquids:** (disinfection and sterilization)		**Toxins:** (sterilization)
Non-ionizing radiation: ultraviolet (UV) (disinfection)			

Gloves are required for all procedures involving exposure to broken skin, blood, and other body fluids. The following are examples of commonly used types of gloves:

- Disposable gloves – used one time and then discarded. They are not allowed to be used if damaged, such as by punctures or tears. There are two types: examination gloves and sterile gloves:

  - Examination gloves – worn when a sterile environment is not required
  - Sterile gloves – worn during sterile procedures, such as surgeries or urinary catheter insertion and removal.

- Utility gloves – used for cleaning procedures, these are stronger in structure than disposable gloves. They can be decontaminated and reused, as long as they are not deteriorated or discolored.

In procedures where the eyes, nose, and mouth may be exposed, protective equipment includes various types of eyewear, face shields, and masks. These types of equipment are common in surgery or blood collection, in which there is a potential for blood to be splashed or sprayed.

Protective gowns, aprons, or laboratory coats are used when there is a strong possibility of blood or body fluids being splashed or sprayed onto the health care worker's normal clothing. Hair or shoe covers may also be required. It is important to always bring another change of regular work clothing in case substances are splashed onto the work clothing you are wearing during a procedure, even while PPE is in place.

Often, more than one type of PPE must be worn simultaneously during a procedure. There is an accepted order of putting on (donning) and taking off (removing) various types of PPE. This includes the following steps for donning, which is reversed when removing PPE:

- Gown
- Mask and/or face shield
- Gloves.

Removal of these items in reverse order helps reduce possibility of cross-contamination.

Antiseptics, disinfectants, and sterilization

Physical agents are generally used for sterilization of objects. Chemicals are usually used for disinfection and antisepsis. Chemicals must be used very carefully in all settings, for safety. They also help prevent microbial growth in food and treat infectious diseases. Chemicals used outside of the human body include:

- Alcohols: extremely widely used as antiseptics and disinfectants. They are bactericidal and fungicidal, but not sporicidal. The most popular alcohol germicides include *ethanol* and *isopropanol*, usually in 70% to 80% concentrations. Sufficient disinfection of small instruments may be achieved by soaking them in either of these agents for only 10–15 minutes.
- Household bleach: effective for disinfecting surfaces that have been contaminated with viruses, including HIV.
- Phenol derivatives: creosols and xylenols.

Disinfection

Disinfection is a process by which pathogenic microorganisms are killed, or their actions are inhibited. It greatly reduces the total microbial population and destroys potential pathogens. Disinfectants are usually chemical agents that are normally used only on inanimate objects, not humans. They are primarily used for large instruments, scopes, and heat-sensitive items that would be damaged by the autoclaving process. Disinfectants do not necessarily sterilize objects, since viable spores and some microorganisms may remain. It is difficult to verify that an object has been fully disinfected.

Many disinfecting agents are available, of varying effectiveness. For each product, health care professionals must follow manufacturers' guidelines for proper use. The product's advantages, disadvantages, and possible sources of errors must be understood. Examples of disinfectants include *household bleach*, isopropyl or ethyl alcohols, and organic *glutaraldehyde*-based formulas.

> ### You should remember
>
> In the home, Lysol® and bleach are common disinfectants that are capable of eliminating certain pathogens. The recommended concentration of bleach solution is one part bleach to nine parts water.

Sanitization

Sanitization decreases microorganisms to safe levels, according to public health guidelines. It is closely related to disinfection. Sanitizers are often used for the cleaning of eating utensils in restaurants. Inanimate objects are usually cleaned, as well as partially disinfected. Cleaning and scrubbing of contaminated objects remove debris, but do not destroy microorganisms. In health care, professionals must wear gloves while performing sanitization. If instruments are sharp or have pointed edges, thick utility gloves should be worn.

Antisepsis is the prevention of infection or sepsis via the use of antiseptics. These are chemical agents applied to body tissues to prevent infection. They kill or inhibit pathogen growth and reduce the total microbial population. Since they must not destroy too much host tissue, antiseptics are usually not as toxic as disinfectants.

> ### You should remember
>
> According to the CDC, in the home, sterilization of water is achieved by boiling it. This is the preferred way to kill harmful bacteria and parasites. Bringing water to a rolling boil for one full minute will kill most organisms. However, chemical contaminants in water are not removed by boiling.

Sterilization

Sterilization is the removal or killing of all microorganisms. It may involve extreme heat, ultraviolet (UV) radiation, and saturated steam under pressure as used in autoclaving. Sterile objects are completely free of viable microorganisms, spores, or other infectious agents. Dry heat sterilization is another common method, using heated dry air at a temperature of 160 to 180°C (320 to 356°F) for between 90 minutes and three hours. *Ethylene oxide* is a gas used for items sensitive to heat; this method is called **gas sterilization**. It requires special equipment and aeration of materials after the gas has been applied. Ethylene oxide is extremely flammable and toxic. Gas sterilization is regularly used in hospitals equipped with room-sized gas sterilization chambers. This method is used to sterilize many prepackaged products for intravenous infusion, as well as bandages.

Most instruments and equipment are sterilized inside an **autoclave** (see Figure 12.8), using pressurized steam, at temperatures higher than the boiling point of water (212°F, or 100°C). Steam autoclaves are preferred over dry heat sterilization since they operate at lower temperatures, and the **moist heat** more quickly permeates the clean and porous wrappings that contain items to be sterilized. The item remains sterile for 30 days if the packaging is kept dry and intact. This period is called the item's *shelf life*.

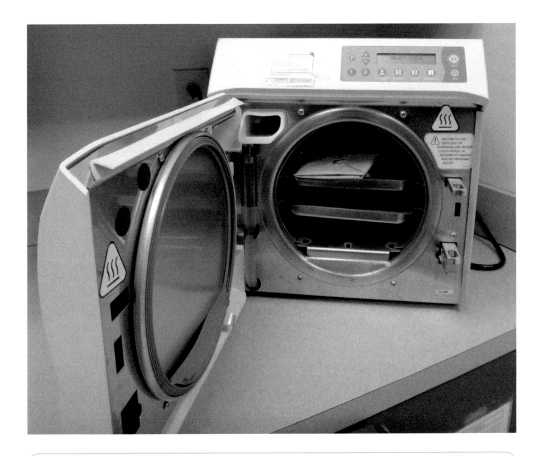

Figure 12.8 An autoclave.

Surgical asepsis

It is important to understand that **surgical asepsis** is distinct from **medical asepsis**. Surgical asepsis completely eliminates microorganisms, while medical asepsis only reduces them. The clear goal of surgical asepsis is to eliminate all microorganisms before they can enter the body. This requires sterilization of surgical instruments before their use and during sterile procedures. The steps of surgical asepsis is as follows:

- Sterile field creation
- Bring sterile items into the sterile field
- Performing surgical scrubs
- Donning sterile gloves
- Equipment sanitization, disinfection, and sterilization.

CASE STUDY

Proper infection control procedures must always be followed exactly as required, or disease and death can result. In a hospital in the United States, a bacterial outbreak killed two infants and caused an infection in three others. It was found that respiratory therapy staff members had washed laryngoscope blades with soap, tap water, and alcohol wipes – instead of following proper sterilization procedures.

1 What are proper methods of sterilization for medical instruments and equipment?
2 Why are sanitization methods insufficient for this type of equipment?
3 What is the term used to describe the type of infection that occurred in this example?

Chapter highlights

This section answers the Objectives found at the beginning of the chapter.

1 **Differentiate between the structures of bacteria and viruses.**

- Bacteria are small unicellular microorganisms lacking a true nucleus or cellular metabolism. They are able to multiply extremely quickly, and are classified according to their shapes. Bacteria may be spherical, coffee bean-shaped, unpaired or paired, oval, in chains, in grape-like clusters, and also may be rod- or spiral-shaped.
- Viruses can only live inside cells, and are the smallest of all microorganisms. They are much simpler than bacteria, and are not usually considered cellular. Their core consists of DNA or RNA that is surrounded by a protein coating. Certain viruses can create an additional coating, or envelope, that protects against attack by the immune system.

2 **Give examples of diseases caused by bacteria and viruses.**

- Examples of bacterial diseases include diarrhea, gonorrhea, pneumonia, sinusitis, and urinary tract infections.
- Examples of viral diseases include the common cold, genital herpes, hepatitis, influenza, measles, the infections caused by HIV, and the West Nile virus.

3 Explain how fungi grow, and in which individuals they primarily cause disease.

- Fungi grow in single cells (such as in yeasts) or in colonies (such as in molds). They mostly cause disease in immunologically impaired individuals.

4 List the ways that protozoal infections spread, and give examples of common protozoal infections.

- Protozoal infections spread through ingestion of food or water that is contaminated, or through insect bites.
- Common protozoal infections include amebic dysentery, gastroenteritis, malaria, and vaginal infections such as *Trichomonas vaginalis*.

5 Identify the six essential links in the chain of infection.

- Causative agent (biological, chemical, or physical)
- Reservoir (where an agent is able to survive)
- Portal of exit (the route by which the agent leaves the reservoir)
- Mode of transmission (contact, airborne, vehicle, vector-borne)
- Portal of entry (the route through which an infectious agent enters a host)
- Susceptible host (any organism that can be affected by an agent).

6 List examples of diseases transmitted by direct contact, and diseases caused by airborne particles.

- Diseases transmitted by direct contact include colds, influenza, and sexually transmitted diseases.
- Diseases transmitted via airborne particles include measles and anthrax.

7 List some factors that influence a host's susceptibility to disease.

- Age, concurrent disease, heredity, immunization/vaccination status, lifestyle, nutritional status, occupation, and stress.

8 List examples of personal protective equipment.

- Personal protective equipment protects against physical hazards, and includes gloves, eyewear such as goggles, face shields, masks, gowns, aprons, laboratory coats, hair covers, and shoe covers.

9 Identify the type of infection control procedure that is the most effective against microorganisms, and examples of how it is utilized.

- Sterilization is the removal or killing of all microorganisms; it may involve extreme heat, ultraviolet (UV) radiation, saturated steam under pressure, or the passage of air or liquids through extremely fine filters; other methods include dry heat sterilization and gas sterilization.
- Most instruments and equipment are sterilized inside an autoclave, using pressurized steam; this method is preferred over dry heat sterilization.

10 Differentiate between surgical asepsis and medical asepsis.

- Surgical asepsis completely eliminates microorganisms, while medical asepsis only reduces them; the clear goal of surgical asepsis is to eliminate microorganisms before they can enter the body – this requires sterilization of surgical instruments before their use and during sterile procedures.

Summary

Infection control is an essential component of safety in the workplace. Potentially harmful pathogens that are linked to infection include bacteria, viruses, fungi, protozoans, and rickettsiae. Various methods are used to classify various types of pathogenic microorganisms. When one of the links in the chain of infection is broken, infection develops. These links include a causative agent, reservoir, portal of exit, mode of transmission, portal of entry, and susceptible host. Infection control involves hand hygiene, antiseptics, disinfectants, personal protective equipment, and sterilization. Infection control is most critical during surgery, in which surgical asepsis – the complete lack of microorganisms – must be achieved.

Review questions

1 What are the classifications of microorganisms?
2 What are the characteristics of viruses?
3 What are three examples of pathogenic fungal conditions?
4 What is the chain of infection?
5 What is personal protective equipment?
6 What are disinfectants and antiseptics?
7 What are the definitions of *sporicidal* and *fungicidal*?
8 What are the indications of sanitizers?
9 When is ethylene oxide used?
10 What is autoclaving?

Bibliography

Association for the Advancement of Medical Instrumentation. 2013. *ANSI/AAMI ST79: Comprehensive Guide to Steam Sterilization and Sterility Assurance in Health Care Facilities, 4th Edition.* Denver: Association of Operating Room Nurses, Inc. Print.

ATI Nursing Education. 2016. Surgical Asepsis: Accepted Practice. Available at: http://atitesting.com/ati_next_gen/skillsmodules/content/surgical-asepsis/equipment.html. Philadelphia: ATI Nursing Education.

Beltz, L.A. 2011. *Emerging Infectious Diseases: A Guide to Diseases, Causative Agents, and Surveillance.* San Francisco: Jossey-Bass. Print.

Booth, K.A., Whicker, L.G., and Wyman, T.D. 2013. *Medical Assisting: Administrative and Clinical Procedures with Anatomy and Physiology, 5th Edition.* New York: McGraw-Hill. Print.

CDC. 2016. Guideline for Disinfection and Sterilization in Healthcare Facilities. Available at: www.cdc.gov/hicpac/disinfection_sterilization/6_0disinfection.html. Atlanta: U.S. Centers for Disease Control and Prevention.

CDC. 2016. Hand Hygiene. Available at: www.cdc.gov/handhygiene. Atlanta: U.S. Centers for Disease Control and Prevention.

CDC. 2016. Infection Control and Prevention. Available at: www.cdc.gov/tb/topic/infectioncontrol/default.htm. Atlanta: U.S. Centers for Disease Control and Prevention.

CDC. 2016. Principles of Epidemiology: Chain of Infection. Available at: www.cdc.gov/ophss/csels/dsepd/SS1978/lesson1/section10.html. Atlanta: U.S. Centers for Disease Control and Prevention.

Gudgin-Dickson, E.F. 2012. *Personal Protective Equipment for Chemical, Biological, and Radiological Hazards: Design, Evaluation, and Selection.* Hoboken: Wiley. Print.

Hubpages. 2016. How Infections Spread in the Workplace: Sites, Causes, Prevention Strategies. Available at: http://hubpages.com/health/how-infections-spread-in-the-workplace-sites-causes-prevention-strategies. Boston: Hubpages.

International Commission on Microbiological Specifications for Foods (ICMSF). 2011. *Microorganisms in Foods: Use of Data for Assessing Process Control and Product Acceptance, 8th Edition.* New York: Springer. Print.

Jarvis, W.R. 2013. *Bennett & Brachman's Hospital Infections, 6th Edition.* New York: Lippincott, Williams, & Wilkins. Print.

Levy, J. 2010. *The World of Microbes: Bacteria, Viruses, and Other Microorganisms (Understanding Genetics).* New York: Rosen Classroom. Print.

McWhorter, B., and Schlafer, L. 2015. *How to Improve Workplace Safety: Learn Why Safety Programs Fail While Others Succeed.* Seattle: Amazon Digital Services, Inc. Digital.

The Microbe World. 2016. Classification of Microbes. Available at: www.edu.pe.ca/southern kings/microclass.htm. Prince Edward Island: Prince Edward Island, Canada Government.

Miller, C.H., and Palenik, C.J. 2013. *Infection Control and Management of Hazardous Materials for the Dental Team, 5th Edition.* Maryland Heights: Mosby. Print.

Occupational Health and Safety. 2016. Infection Prevention: Why It Matters in the Workplace. Available at: https://ohsonline.com/blogs/the-ohs-wire/2014/04/infection-prevention-why-it-matters-in-the-workplace.aspx. Dallas: Occupational Health and Safety – 1105 Media Inc.

Rideal, S. 2012. *Disinfection and Disinfectants (Chemical Substances Used as Antiseptics and Preservatives).* Seattle: Ulan Press. Print.

Safety Works! Maine Department of Labor. 2016. Create a Safe and Healthy Workplace. Available at: www.safetyworksmaine.com/safe_workplace. Bangor: Maine Department of Labor.

Sandle, T. 2015. *Pharmaceutical Microbiology: Essentials for Quality Assurance and Quality Control.* Sawston, UK: Woodhead Publishing. Print.

Smith, D. 2011. *Hand Hygiene: Guidelines for Best Practice.* Chipping Campden, UK: Campden BRI. Print.

Todar, K. 2016. Control of Microbial Growth. Available at: www.textbookofbacteriology.net/control.html. Madison: University of Wisconsin Department of Bacteriology.

U.S. Department of Labor, Occupational Safety and Health Administration. 2014. *Personal Protective Equipment.* Seattle: CreateSpace Independent Publishing Platform. Print.

U.S. Department of Labor. 2016. Personal Protective Equipment. Available at: www.osha.gov/sltc/personalprotectiveequipment. Washington, D.C.: U.S. Department of Labor.

Weston, D. 2008. *Infection Prevention and Control: Theory and Practice for Healthcare Professionals.* Hoboken: Wiley-Interscience. Print.

Weston, D. 2013. *Fundamentals of Infection Prevention and Control: Theory and Practice, 2nd Edition.* Hoboken: Wiley-Blackwell. Print.

Zelman, M., and Milne-Zelman, C. 2013. *Infection Control and Safety.* Upper Saddle River: Prentice Hall. Print.

Zollinger, R., and Ellison, E. 2010. *Zollinger's Atlas of Surgical Operations, 9th Edition.* New York: McGraw-Hill Education. Print.

Chapter 13

Occupational Safety and Health Administration (OSHA) standards

Objectives

After study of the chapter, readers should be able to:

1 Explain how hepatitis B and C are transmitted in the health care setting.
2 Describe components of the OSHA standard.
3 Explain the purpose of OSHA.
4 Describe an exposure control plan.
5 Explain the purpose of OSHA labeling requirements.
6 Detail what should be included in a fire safety and emergency plan.
7 List examples of potential fire hazards.
8 Explain what is contained on a chemical safety data sheet.
9 Explain ergonomics.
10 List measures used to reduce radiation hazards.

Overview

Accidents can happen at any time in any location, and are not uncommon in health care. Every health care professional has the critical responsibility to correct or remove chemical and physical hazards, as well as biohazardous materials, in order to prevent injuries to patients, health care workers, and other staff members. In the workplace, safety issues are of critical importance. Environmental protection measures were designed to minimize risks of occupational injuries, by removing or isolating mechanical or physical health hazards. The Occupational Safety and Health Act was passed by Congress in 1970. Its focus was the prevention of diseases and injuries in the workplace. This Act also established the Occupational Safety and Health Administration (OSHA). Previously, workplace injuries were common, and there was little government regulation that protected employees from harm.

Nearly every employer in the United States is impacted by the rules of OSHA, and must make stringent efforts to ensure employee health and safety. OSHA regulates many things in the workplace, including equipment, machinery, first aid, and materials used on the job. The working environment must be free of hazards such as extreme temperatures, excessive noise, dangerous machinery, toxic chemicals, and unsanitary conditions. The Occupational Health and Safety Review Commission oversees all OSHA standards.

OSHA Bloodborne Pathogens Standard

The Bloodborne Pathogens Standard was established by OSHA in 1991 to reduce occupational exposures to the *human immunodeficiency virus (HIV)* and the *hepatitis B virus (HBV)*. This standard identified certain health care professionals as *Category I employees*, meaning that they are at highest risk of exposure to communicable diseases from body fluids and other potentially infectious materials in the workplace. The following requirements are listed in the Bloodborne Pathogens Standard:

- Determining steps to take for various types of exposure
- Development of exposure control plans
- Follow-up procedures after exposures occur
- Proper biologic waste labeling and disposal
- Free hepatitis B vaccinations for all employees
- Standards concerning housekeeping and laundry
- Personal protective equipment standards
- Record-keeping standards
- Employee training about bloodborne pathogens and related practices
- The use of universal precautions
- Work practice standards.

You should remember

If an exposure occurs, the area of injury should immediately be washed very thoroughly, and a supervisor must be informed. A written incident report is then completed, and the injured employee must receive adequate medical testing and evaluation, as well as any needed post-exposure treatments. Failures of employers to comply with OSHA standards may result in penalties as high as $7,000 for each violation.
Source: www.osha.gov/pls/oshaweb/owadisp.show_document?
p_table=oshact&p_id=3371.

HIV and AIDS

The *human immunodeficiency virus* (HIV) attacks the immune system by destroying CD4 positive T-cells. These cells are vital for the body to fight off infection. When they are destroyed, an HIV-positive person becomes vulnerable to other infections, diseases, and various complications. *Autoimmune deficiency syndrome (AIDS)* is the final stage of HIV infection.

The HIV virus can be spread in several different ways, including:

- Unprotected sex, mostly through vaginal or anal intercourse
- Through the blood, such as by transfusion, accidental needlesticks, or by sharing needles
- The transplantation of infected tissue or organs
- Mother-to-child transmission via the placenta during birth or, rarely, via breastfeeding.

If HIV-positive blood is transfused, the recipient has a 90% chance of being infected. Needle sharing is the second most efficient method of spreading HIV, followed by sexual transmission. The virus is more easily transmitted from an infected male to an uninfected female than the reverse. There is about a 30 times greater chance of transmitting the virus through anal intercourse than through vaginal intercourse. The number of pregnant women living with HIV is 1.5 million (source: www.aids.gov/hiv-aids-basics/hiv-aids-101/global-statistics/index.html).

Initially, HIV was spread through unprotected sex between homosexual men, though in Africa it spread between men and women very quickly. In China, HIV spread at first due to infected blood transfusions, then through heterosexual sex and by sharing needles.

HIV attacks the immune system over time. After becoming infected with the virus, about half of all individuals will be diagnosed with AIDS within ten years. During the initial period of infection, the infectiousness of the virus is high. It also increases as the immune system becomes weakened and if there are any other sexually transmitted infections present. Deterioration of the immune system results in a series of opportunistic infections. Untreated HIV patients may develop herpes, tuberculosis, various cancers, toxoplasmosis, cryptococcal meningitis, or other infections.

To combat the spread of HIV and AIDS, there has been an increased effort to promote the use of condoms as well as the treatment of affected individuals with *antiretroviral* medications. Worldwide, of all adults living with HIV, 38% received antiretroviral therapy (ART), but only 24% of children living with HIV receive the same.

HIV and AIDS is more prevalent in sub-Saharan Africa than in any other region of the world. It is most common in people between the ages of 15 and 59. Today, more than 4.7% of adults in this part of Africa between the ages of 15 and 49 are HIV-positive. The HIV and AIDS epidemic is changing, and now ranks higher as a cause of death for African women than for men, whereas previously the reverse was true.

In 2012, 39% of new HIV infections worldwide occurred in people between the ages of 15 and 24. Knowledge of the disease and treatment in high-income countries has greatly reduced transmission of the virus between mothers and children. Overall, the number of infected children was reduced by 35% between 2009 and 2012. New HIV infections peaked globally in 1999. While HIV was the sixth leading cause of death for all age groups throughout the world in 2010, it was the second leading cause of death in sub-Saharan Africa, and in the 15- to 49-year-old age group, the *leading* cause of death.

Stopping or slowing the spread of HIV involves preventing new infections from occurring since there is no therapeutic vaccine available. Prevention efforts combine surveillance, education, communication, information, counseling and testing on a voluntary basis, condom promotion, screening and treatment for sexually transmitted infections, voluntary circumcision for males, antiretroviral treatment and avoidance of pregnancy for HIV-positive mothers, and efforts to stop transmission between high-risk and low-risk populations. Universal precautions in health care settings, blood safety practices, and measures to stop sharing of needles between injectable drug users are also proving successful.

The goals of worldwide HIV and AIDS prevention include the 90/90/90 plan, targeted to be achieved by the year 2020:

- 90% of HIV-positive individuals will know their status
- 90% of HIV-positive individuals will be receiving antiretroviral therapy
- 90% of individuals being treated will have suppressed viral loads.

You should remember

The risk of health care workers being exposed to HIV on the job is very low, especially when they use protective practices and equipment. The primary risk of HIV transmission is from being stuck with an HIV-contaminated needle or other sharp object. If such an exposure occurs, the CDC recommends immediate treatment with a short course of anti-retroviral drugs to prevent infection.

Focus on AIDS

As of 2016, there were 36.9 million people worldwide currently living with HIV/AIDS. In the United States, more than 1.2 million people have the HIV infection, and almost one in eight (12.8%) do not know they have it.
Sources: http://files.kff.org/attachment/fact-sheet-the-global-hivaids-epidemic; www.cdc.gov/hiv/statistics/overview/

Viral hepatitis

Hepatitis is inflammation of the liver, most commonly caused by viruses, but which may also be caused by other microorganisms, alcohol, drugs, or poisonous substances. There are six forms of viral hepatitis, which are signified with the letters A, B, C, D, E, and G. Many of these forms are extremely communicable. Fortunately, epidemics may be prevented through the use of vaccines. The biggest threats to health care employees from occupational exposure are the hepatitis B virus (HBV), hepatitis C virus (HCV), and HIV.

Hepatitis A

Hepatitis A is caused by the hepatitis A virus (HAV), and is the least serious. Most patients (98%) recover from hepatitis A. This disease is spread by the fecal–oral route, with the virus being spread through fecally contaminated food or water. The infection usually occurs in young adults, and is most commonly followed by complete recovery. Duration of the disease is from 15 to 45 days. In 15% of patients, relapses occur 6 to 12 months after the initial diagnosis. Prophylaxis with immune globulin is effective for household and sexual contact with the virus.

A vaccine for immunization is readily available, and is recommended for people who live in or travel to areas of the world that have poor sanitation and overcrowded conditions. It is also called *acute infective hepatitis*. The vaccine for hepatitis A is given in two separate doses. Table 13.1 lists the most important facts about various types of viral hepatitis.

Table 13.1 Viral hepatitis

Type	Incubation period	Transmission	Epidemiology	Infectivity
Hepatitis A virus (HAV)	15–20 days (average 28)	Fecal–oral (fecal contamination and oral ingestion)	Crowded conditions; poor personal hygiene or sanitation; contaminated food, milk, water, shellfish; subclinical infections; infected food handlers; sexual contact	Usually, 2 weeks before onset of symptoms; infectious 1–2 weeks after symptoms begin
Hepatitis B virus (HBV)	45–180 days (average 56–96)	Parenteral or mucosal exposure to blood or blood products; sexual contact; perinatal transmission	Contaminated needles, syringes, blood products; sexual contact; asymptomatic carrier contact; tattoos or body piercing with contaminated needles; bites	Infectious before and after symptoms appear, for 4–6 months; in carriers, continues throughout life
Hepatitis C virus (HCV)	14–180 days (average 56)	Parenteral or mucosal exposure to blood or blood products; high-risk sexual contact; perinatal transmission	Blood and blood products, needles, syringes, sexual contact	1–2 weeks prior to symptoms, continues during clinical course; 75–85% develop chronic hepatitis
Hepatitis D virus (HDV)	2–26 weeks; HBV must precede HDV; chronic HBV carriers always at risk	Only causes infection when HBV is present, with same routes of transmission	Same as HBV	Blood is infectious at all stages of HDV infection

continued

Table 13.1 Viral hepatitis

Type	Incubation period	Transmission	Epidemiology	Infectivity
Hepatitis E virus (HEV)	15–64 days (average 26–42)	Fecal–oral; outbreaks linked to contaminated water in developing countries	Contaminated water; poor sanitation; occurs in Asia, Africa, Mexico but not common in USA and Canada	Not known; may be similar to HAV
Hepatitis G virus (HGV)	Unknown	Blood, sexual contact; only rare perinatal transmission	Sharing needles, hemodialysis patients, transfusion and organ transplant recipients, sexual contact	Infection reported in 10–20% of people with chronic HBV or HCV infection

Source: www.cdc.gov/hepatitis/resources/professionals/pdfs/abctable.pdf.

> **You should remember**
>
> Those at highest risk of contracting hepatitis A include travelers to countries with higher prevalence of the virus, male homosexuals, users of both injection and non-injection illegal drugs, people with clotting factor disorders, and people who work in zoos or research involving contact with monkeys or apes.

Hepatitis B

The hepatitis B virus (HBV) damages the liver, and may be acute or chronic. In fact, it is a leading risk factor for certain cancers of the liver, along with the hepatitis C virus. The hepatitis B virus is transmitted through contact with an infected person's blood or body fluids. Some 95% of patients clear the infection and develop antibodies to HBV. The remaining 5% who are unable to clear the virus develop chronic infections that put them at risk for long-term complications. Severe infection may cause prolonged illness.

Hepatitis B is also called *serum hepatitis*. Approximately 240 million people worldwide are chronically infected with HBV. Prevalence is highest in South Africa and Eastern Asia, where between 5 and 10% of adults are chronically infected. Over 780,000 people around the world die annually because of complications of HBV, which include cirrhosis and liver cancer. Hepatitis B is an important occupational hazard for health care workers, since it can survive outside the body for at least seven days. However, its survival depends on factors such as temperature, humidity, and sunlight. The virus has very low infectivity outside of body fluids.

In highly endemic areas, hepatitis B is often spread from mother to child at birth, or through exposure to infected blood, especially between infected and uninfected children during the first five years of life. The virus is also spread by percutaneous or mucosal exposure to infected blood or body fluids, which include saliva, menstrual, vaginal, and seminal fluids. Most infected people have no symptoms during the acute phase. Some develop symptoms that last for several weeks, including jaundice, dark urine, extreme fatigue, nausea, vomiting, and abdominal pain. Fortunately, over 90% of healthy adults naturally recover from the hepatitis B virus within one year.

Laboratory confirmation of HBV is essential, and there are many blood tests available that can also distinguish between acute and chronic infections. The World Health Organization recommends that all blood donations be tested for HBV. Once confirmed in a patient, there is no specific treatment for HBV infection. Care includes adequate nutrition, fluid replacement, and oral antiviral agents (for chronic cases), including the drugs tenofovir or entecavir. For most people, treatment for HBV will continue throughout life. Unfortunately for many people throughout the world, limited access to diagnosis means that they are diagnosed only when they have already developed advanced liver disease.

When an infant is born to a mother who has hepatitis B, the infant must receive the HBV vaccine and immune globulin within 24 hours. Additional HBV vaccines must be administered to the infant after one month, and then at six months. All children and adolescents younger than 18 years of age, and not previously vaccinated, are recommended to receive the HBV vaccine if they live in countries with low or intermediate occurrence of hepatitis B. Unfortunately, in many of these countries, access to the vaccine is very limited, if it is available at all.

High-risk individuals should also receive the HBV vaccine, which is given in three doses. They include:

- Those who are in contact with blood or body fluids of infected people, including physicians, dentists, dental hygienists, nurses, and laboratory personnel
- Those often requiring blood or blood products
- Dialysis patients
- Recipients of solid organ transplants
- People who are imprisoned or work in prisons
- Injectable drug users
- Those with casual or sexual contact with people who have chronic HBV
- Those with multiple sexual partners
- Health care workers and others who may be exposed to blood or blood products
- Travelers who have not received a hepatitis B vaccination series.

The hepatitis B vaccine, first developed in 1982, has been successful in preventing hundreds of thousands of deaths annually, including those from cirrhosis and liver cancer. The vaccine is 95% effective, and was the first vaccine to protect against a major cause of cancer.

OSHA requires that all health care professionals be immunized against hepatitis B since they are at risk for exposure to bloodborne pathogens. The HBV vaccine must be available at no cost to these professionals, regardless of whether they work part time or full time, within ten days of beginning employment. Each employee may decline the immunization but must sign paperwork, which will be kept in their records, indicating that they did not receive the immunization. If the employee decides at a later time to receive the immunization, it is still administered without charge. The hepatitis B vaccine is available in various formulations and trade names. Over one billion doses of the hepatitis B vaccines have been administered worldwide, and the rate of chronic infection in most countries has been greatly reduced. As of 2013, more than 81% of children in 183 countries have received the vaccine.

You should remember

In the United States, President Bill Clinton signed a law that all children could receive free hepatitis B vaccines prior to age 18.

Hepatitis C

The hepatitis C virus (HCV) can cause both acute and chronic hepatitis infections, which range from mild to severe, and can last from a few weeks to an entire lifetime. The blood-borne hepatitis C virus is most often transmitted through sharing needles by intravenous drug users, inadequate sterilization of medical equipment, and transfusion of unscreened blood and blood products. Almost 80% of infected people remain asymptomatic for 10–20 years. There is no vaccine currently available for hepatitis C. However, because hepatitis C carriers are vulnerable to severe hepatitis if they contract hepatitis A or B, vaccination against hepatitis A and B is recommended. Hepatitis C is also called *parenterally transmitted non-A non-B hepatitis*. Remember that the term *parenteral* refers to the piercing of the skin or mucous membranes.

Between 130 and 150 million people throughout the world have chronic hepatitis C infection. Many of these people will develop cirrhosis or liver cancer. Nearly 500,000 people die annually from hepatitis C-related liver diseases.

Focus on chronic hepatitis C

People with hepatitis C have significant chances of developing serious complications. Chronic infection develops in 75–85% of patients, and 60–70% will develop chronic liver disease. Cirrhosis will occur in 5–20% of patients, and 1–5% will die from consequences of chronic infection, which include liver cancer and cirrhosis.

Source: https://consumer.healthday.com/encyclopedia/
hepatitis-c-23/hepatitis-news-373/what-can-i-expect-
over-time-with-hepatitis-c-645180.html.

Hepatitis D

The hepatitis D virus is also known as the *delta hepatitis*. It cannot replicate without the hepatitis B virus being present. Together, the hepatitis B and D viruses can cause worsening of symptoms and an increased risk of the development of chronic hepatitis with sudden and severe signs and symptoms. The hepatitis D virus is transmitted sexually and through needle sharing. The only treatment is the prevention of HBV. While uncommon in the United States, hepatitis D is most prevalent in Italy and the former country of Yugoslavia. There is no vaccine currently available for hepatitis D.

Hepatitis E

The hepatitis E virus is spread through the fecal–oral route, which often occurs because of contaminated food or water. It is a self-limited type of hepatitis occurring primarily in Asia and Africa. This type of hepatitis does not cause chronic hepatitis. However, it can be fatal to women who are pregnant. Outbreaks of epidemic hepatitis E occur most often after heavy rainfall or monsoons, due to disruption of water supplies. There is no vaccine currently available for hepatitis E.

Hepatitis G

The hepatitis G virus is linked to blood transfusions, but is also transferred through sexual intercourse and pregnancy. Infection is of widespread occurrence and patients are either asymptomatic or have mild symptoms. Hepatitis G is seen in patients after drug transfusions, in those undergoing hemodialysis, and in IV drug abusers. It is also seen in infants born to infected mothers. The virus is not primarily replicated in the liver. This form of hepatitis may be carried throughout life. There is no vaccine currently available for hepatitis G.

Focus on immunization of health care workers

The hepatitis A and hepatitis B vaccines are extremely safe.

- The hepatitis A vaccine is administered in one intramuscular dose, followed by an individual dose 6–18 months later.
- The hepatitis B vaccine is administered in one intramuscular dose, followed by additional doses at one and six months later.

Components of the OSHA Standard

The components of the OSHA Bloodborne Pathogens Standard begin with universal precautions, and include a written exposure control plan that addresses how to handle exposure incidents, labeling requirements, and accurate record-keeping.

Universal precautions

In the health care setting, universal precautions are used in the control of infection. Employees and employers must assume that all blood, blood products, tissues, and most body fluids are infectious for pathogens such as HIV and HBV. Fluids that may contain pathogens also include fluids with visible blood, semen, cerebrospinal fluid, vaginal secretions, amniotic fluid, pleural fluid, synovial fluid, peritoneal fluid, pericardial fluid, feces, urine, nasal secretions, sputum, breast milk, tears, saliva, and vomitus. Universal precautions are also required when dealing with broken skin and all mucous membranes.

Health care facilities utilize *Standard Precautions*, which combine universal precautions with rules designed to reduce disease transmission in relation to moist body substances. These rules are known as *Body Substance Isolation (BSI) guidelines*. Standard precautions are extremely important, and are used for the care of all patients. They apply to the following:

- Blood
- Mucous membranes
- Non-intact skin
- All body fluids, secretions, and excretions – except sweat.

Standard precautions help protect against pathogens being transmitted when infected blood contacts another individual's skin – especially when the skin has been punctured or wounded, as well as when infected blood contacts another individual's mucous membranes. Therefore, standard precautions reduce the likelihood of disease transmission between all individuals, including patients and health care professionals.

The safeguards that must be applied for each specific medical procedure or *task* are based on the unique level of risk involved, which concerns the amount of likely exposure to potentially infectious substances. OSHA outlines the levels of risk and the safeguards that must be applied, which include:

- Hand washing
- Gloves
- Mask and protective eyewear or face shield
- Laboratory coat or gown
- Reusable sharps containers
- Sharps disposal
- Biohazardous waste containers
- Disinfection.

The three categories of *task* designated by OSHA, in relation to Standard Precautions, are as follows:

- *Category I* – The health care professional may be exposed to blood, body fluids, or tissues.

  - The task being performed may have a chance of spilling or splashing, such as minor surgical procedures.
  - Specific protective measures are required, which include hand washing, gloves, mask, protective eyewear or face shield, protective clothing, handling disposable and non-disposable sharps, and decontaminating work surfaces.

- *Category II* – No special protection is usually required since there is often no visible blood, but there may be exposure in certain situations.

  - The task being performed may require mouth-to-mouth resuscitation, saliva exposure.
  - Protective measures may include gloves, disposable airway equipment, or resuscitation bags.
  - The particular concern is transmission of HIV or hepatitis B.

- *Category III* – No special protection required since there is no exposure to blood, body fluids, or tissues; however, you should check for any open wounds before performing any procedure.

  - The task being performed may require taking blood pressure, instilling medicated nose drops, instructing a patient about using medical equipment, taking care of a cast, or other procedures.
  - Protective measures may include hand washing.

Written exposure control plan

OSHA requires every medical facility to have a *written* exposure control plan, which is a procedure about how people should be treated after exposure to biohazardous or other harmful substances. It is designed to minimize risks of exposure and must be updated as necessary. All employees must have access to the plan if they are at risk of bloodborne exposure. Each new employee whose job may put them at risk must review the plan when they begin employment. All at-risk employees must review exposure control plans on an annual basis. Written copies must be supplied to any employee requesting them. Every written exposure control plan must include the following information:

- *Employee exposure determination* – this identifies employees requiring training, protective equipment, hepatitis immunization, and other OSHA-required protections; it must list all job classifications for every employee likely to have occupational exposures, as well as those classifications in which only certain employees are likely to have occupational exposures.
- *Exposure control method implementation* (also known as *method of compliance*) – this documents specific measures that can be taken to eliminate or minimize risks of occupational exposure, including:
  - Engineering and work practice controls
  - Housekeeping
  - Personal protective equipment
  - Universal precautions.
- *Vaccination for hepatitis B.*
- *Post-exposure evaluation, and procedures for follow-up* – this specifies procedures to follow when an occupational exposure occurs, how it should be documented and investigated, and how it must be followed up.
- *Employee hazard communication and training.*
- *Record-keeping.*

Focus on employee OSHA training

Medical employers must provide training for all employees who are at risk for occupational exposures. The training must be provided the first time an employee is assigned to tasks that could result in exposure, and at least once per year of employment after that.

Exposure incidents

An *exposure incident* occurs when an employee believes he or she has come into contact with a potentially infectious substance, despite all precautions. Exposure incidents are handled according to the OSHA Bloodborne Pathogens Standard. In health care, most exposure incidents involve needlesticks and other types of skin puncture. Serious infections including HIV and HBV must be taken into account.

When an exposure incident occurs, the employer must be notified immediately in order to reduce the likelihood of the injured employee developing a disease. The employer can take steps so that the employee receives prompt treatment, to ensure others are not infected. Prompt reporting also helps to prevent the same exposure incident from happening again. The employer must offer a free medical evaluation to the employee. A licensed health care provider can then counsel the employee about the incident and preventing the spread of a potential infection. A blood sample will be taken and an appropriate treatment will be prescribed. Employees do have the right to refuse medical evaluation and treatment, but this refusal must be documented. In most cases, the employee should be tested for HBV and receive the vaccination if necessary. For example, if a patient's blood has potentially exposed a health care professional to infection, the patient should be tested for HBV and the health care professional notified of the test results. If the patient in this case did not wish to be tested, the health care professional should be tested. If the health care professional does not wish to be tested, a blood sample must be kept for 90 days should symptoms of infection develop.

When a post-exposure evaluation has been completed, the employer must receive a written report that states if HBV vaccination was recommended and received. The report must also state if the employee was informed of the results of any blood tests performed. All additional information must be kept confidential.

Health care professionals must also be evaluated for exposure to HCV or HIV. The estimated risk of infection after a needlestick or other exposure to HCV-infected blood is approximately 1 in 50. Risks following a blood splash to mucous membranes are unknown, but believed to be very small. Evaluation after exposure to HCV or HIV may consist of one or several blood tests, along with patient history. The average risk for HIV infection after a needlestick or other exposure to HIV-infected blood is approximately 1 in 300. The risk after exposure of the mucous membranes is estimated to be about 1 in 1,000.

Labeling requirements

Biohazard warning labels must be applied to anything containing biohazardous materials. These include containers of regulated waste, freezers or refrigerators that store blood or other potentially infectious materials, and any containers or bags used to store, transport, or ship these materials. Red bags or containers are acceptable substitutes for biohazard warning labels. Biohazard and hazard labels are discussed in detail below.

Record-keeping

The OSHA Bloodborne Pathogens Standard requires two types of records to be maintained, as follows:

- *An accurate OSHA medical record* – maintained by the employer, for every employee at risk for occupational exposure. This is kept confidential, for review by OSHA officials, and as required by law. This record must contain the employee's name, social security number, hepatitis B vaccination status with dates of vaccination, post-exposure examination results, medical tests, follow-up procedures, and a written evaluation of exposure incidents with their exposure incident reports. This record must be kept by the employer for the duration of each applicable individual's employment, plus 30 years.
- *A sharps injury log* – this is required for employers who have more than ten employees who are at risk of occupational exposures from contaminated sharps. This log must protect confidentiality of injured employees by removing all personal identification. It is designed to help employers and employees track all needlestick injuries, and to identify problem areas requiring attention and devices that may be ineffective and need replacement. The sharps injury log must contain the type and brand of device involved in injury, location inside the work area where the incident occurred, and an explanation of what happened.

OSHA Hazard Communication

The OSHA Hazard Communication standard requires all employees to be trained in workplace hazards. This training must include methods to read and understand the documents that accompany hazardous substances and how to handle exposures. Each hazardous material must be labeled correctly. Every employee must be able to access all related documentation, including the steps to take in order to protect themselves from being harmed.

Biohazard labels

Biohazard labels, containing the biohazard symbol, must be applied to every container that stores waste products, blood or blood products, and other specimens that may be contaminated with bloodborne pathogens, since these are considered to be *biohazardous*. The biohazard symbol is bright orange-red in color. It has clear lettering that states "biohazard" at the top and "infectious waste" at the bottom. Biohazard labels must always be securely attached to containers. Facilities that have biohazardous materials present must also post warning signs that alert individuals to the presence of these materials. The warning signs must also list important safeguards to follow in relation to eating, drinking, smoking, mouth pipetting, application of cosmetics or lip balm, and touching of contact lenses.

Hazard labels

Every hazardous substance in the workplace must be identified with *hazard labels* as well as material safety data sheets (MSDS). A hazard label is a shorter version of the MSDS, and is permanently attached to containers that store hazardous substances. According to OSHA, each hazard label must list the chemical or trade name of the biohazardous material and a short statement of its hazardous effects. No color-coding or numbering system that requires training is specified by OSHA. If a hazard label does have color-coding or numbering, you must contact the manufacturer for an explanation of this information, since such information is not consistent between manufacturers.

Hazardous waste management

Hazardous wastes may be in a variety of forms, including gases, liquids, solids, and semi-solids. These substances are not clean, disinfected, or sterilized. Hazardous wastes may be classified as having any of the following properties:

- Caustic – able to cause burns or other damage to body tissues
- Corrosive – able to destroy metal
- Cytotoxic – able to kill cells
- Ignitable – able to create fires
- Radioactive
- Reactive – able to cause explosions or fumes because of instability
- Toxic.

The Environmental Protection Agency (EPA) classifies hazardous wastes as either *F-list* (in which there is no specific source), *K-list* (in which there is a specific source), or *P-list*, also called *U-list* (which includes discarded commercial chemicals).

It is absolutely essential that hazardous wastes are handled safely, at all times. To minimize possible contact, proper protective handling equipment must be worn when hazardous materials are handled. There are strict regulations in place concerning hazardous wastes, which cover air emissions, closure of containers, groundwater monitoring, proper clean-up procedures, land disposal restrictions, and highly controlled permitting procedures.

Focus on regulated medical waste

In the medical office, waste products are generated during regular activities in treating patients. Some of these waste products are referred to as *regulated medical waste* because of specific characteristics, which include:

- Liquid or semi-liquid blood products or other potentially infectious materials (OPIM)
- Items contaminated with blood products or OPIM, which could be released if compressed (squeezed)
- Items with dried blood products or OPIM, which could be released during handling procedures
- Contaminated sharps
- Pathologic or microbiologic wastes containing blood products or OPIM.

Disposal of hazardous wastes

All materials that have come into contact with blood or body fluids must be treated as hazardous wastes, which may consist of used needles, as well as linen or clothing contaminated with blood or body fluids. In order to avoid risk of contact exposures, these items must be properly contained. Leak-proof, puncture-proof containers are used to contain sharps such as needles, scalpels, glass slides, or disposable syringes (see Figure 13.1). These containers are labeled with the *biohazard symbol*, which informs anyone working with them that the contents are hazardous.

Plastic biohazard bags are used to contain soft materials such as dressings, gloves, and paper towels. These bags are also labeled with the biohazard symbol. Figure 13.2 shows a biohazard container, with a biohazard bag, for contaminated soft items such as gauze and gloves.

The removal and disposal of hazardous wastes are usually handled by specialized companies. Cleaning staff of facilities that have hazardous waste containers must be instructed never to empty them. When hazardous waste bags are changed, employees who handle them must wear personal protective equipment that includes gloves, eyewear, and masks. Hazardous waste bags must be closed securely. If there is any possibility of leakage, they must be placed inside a second hazardous waste bag, which must also be closed securely. This *double-bagging technique* is the best way to safely remove contaminated items. Anyone removing such items should wear proper personal protective equipment. Bags should be appropriately labeled as to what they contain, with hazardous waste or linen markers so that others are alerted that they require special handling.

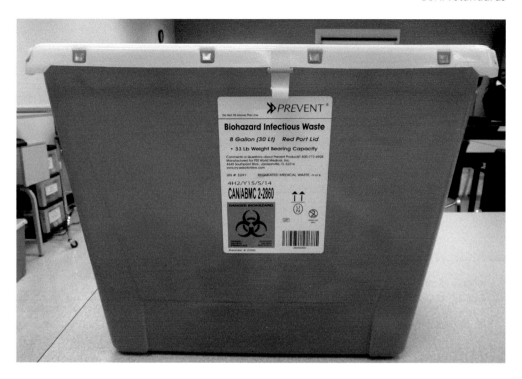

Figure 13.1 Sharps container.

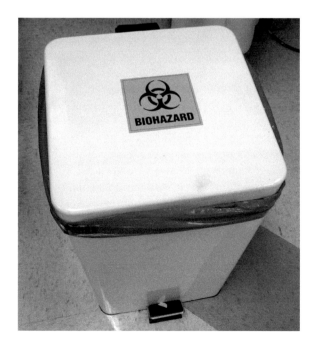

Figure 13.2 Biohazard container for soft items.

Use of personal protective equipment

Personal protective equipment (PPE) is used regularly by many health care professionals. This equipment may include face shields, gloves, goggles, gowns, hair covers, masks, shoe covers, and surgical gowns with cuffs. All of these barrier precautions are designed to protect employees from exposure to pathogenic microorganisms and other hazards. They create a barrier between skin, mucous membranes, or non-intact skin and possibly harmful or infectious materials. The term *non-intact* refers to skin that has a break in its surface, and includes abrasions, burns, chapping, cuts, hangnails, and conditions such as acne or dermatitis.

Each type of personal protective equipment has specific uses. For example, if there is a possibility of body fluids being splashed or splattered, employees should wear face shields, goggles, and masks. When gowns, lab coats, or scrubs are worn while working, they must be left in the work facility in a special area designed to store them. Gloves, either latex or non-latex, are commonly worn on a regular basis by most health care professionals while at work. Proper glove guidelines include the following:

- Keep fingernails trimmed short to reduce risk of tearing gloves
- Always wear the correct glove size
- Avoid oil-based hand lotions or creams; these can deteriorate natural rubber latex gloves
- Never store gloves in extremely warm or cold areas, because they may be deteriorated by these conditions.

Fire safety and emergency plan

To comply with OSHA, a fire safety and emergency plan must have written procedures that clearly detail building exits, clearly labeled fire doors and escape routes, fire alarm pull boxes, smoke detectors, and fire extinguishers. Fire alarm pull boxes must be located high enough on walls for easy use by most employees. They are activated by pulling down on their handles. Fire sprinklers should be mounted on ceilings throughout the building. Clear escape routes must be posted around the facility where employees can easily see them (see Figure 13.3), and employers must provide fire prevention training. Emergency phone numbers must be posted near all telephones. Hallways should free from excessive items that may impede safe evacuation. Periodic fire drills must also be conducted, and both fire alarm and sprinkler systems must be tested. Daily work schedules should be used so that everyone inside the facility can be accounted for in case of emergency.

Part of the emergency and fire training that employees should be aware of is to always avoid using an elevator to exit the building and instead use the stairs. Employees should also be trained how to correctly report a fire or other emergency. Fire containment should be practiced, as well as how to ascertain that an "all clear" can be given and employees can return to work.

Fire hazards include electrical wires, improperly grounded plugs, overloaded circuits, paper, matches, rags, lighters, other flammable items, insufficient protective measures when oxygen is in use, and smoking in the facility. All potential fire hazards must be regularly reported and corrected. Smells of smoke or burning must also be reported immediately. Wastepaper cans must always be emptied into accepted receptacles on a regular basis. Supplies must never be stacked so high that they are less than 18 inches from the ceiling – this prevents the fire sprinklers from working effectively. Fire prevention takes into account three major components: a source of ignition, presence of oxygen, and enough heat to ignite a fire.

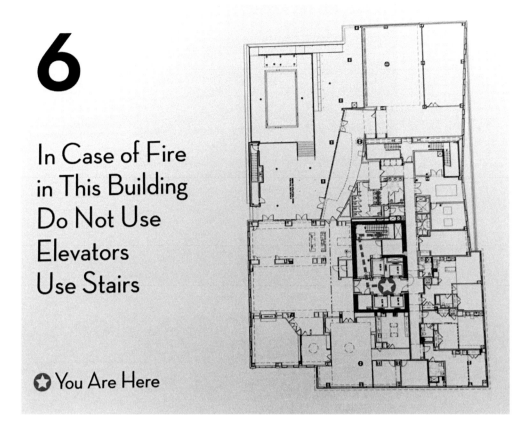

6

In Case of Fire
in This Building
Do Not Use
Elevators
Use Stairs

⭐ You Are Here

Figure 13.3 Clear escape route indicated, as part of a fire safety plan.

If an employee discovers a fire before an alarm has been sounded, he or she should attempt to extinguish it. However, if this is not possible, the alarm should be sounded. All employees should exit the building, closing doors behind them as they leave. This helps to isolate any fires and keep them from spreading quickly. Fire extinguishers are of three primary types: A, B, and C. They use either carbon dioxide (in types B and C), water (in type A), a multi-purpose dry chemical (in all three types), or a regular dry chemical (in types B and C). An example of a fire extinguisher is shown in Figure 13.4.

Oxygen hazards

The administration of oxygen is commonly used when a patient cannot breathe in enough oxygen normally. Devices used for oxygen delivery, along with the amount administered and length it is required, are determined by the physician. The use of oxygen requires special precautions because it is highly flammable. These special precautions include the following:

● *Electrical sparks* – electrical appliances, equipment, and even toys should be kept out of areas where oxygen is in use because they can cause sparks, which could trigger an explosion; examples of these items include computer games, electric shavers, fans, hair-dryers, heating pads, radios, and space heaters.

319

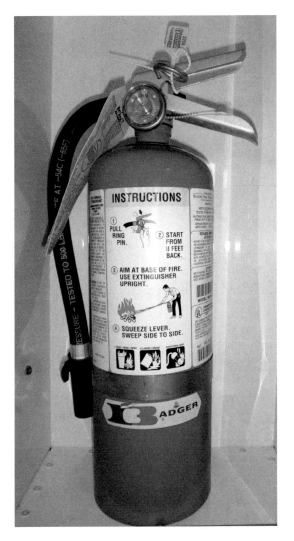

Figure 13.4 A fire extinguisher.

- *Flammable liquids* – these include adhesive tape remover, alcohol, nail polish or nail polish remover, and various oils.
- *Proper use of oxygen tanks* – tanks must be secured so that they do not fall over, and must not be placed near heat or in the sunlight; valves and stems on oxygen tanks must be handled with care to avoid sudden release of pressure.
- *Smoking* – no smoking is allowed anywhere near the use of oxygen; therefore, no smoking materials, including matches and open flames, are allowed.
- *Special signs* – "oxygen in use" signs should be posted when oxygen is being used, according to the facility's policies and procedures manual.
- *Static electricity* – since this can create sparks, no synthetic or wool materials should be used, including clothing, blankets, and gowns; cotton is the preferred fabric since it does not create sparks.

Fire prevention

In health care facilities, safe practices to prevent fires are essential. A great deal of medical equipment requires high voltage, and can be a potential fire hazard. Additional fire hazards include flammable chemicals such as alcohol, certain disinfectants, as well as oxygen and other types of gases. Flammable liquids must always be kept away from heat sources. Material safety data sheets provide detailed information on the flammability of each chemical in the workplace. It is crucial for all health care professionals to understand and practice proper fire-prevention techniques. Paper products such as table coverings may also be fire hazards. All flammable items must be stored properly and disposed of in specific ways to minimize these potential hazards.

No smoking is permitted in medical facilities, because it is both a fire hazard and a health hazard. Therefore, "No Smoking" signs are displayed throughout health care practices of all types. Smoke detectors must be working properly, with batteries changed on a regular basis. Preferred smoke detectors have both sound and visual modes that quickly alert everyone in the facility to the presence of smoke.

In certain facilities, open flames are used for medical procedures. If this is required, it is important to extinguish the flames immediately after finishing the procedure, and keep hair and clothing away from the source of the flame. Any chemicals being used during an open-flame procedure must be verified concerning flammability. Fire extinguishers should be nearby whenever open flames are being used. It is important never to lean over an open flame or to leave it unattended. When finished, gas valves that supply the fuel for the flame must be turned off completely. Adequate ventilation is required whenever open flames are used.

You should remember

When a fire occurs in the workplace, your basic response procedures should be as follows, using the "R-A-C-E" acronym:

Rescue anyone who is in immediate danger
Activate the fire alarm or fire code system, notifying appropriate people
Confine the fire by closing windows and doors
Evacuate people to a safe location, and/or **extinguish** the fire if possible.

Focus on emergency situations

It is critical to remain calm when an emergency situation occurs. This allows you to think clearly and make critical decisions that will be more focused on what is required to make the best of what is happening. For example, many fires can be easily extinguished before they become larger and more dangerous. Therefore, it is important to know the location and proper use of fire extinguishers and all equipment that is available for emergency use.

Chemical hazards and safety

Chemical hazards may have a variety of harmful effects, and are under strict OSHA controls when used in the workplace. Employers must strive to protect their employees from exposure to hazardous chemicals. Exposure to chemicals can occur through direct absorption via the skin or breaks in the skin, inhalation, entry through mucous membranes, and ingestion. All employees must receive information and training about safe work practices concerning chemicals. If special equipment or conditions are required when using the chemical, all individuals must comply.

OSHA requires a safety data sheet for each hazardous chemical present in the workplace (see Appendix A). These sheets contain the chemical's trade name, chemical name, synonyms, chemical family, manufacturer information, emergency telephone number, hazardous ingredients, physical data, fire and explosion data, health hazard information, and protection information. Chemical containers must also be tightly sealed in between usages. Chemical spill clean-up kits must be present close to areas where chemicals are being used.

Examples of chemical hazards include those that are:

● Carcinogenic – able to cause cancer
● Caustic – able to cause corrosion or burning of body tissues
● Flammable – able to start a fire
● Poisonous – able to cause illness or death if ingested
● Teratogenic – able to cause birth defects.

All hazardous substances must be stored below eye level to reduce risks of being spilled into the eyes of employees. Protective gear must be worn to protect from harm or damage to clothing – this gear must be removed before leaving the workplace. Chemical containers must be carried with both hands for safety. Hazardous chemicals must be used only in properly ventilated areas.

Important steps that must be followed when working with chemicals include the following:

● If safety data sheets indicate, wear a personal ventilation device when working with specific chemicals.
● If you must smell chemicals that you use, hold them a few inches away from your nose and fan them toward you – never hold them directly under your nose.
● If the chemical's vapor may be hazardous, work inside a fume hood.
● Never combine chemicals in any way not specified as safe.
● Never use mouth pipetting with chemicals.
● Acids, when being combined with other chemicals, must always be added to the other chemicals. This is because adding substances to an acid increases splashing risks.
● If there is an unknown chemical spilled, never pour another chemical onto it. It must be cleaned up following the facility's hazardous waste control procedures. Never touch any unknown substance with your hands.

Everyone working in the facility must understand all hazardous chemicals present, their health risks, and the information contained on their safety data sheets and hazard labels. All potentially hazardous chemicals must have hazard labels. Employers must also have a *chemical hygiene plan* outlining all chemicals, their safe handling, and their disposal procedures.

Employees must be fully trained about chemical exposures, chemical hygiene, and safety procedures. In case of emergency chemical exposure situations, as well as exposures to body fluids, the work environment must have *eyewash stations* available for employees (see Figure 13.5). Employees must be trained in their proper usage. Also, *every* health care facility is required by law to provide these stations. Eyewash stations are used when anyone is exposed to chemicals or body fluids. They allow the employee to flush out the eyes or mucous membranes with water as quickly as possible after contact with a potentially hazardous substance. Eyewash stations must be located in areas that are easy to access, in spite of limited vision or no vision. They must be checked monthly to verify that they are working correctly.

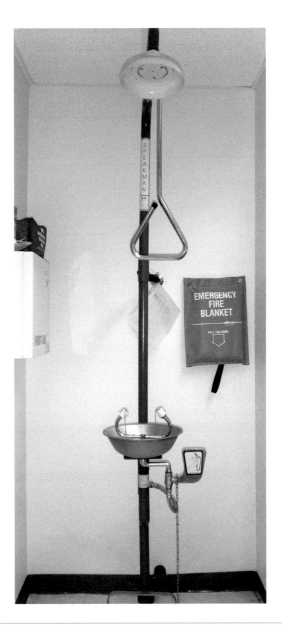

Figure 13.5 Eyewash station.

> ## Focus on eyewash stations
>
> Eyewash stations are designed to allow for rinsing of the eyes after contact with a potentially harmful substance. Prior to using them, contact lenses should be removed, and the injured individual should not rub his or her eyes in order to avoid further absorption of the substance. The eyes should be washed for a minimum of 15 minutes. After this, the injured individual should be taken to the emergency department of the local hospital.

> ## Focus on chemical hazards
>
> Examples of potentially hazardous chemicals in the workplace include alcohol, anesthetic substances, chemotherapeutic agents, cleaning solutions, dermatologic agents, disinfectants, immune agents, neurotoxic substances, sensitizers, and agents that may have pneumoconiotic (dust inhalation) dangers.

Physical safety

All appropriate steps must be taken to ensure physical safety in the medical office. Emergency phone numbers must be posted in multiple locations so that they can be easily accessed. Emergency numbers should be verified that they are accurate and up-to-date every three months. Common-sense steps to assure physical safety include:

- Keeping floors clear of objects
- Not allowing anyone to run in the facility, only walk
- Cleaning up spills immediately after they occur
- Carpet that is in good condition, without damaged areas that could cause people to trip
- Immediate disposal of all medications accidently dropped on the floor
- Careful carrying of items, especially near corners of hallways
- Keeping all drawers, cabinets, doors, and desks closed when not in use
- Regular inspection of furniture to prevent sharp corners or rough edges
- Taping down and fastening of all cables and cords that run along walls
- Avoiding use of cracked, chipped, or otherwise damaged supplies or equipment.

In laboratories, additional physical safety practices include:

- Avoiding eating or drinking, as well as the storage of food; also, laboratory beakers and other containers should never be used for eating or drinking
- Avoiding putting anything into the mouth while working, since it could be contaminated by chemicals or other substances
- Never inserting contact lenses, applying lip balm, or applying make-up in the laboratory
- Making sure everyone knows where first-aid kits are located, and that they are fully stocked with supplies; all medications in the kit must not have passed their expiration dates
- Making sure everyone knows the location and proper operation of eyewash and/or shower stations in the facility

- Wearing of appropriate protective gear and clothing, including heat-resistant hand protection and closed-toed shoes with rubber soles
- Avoiding the wearing of loose clothing or dangling jewelry
- Keeping the hair pulled back or covered
- Waiting for centrifuges to stop spinning before opening
- Never grasping containers if they, or your hands, are wet
- Closing containers immediately after being used
- Cleaning up broken glass with a broom and dustpan in order to avoid handling it – if the spilled material is biohazardous, use tongs or forceps to pick it up and put the broken pieces into a proper container that is labeled to identify its contents.

Latex allergy

Gloves are extremely important during most medical procedures, and especially during surgery. The gloves you wear must be of proper size, and made of nitrile, vinyl, or latex. Gloves that are too big can catch on equipment or instruments and result in accidents. The wearing of gloves is required during any procedure in which there may be exposure to potentially infectious or hazardous materials. Gloves also help to protect the patient from any infectious organisms on the hands of the health care professional.

For many years, latex gloves were preferred in the health care industry. This has changed because of the increased occurrence of latex allergies among health care professionals. Reactions to latex most commonly involve allergic contact dermatitis and, less commonly, irritant contact dermatitis. When an allergic reaction to latex is extremely serious, immediate hypersensitivity occurs, which can cause shock and even death. The powder in latex gloves, which makes them easier to put on, is one of the primary sources of latex allergy, since the latex protein that causes the allergy mixes with the powder. When the gloves are removed, the powder containing the latex protein enters the air and is inhaled. Therefore, many health care facilities have switched to hypoallergenic low-powder or powderless latex-free gloves (see Figure 13.6). Latex, which is derived from rubber trees in Brazil, causes allergic responses in 8–12% of individuals. Other products containing latex include blood pressure cuffs, catheters, stethoscopes, and wound drains.

Ergonomics

A term known as *human engineering*, or ergonomics, is the science concerned with the design of equipment and environments for human needs. Ergonomics is focused on increasing the comfort, performance, and well-being of workers. When chairs and desks are ergonomically designed, they help to reduce discomfort and fatigue. To prevent muscle fatigue of the upper extremities, the computer keyboard should be placed at a level that is lower than that of a conventional desk. An adjustable chair with adequate back support should be used to attain the correct typing height for each individual working with a computer (see Figure 13.7). When an employee is suffering from extreme fatigue, it affects his or her ability to respond appropriately, resulting in faulty decision-making and poor problem-solving. Employers should follow the OSHA ergonomic standards when they design their workplace environments. Ergonomics also extends into physical movements while working that help to avoid injury, such as using the legs to support lifting a heavy weight, rather than using the lower back.

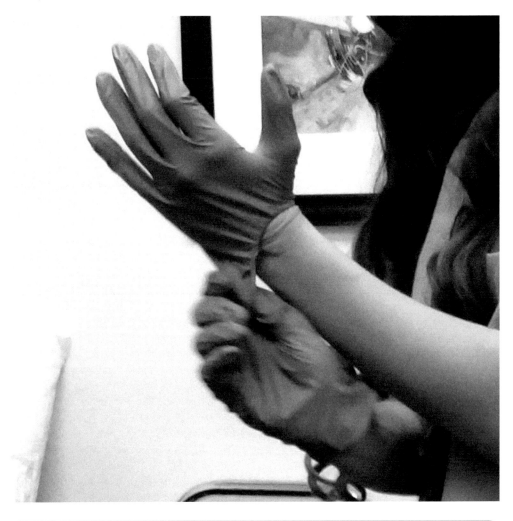

Figure 13.6 Latex-free gloves.

Employers must provide printed information to their employees concerning work-related musculoskeletal disorders. This includes common disorders, common hazards, how to report these disorders, the signs and symptoms of these disorders, why it is important to report them early, and a summary of OSHA standards and requirements. Steps to decrease risks of injury when lifting include:

- Plan how you will lift the load, and test it
- Ask for help to lift the load
- Make sure you have a firm footing
- Bend your knees
- Tighten your abdominal muscles
- Use your legs to lift
- Keep the load close when lifting
- Keep your back straight and upright.

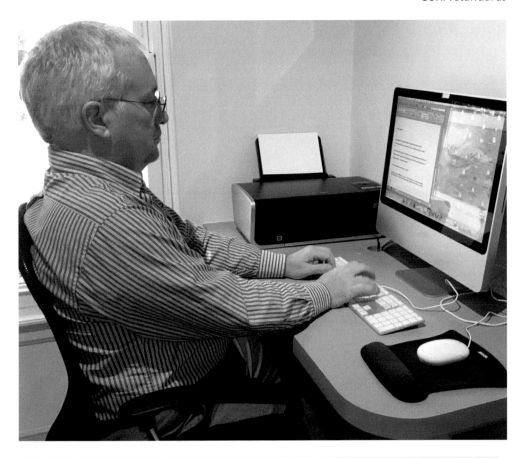

Figure 13.7 Keyboard ergonomics.

You should remember

Ergonomics can greatly help to reduce strain upon the body, as well as any resulting injury. It accomplishes this by improving posture and encouraging habits of following proper body mechanics. Good ergonomic measures include safe workplace design, appropriate tools and equipment, adequate lighting, and protection against excessive noise and vibrations.

Focus on decreasing accidents in the workplace

There are many steps that can be taken to reduce the likelihood of workplace accidents, including always using equipment correctly, avoiding the use of electrical cords that lack the third *grounding prong*, immediately reporting any signs of abnormal equipment operation, and staying alert for wet or slippery surfaces.

Radiation hazards

In certain workplaces, the use of radiation requires procedures to protect against related hazards. For example, *radiopharmaceutical substances* used in chemotherapy are able to harm body tissues if a health care worker is exposed. Measures to reduce radiation hazards include increased distances between the radiation source and workers, a decreased amount of time spent working with radioactive substances, the use of film badges to monitor exposure, proper labeling of all materials, and the use of effective radiation shields.

Radiation safety standards concern radiation dose limits, levels in work areas, and concentrations in the air, water, and in disposed wastes. The United States Nuclear Regulatory Commission enforces precautionary procedures and imposes serious regulations concerning radiation. The Food and Drug Administration regulates radiopharmaceuticals. Specialized training is required to work with these substances.

> ### You should remember
>
> All forms of ionizing radiation have enough energy to destabilize molecules within body cells and lead to tissue damage. Ionizing radiation is either *particulate* (alpha, beta, neutrons) or *electromagnetic* (X-rays, gamma rays). Non-ionizing radiation is electromagnetic radiation that ranges from extremely low frequency to ultraviolet radiation.

Workplace violence

In health care settings, most workplace violence is related to assault. It is important for employers to have strong violence-prevention programs in place. These focus on employees as well as patients or other clients. Employees should participate in prevention programs. Other measures that help to reduce workplace violence include alarm systems, security cameras, adequate exits, barriers, and "safe" areas. To reduce the likelihood of violence, employees are encouraged to state the expectations of patients and clients, have a good relationship with security personnel and law enforcement representatives, have enough staff to cover workflow needs, and develop policies to deal with anyone who becomes upset, angry, or aggressive.

Employee responsibilities

Employees are required to comply with all OSHA standards, though they are not individually penalized by OSHA for failure to comply. Instead, OSHA penalizes the employer for not ensuring employee compliance. As well as federal OSHA regulations, some states have their own safety and health programs that employees and employers must follow. To follow such guidelines, it is important the employees do the following:

- Read OSHA posters in the workplace and comply with all standards that apply to their work.
- Follow all safety and health guidelines set out by the employer, such as wearing correct protective equipment while working.

- Report hazards to the employer.
- Report injuries or illnesses related to the job and seek prompt treatment.
- If an OSHA inspector comes to the workplace, cooperate by answering all questions about workplace health and safety conditions.
- Exercise employee rights under OSHA responsibly.

You should remember

OSHA standards are essential in protecting employees from harm in the workplace. For example, more than 1,000 eye injuries are estimated to occur daily in American workplaces. The chief reasons for these injuries come from employees who do not follow required OSHA guidelines. These reasons include not wearing eye protection, or wearing the wrong kind of eye protection. Most injuries occur from contact with particles in the air, or with chemicals, when working with industrial equipment.

Source: www.iatse122.com/safety/osha_tips/tips03.html.

CASE STUDY

Marie has been treated for chronic back pain for more than one year. She was recently hired by a government agency, where she is required to work at a computer desk for most of each workday, but also to deliver intra-office correspondence to more than 50 other employees.

1 What can Marie's employer do to make sure that her computer desk and work area are as ergonomic as possible?
2 What could be provided to assist Marie in delivering intra-office correspondence to the other employees?
3 What can Marie do that will most benefit her body while at work, and potentially reduce or prevent any discomfort?

Chapter highlights

This section answers the Objectives found at the beginning of the chapter.

1 Explain how hepatitis B and C are transmitted in the health care setting.

- The hepatitis B virus is transmitted through contact with an infected person's blood or body fluids that contain blood or semen. It is an important occupational hazard for health care workers, since it can survive outside the body for up to seven days (though this is unlikely). Injury can occur during medical procedures, including blood transfusion, dialysis, organ transplant, and handling of blood and body fluids for testing.
- The hepatitis C virus can be transmitted through inadequate sterilization of medical equipment as well as the same procedures through which hepatitis B may be

transmitted. Any piercing of the skin or mucous membranes that involves contact with infected blood or body fluids is able to transmit the HCV virus. Unlike HBV, there is no vaccine currently available for hepatitis C.

2 Describe components of the OSHA standard.

- Universal precautions – employers and employees must assume that all blood, blood products, tissues, and most body fluids are infectious for pathogens such as HIV and HBV. Universal precautions are also required when dealing with broken skin and all mucous membranes.
- Written exposure control plan – this must address how to handle exposure incidents, for all employees at risk of bloodborne exposure. All at-risk employees must review this plan annually, and written copies must be supplied to any employee requesting them.
- Labeling requirements – including biohazard and hazard labels, containers, and bags
- Accurate record-keeping – including an OSHA medical record and a sharps injury log.

3 Explain the purpose of OSHA.

- The Occupational Safety and Health Act was passed to prevent diseases and injuries in the workplace. It also established the Occupational Safety and Health Administration (also called OSHA). Because of OSHA, equipment, machinery, first aid, and materials are regulated in the workplace. Working environments must be free of extreme temperatures, excessive noise, dangerous machinery, toxic chemicals, and unsanitary conditions.

4 Describe an exposure control plan.

- A written procedure about how people should be treated after exposure to biohazardous or other harmful substances. It is designed to minimize risks of exposure and must be updated as necessary.
- Exposure control plans must include employee exposure determinations, exposure control method implementation (method of compliance), hepatitis B vaccinations, post-exposure evaluation, and procedures for follow-up, employee hazard communication and training, and record-keeping.

5 Explain the purpose of OSHA labeling requirements.

- Biohazard warning labels must be applied to anything containing biohazardous materials, including regulated waste containers, freezers, refrigerators, and any containers or bags used to store, transport, or ship these materials. The purpose of biohazard labels is to alert people to the presence of biohazardous materials and important safeguards to follow regarding their presence in the workplace.

6 Detail what should be included in a fire safety and emergency plan.

- To comply with OSHA, a fire safety and emergency plan must have written procedures that clearly detail building exits, clearly labeled fire doors and escape routes, fire alarm pull boxes, smoke detectors, and fire extinguishers.

7 List examples of potential fire hazards.

- Fire hazards include electrical wires, improperly grounded plugs, overloaded circuits, paper, matches, rags, lighters, other flammable items, insufficient protective measures when oxygen is in use, and smoking in the facility.

8 **Explain what is contained on a chemical safety data sheet.**

- As required by OSHA, a chemical safety data sheet contains the chemical's trade name, chemical name, synonyms, chemical family, manufacturer information, emergency telephone number, hazardous ingredients, physical data, fire and explosion data, health hazard information, and protection information.

9 **Explain ergonomics.**

- Ergonomics, or human engineering, is the science concerned with the design of equipment and environments for human needs. Ergonomics is focused on increasing the comfort, performance, and well-being of workers. When chairs and desks are ergonomically designed, they help to reduce discomfort and fatigue. Ergonomics also extends into physical movements while working that help to avoid injury, such as using the legs to support lifting a heavy weight, rather than using the lower back.

10 **List measures used to reduce radiation hazards.**

- Measures used to reduce radiation hazards include increased distances between the radiation source and workers, a decreased amount of time spent working with radioactive substances, the use of film badges to monitor exposure, proper labeling of all materials, and the use of effective radiation shields.

Summary

Health care professionals must always follow OSHA standards, as well as the policies and procedures of their employers. To control infection, health care professionals use universal precautions when handling blood and all body fluids. The two most significant diseases related to universal precautions are HIV and HBV. Each health care facility must have a clearly designed fire safety and emergency plan that details escape routes and fire equipment. Health care professionals must be trained to handle fires and other emergencies, as well as how to recognize potential hazards. Workplaces must provide clean air that is sufficiently filtered. Potential allergens such as latex gloves should be replaced with non-allergenic alternatives.

Ergonomic practices should be used to reduce discomfort while working, and to improve well-being and employee performance. Chemical and radiation hazards should be reduced or eliminated if possible, and proper documentation of all hazards must be available for employees. Another area of concern is workplace violence, which must be dealt with by establishing strong violence-prevention programs. Employees are required to comply with all OSHA standards, and OSHA penalizes employers who do not ensure this compliance.

> ### Review questions
>
> 1 What are universal precautions?
> 2 What are the most important factors concerning bloodborne pathogens?
> 3 What are the classifications of viral hepatitis?
> 4 What immunizations are recommended in relation to bloodborne pathogens?
> 5 Why may latex gloves cause an allergic reaction?
> 6 What does fire safety mean?
> 7 What does ergonomics mean?
> 8 What are the differences between chemical hazards and radiation hazards?
> 9 What is an exposure control plan?
> 10 What are employee responsibilities in relation to OSHA standards?

Bibliography

Advisory Committee on Dangerous Pathogens. 2003. Infection At Work: Controlling the Risks. Available at: www.hse.gov.uk/pubns/infection.pdf. Colegate: U.K. Advisory Committee on Dangerous Pathogens.

CDC. 2016. Bloodborne Infections Diseases. Available at: www.cdc.gov/niosh/topics/bbp/universal.html. Atlanta: U.S. Centers for Disease Control and Prevention.

CDC. 2016. HIV/AIDS Statistics. Available at: www.cdc.gov/hiv/statistics/overview/. Atlanta: U.S. Centers for Disease Control and Prevention.

CDC. 2016. The ABCs of Hepatitis. Available at: www.cdc.gov/hepatitis/resources/professionals/pdfs/abctable.pdf. Atlanta: U.S. Centers for Disease Control and Prevention.

Center for Chemical Process Safety. 2008. *Guidelines for Hazard Evaluation Procedures, 3rd Edition*. Hoboken: Wiley/American Institute of Chemical Engineers. Print.

Cobb, J. 2014. *Urban Emergency Survival Plan: Readiness Strategies for the City and Suburbs*. Iola: Living Ready. Print.

Creekmore, M.D. 2012. *Thirty-One Days to Survival: A Complete Plan for Emergency Preparedness*. Boulder: Paladin Press. Print.

Della-Giustina, D.E. 2014. *Fire Safety Management Handbook, 3rd Edition*. Boca Raton: CRC Press. Print.

Ergonomics.org – Posture, Motion, and Ergonomics. 2016. Ergonomics.Posture.The Problem.A Solution. Available at: http://ergonomics.org. London: Ergonomics.org.

Field, R.I. 2006. *Health Care Regulation in America: Complexity, Confrontation, and Compromise*. New York: Oxford University Press. Print.

Field, R.I. 2016. Why is Health Care Regulation So Complex?. Available at: www.ncbi.nlm.nih.gov/pmc/articles/PMC2730786. Bethesda: National Center for Biotechnology Information.

Fife, B. 2009. *Health Hazards of Electromagnetic Radiation, 2nd Edition*. Colorado Springs: Piccadilly Books, Ltd. Print.

Fowler, D. 2013. *Violence in the Workplace: Education, Prevention & Mitigation*. Coeur d'Alene: Personal Safety Training Inc. Print.

Hill, M.K. 2010. *Understanding Environmental Pollution, 3rd Edition*. New York: Cambridge University Press. Print.

Jaret, P. 2016. What Can I Expect Over Time with Hepatitis C?. Available at: https://

consumer.healthday.com/encyclopedia/hepatitis-c-23/hepatitis-news-373/what-can-i-expect-over-time-with-hepatitis-c-645180.html. Norwalk: HealthDay – News for Healthier Living.

KFF.org. 2016. The Global HIV/AIDS Epidemic. Available at: http://files.kff.org/attachment/fact-sheet-the-global-hivaids-epidemic. Menlo Park: Kaiser Family Foundation.

Konieczny, M. 2012. *The Latex Allergy Crisis: A Forgotten Epidemic – What Happened, Why It Happened, and What Happened to Me.* Houston: K and K Publishing. Print.

Mancomm Inc. 2015. *OSHA General Industry Regulations CFR 1910.* Davenport: Mancomm Inc. Print.

McCauley-Bush, P. 2011. *Ergonomics: Foundational Principles, Applications, and Technologies.* Boca Raton: CRC Press. Print.

Moran, M.M., and Moran, C. 2014. *The OSHA Answer Book for General Industry, 12th Edition.* Jacksonville: Moran Associates. Print.

National Fire Protection Association. 2011. *NFPA 70E: Standard for Electrical Safety in the Workplace, 2012.* Quincy: NFPA. Print.

National Fire Protection Association. 2016. Public Education – Escape Planning. Available at: www.nfpa.org/safety-information/for-consumers/escape-planning. Quincy: National Fire Protection Association.

National Institute of Occupational Safety and Health. 2007. *NIOSH Pocket Guide to Chemical Hazards.* Seattle: CreateSpace Independent Publishing Platform. Print.

Rieuwerts, J. 2015. *The Elements of Environmental Pollution.* London: Routledge. Print.

Safian, S.C. 2009. *Essentials of Health Care Compliance (Health Care Administration).* Boston: Delmar Cengage Learning. Print.

Salvendy, G. 2012. *Handbook of Human Factors and Ergonomics, 4th Edition.* Hoboken: Wiley. Print.

Statkiewicz-Sherer, M.A., et al. 2013. *Radiation Protection in Medical Radiography, 7th Edition.* Maryland Heights: Mosby. Print.

Summit Training Source. 2012. *Bloodborne Pathogens: Universal Precautions Employee Handbook.* Seattle: Amazon Digital Services, Inc. Print.

TakeOneStep – Wellness At Work. 2016. Workplace Hazards. Available at: www.takeonestep.org/Pages/yoursafety/safenotsorry/workplacehazards.aspx. Boston: TakeOneStep.org.

U.S. Department of Health and Human Services. 2016. Laws and Regulations. Available at: www.hhs.gov/regulations/index.html. Washington, D.C.: U.S. Department of Health and Human Services.

U.S. Department of Labor. 2016. Chemical Hazards and Toxic Substances. Available at: www.osha.gov/SLTC/hazardoustoxicsubstances. Washington, D.C.: U.S. Department of Labor.

U.S. Department of Labor. 2016. Emergency Action Plan. Available at: www.osha.gov/SLTC/etools/evacuation/eap.html. Washington, D.C.: U.S. Department of Labor.

U.S. Department of Labor. 2016. Eye Protection in the Workplace. Available at: www.iatse122.com/safety/osha_tips/tips03.html. Washington, D.C.: U.S. Department of Labor.

U.S. Department of Labor. 2016. Occupational Safety and Health Act 1970: Penalties. Available at: www.osha.gov/pls/oshaweb/owadisp.show_document?p_table=oshact&p_id=3371. Washington, D.C.: U.S. Department of Labor.

U.S. Department of Labor. 2016. Online Environmental Safety Courses. Available at: www.osha.com/courses/environmental.html. Washington, D.C.: U.S. Department of Labor.

U.S. Department of Labor. 2016. OSHA Standards and Regulations. Available at: www.osha.net/osha-standards-and-regulations. Washington, D.C.: U.S. Department of Labor.

U.S. Department of Labor. 2016. OSHA: Latex Allergy. Available at: www.osha.gov/SLTC/latexallergy/index.html. Washington, D.C.: U.S. Department of Labor.

U.S. Department of Labor. 2016. OSHA: Radiation. Available at: www.osha.gov/SLTC/radiation. Washington, D.C.: U.S. Department of Labor.

U.S. Department of Labor. 2016. OSHA: Workplace Violence. Available at: www.osha.gov/ OshDoc/data_General_Facts/factsheet-workplace-violence.pdf. Washington, D.C.: U.S. Department of Labor.

Washtenaw County Public Health. 2012. Fact Sheet: Universal Precautions. Available at: www.ewashtenaw.org/government/departments/public_health/disease_control/cd_fact_ sheets/universal_precautions.pdf. Ypsilanti: Washtenaw County Public Health Department.

Workplace Safety Experts / Robson Forensic. 2016. Latex Allergies in the Workplace. Available at: http://workplacesafetyexperts.com/first-aid/latex-allergies-in-the-workplace. Lancaster: Robson Forensic.

Unit VI

Communication in the health care profession

Contents

14 The communication process   337

Overview   337
Maslow's hierarchy of human needs   338
Steps of the communication process   339
Types of communication   340
Improving your communication skills   343
Therapeutic communication   345
Interprofessional communication   347
Methods of communication   347
Barriers to communication   349
Written communication   350
Defense mechanisms   351
Dealing with conflict   353
Case study   353
Chapter highlights   354
Summary   355
Review questions   356
Bibliography   357

15 Computers and technology in health care   358

Overview   358
Types of computer   359
Computers in health care   362
Computer security   371
Case study   372
Chapter highlights   372
Summary   374

Review questions   374
Bibliography   375

16 Record-keeping   377

Overview   377
Contents of the medical record   378
Types of medical records   379
Electronic health records   381
Personal health records   382
Medical documentation   383
HIPAA and the medical record   384
Case study   386
Chapter highlights   386
Summary   388
Review questions   389
Bibliography   390

Chapter 14

The communication process

After study of the chapter, readers should be able to:

1 Describe the communication process.
2 Briefly explain the five Cs of communication.
3 Differentiate between open and closed feedback.
4 Compare verbal with non-verbal communication.
5 Describe the importance of therapeutic communication.
6 Discuss examples of negative communication.
7 Describe barriers to communication.
8 Explain why defense mechanisms may be used.
9 Define the terms compensation, displacement, dissociation, and rationalization.
10 Describe how to deal with conflict.

Overview

In all areas of health care, communication is essential. The health care professional must be able to communicate effectively with patients, caregivers, and other professionals. Communication must always be professional and courteous. Health care professionals must be caring, competent, presentable, and knowledgeable, in both verbal and non-verbal modes of communication. This includes face-to-face communication, as well as telephone, computer, fax, and written communication.

Maslow's hierarchy of human needs

Abraham Maslow was a human behaviorist who classified behaviors into a *hierarchy of human needs* (see Figure 14.1). His theory states that specific lower needs must be satisfied before higher needs can be met. Maslow believed that people are basically able to conduct their behaviors in a positive, honest manner as they continually grow and develop healthy relationships with others. He also stated that negative or violent behaviors only happen when human needs are not being met. Maslow's hierarchy of needs are summarized from lowest to highest, as follows:

- *Basic needs* – also called "deficiency needs," these include physiological, safety, love and belonging, and esteem needs.

  - *Physiological* – air, water, food, sleep, warmth, shelter, sexual intimacy. Lack of fulfillment of these needs may cause illness, pain, discomfort, and irritation. *Homeostasis* is established when these needs are met, and then other needs can be addressed.
  - *Safety* – stability and consistency in life, including security, shelter, order, law, and a safe environment.
  - *Love and belonging* – the need for family, social, and work groups that provide love and acceptance. Humans have a strong need to "belong" in society.
  - *Esteem* – the need to feel important and valuable to others

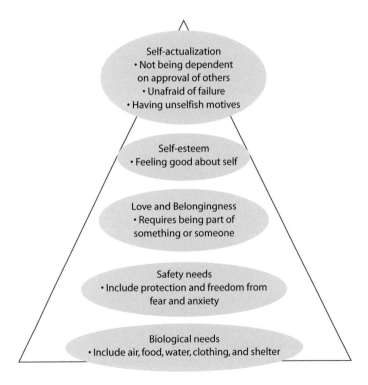

Figure 14.1 Maslow's hierarchy of needs.

Source: www.deepermind.com/20maslow.htm.

- First type of esteem: Competence in tasks, education, training
- Second type of esteem: Attention and recognition from others for accomplishments.

- Self-actualization – Self-fulfillment and realization of total potential. It is based on education, a rewarding career, and balanced personal relationships. Once self-actualized, individuals are usually comfortable with themselves, achieve personal growth, and understand their strengths and weaknesses.

Focus on understanding patient needs

Maslow's hierarchy of needs can be applied when working with patients. You must adjust your communication style in order to take into account what each patient's needs are, based on what they have achieved or lost in life. Examples include an elderly patient who is deficient in the need for love due to loss of a spouse, or a younger patient who is deficient in self-esteem because of divorce or break-up of a family unit.

Steps of the communication process

Communication means sharing thoughts, ideas, information, and feelings. The steps of the communication process involve two or more individuals and the exchange of information between them. The five basic steps in communication include: a sender or source, a message, a channel or mode of communication, a receiver, and feedback (see Figure 14.2).

The person who sends a message, through various channels, is the *sender*. The sender must choose how to transmit the message. The channels used may be spoken words, written messages, and even non-verbal **body language**. The message is encoded by the sender, which means that the specific expression is made through certain words and other channels.

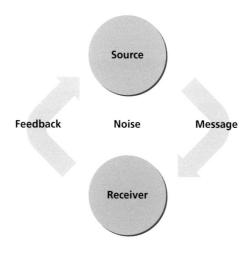

Figure 14.2 Steps of the communication process.

There are five Cs of communication: *complete, concise, clear, cohesive,* and *courteous.* The message contains complete information, which means everything that is necessary to be communicated. It must be concise, and not contain any unnecessary information. It also must be clear, and not be obscure or ambiguous. The message must be cohesive, which requires organization and logic. It must also be courteous to others, showing respect and consideration.

The path between the sender and receiver is the *channel.* It is considered to be downward, upward, or horizontal. A downward channel is one from a superior to an employee. An upward channel is from an employee to a superior. A horizontal channel is between people with similar responsibility levels. The *receiver* of the message decodes it, based on his or her understanding. Sometimes, a message is decoded incorrectly, often due to noise or other interference. There are two forms of noise: *external,* which is from the environment, and *internal,* which is from the receiver's own thoughts.

Feedback involves body language or verbal expressions, and expresses understanding from the receiver about the message that was received. You should always look for feedback when communicating information. Feedback must be clear, positive, specific, and focused. It should refer to changes that might occur and should be descriptive. When giving feedback, you should use statements referring to yourself and your understanding of the message. Try to be careful giving advice so that the feedback you give sounds helpful, not critical. When used correctly, feedback assists the sender and the receiver, helping to make the communication more effective.

Positive (open) styles of feedback are encouraged to be used by the sender. These may be described as accepting, engaged or interactive, interested, open or non-interrupting, responsive, respectful, sincere, thoughtful, and active listening. Taking notes about the feedback that is received is helpful, especially when involved in group communication. In this way, all of the feedback that was given can be acted upon. Feedback is most effective when it is given at the proper time and in the proper way.

There are also negative (closed) styles of feedback that must be avoided by the sender. These may be described as attacking, closed or ignoring, defensive, denying, disrespectful, patronizing, rationalizing, superficial, and inactive listening. All of these take a negative approach to reacting to the feedback being given. They show the receiver of the message that his or her thoughts, in the form of feedback to the sender, are not welcomed, important, or of value. This is a true barrier to effective communication.

It is also possible to give feedback *about* feedback. In this way, the person who receives the feedback is able to express his or her thoughts about it, helping to react even more constructively. If there are any problems with the feedback and how to handle reactions to it, these can be discussed. Feedback is best when it is honest but not overly critical. It can then improve the communication process by encouraging changes that will help make future communications better. Both speakers and receivers can then continually learn and become more skillful communicators.

Types of communication

There are various types of communication that are used every day in the health care field. These include verbal, non-verbal, and written communication. Each of these types can be positive or negative. In order to communicate effectively, you must be familiar with each of the different types of communication.

Verbal communication

In verbal communication, it is not only our words that are exchanged, but also vocal quality and inflections, tone, and pitch. Along with these, non-verbal communication is used, including body posture, facial expressions, and various behavioral responses. Communications between patients and health care professionals go a long way toward determining treatment outcomes and patient compliance.

Phrasing also communicates its own message, and refers to both the style of speaking and the chosen words. The way words are pronounced and how they are presented in conversation affect how the receiver understands them. For clear, accurate verbal communication, your diction and enunciation must be of very high quality. Solid communication skills also involve accurate listening, comprehension, sharing information with others, feedback, and documentation of the feedback.

> ### You should remember
>
> The use of encouraging words along with non-verbal gestures helps to reinforce openness in others when communicating. These non-verbal gestures include head nods, eye contact, and a pleasant, friendly facial expression.

Non-verbal communication

Non-verbal communication is also known as body language. In many cases, body language conveys a person's true feelings when words may not. Be aware of your own body language and pay attention to the body language of others. Vocal tone, inflection, and pitch may play a greater role in communication even than the actual words that are used. In fact, most spoken communication involves non-verbal transmission. Body language is the key component of non-verbal communication, and includes eye contact, facial expressions, grooming, hand gestures, the clothes we wear, the space we create between ourselves and others, posture, tone of voice, touching of other people, and many other aspects.

- *Eye contact* – Making good eye contact when communicating is the most important form of non-verbal communication. It shows interest and attentiveness to the person you are communicating with, as well as the message itself. However, people from different cultures may not practice the same level of eye contact when communicating, feeling that it is a rude behavior. The health care professional should be able to discern this situation and change behavior accordingly.
- *Facial expressions* – When used with direct eye contact, facial expressions assist in communication by reinforcing or conflicting with the message. Your face helps you to show your interest, concern, and care for the patient. If the facial expression shows negativity in any form, the receiver of the message may feel that you are being judgmental or disapproving of them. Head movements also influence communication, such as slightly shaking the head back and forth, which seems to indicate a negative response even though the words being used may sound positive.
- *Grooming* – This influences how others view us, and may cause another person to make preconceived judgments. Overall appearance is a crucial part of non-verbal communication. A person who is not well groomed, according to another person, may be treated with less respect or seriousness. It is difficult not to form opinions based on a person's overall appearance.

- *Hand gestures* – Most people use their hands to emphasize important concepts when speaking. The use of the hands may differ widely among certain cultures, and some people may not appreciate certain movements the way they might have been intended by the speaker.
- *Clothing* – Like grooming, the clothes we wear and how they appear may convey various things to other people. Clothing may identify you as a person who is completely different from your personal values and beliefs. Some people make poor judgments about others based on the clothing being worn.
- *Personal space* – When communicating with others, it is important to be aware of the concept of personal space, which is an area that surrounds an individual. By not intruding on a patient's personal space, you demonstrate respect for his or her feelings of privacy. In most social situations, it is common for people to stand four to 12 feet from each other. For personal conversations, people usually stand between one and four feet apart. Some patients feel uncomfortable and become anxious when another person stands or sits too close to them. Others feel reassured when people are close to them when they speak. It is important to observe each patient carefully. If patients lean back when you lean forward, or if they fold their arms or turn their head away, you may be invading their personal space. Personal space varies among people from different cultures. While many people are comfortable within a very close proximity to others, Americans usually require more personal space in most situations. The reverse may also be true. Too much space between people who are communicating may be seen as impersonal or even insulting. We must attempt to be aware of how other people perceive their personal space in order for communication to be as effective as possible.
- *Posture* – The way you hold or move your head, arms, hands, and the rest of your body can project strong non-verbal messages. During communication, posture can usually be described as open or closed. Posture is determined and controlled by the skeletal muscles as well as our sense of equilibrium. An overly relaxed posture may communicate to certain people a lack of attention or seriousness about what they are saying. A rigid posture may indicate a nervous or alarmed disposition. An open posture signifies friendliness and receptiveness, in which the arms are kept comfortable in the lap or at the sides. The receiver faces the speaker and leans forward, showing interest in what is being said. A closed posture may signify a lack of receptiveness, anger, or that the receiver is upset. The arms may be folded across the chest or held rigidly. Leaning back away from the speaker, avoiding eye contact, or slouching all exemplify closed posture.
- *Tone of voice* – This is also crucial because it can show respect, caring, and understanding when used correctly. Good tone of voice shows a positive, helpful attitude. The voice should always sound calm and confident during professional communications. Negative communication can be increased if the tone of voice sounds impatient, bored, sarcastic, hesitant, parental, bullying, or weak.
- *Touch* – This is a powerful form of non-verbal communication. A touch on the arm or a hug can be a way of saying hello, sharing condolences, or expressing congratulations. The perception of touch is influenced by culture, age, family background, and gender. Some people welcome a touch or think nothing of it while others may view touching as an invasion of their privacy. Usually, it is acceptable in the medical setting to express interest or concern by touching another person on the shoulder, forearm, or back of the hand (see Figure 14.3). Examples of correct touching include the demonstration of how to apply a medication or the palpation of a body part for evaluation of a potential abnormality. If any hands-on approach is required, it is vital to explain what needs to be done and ask for permission to do so.

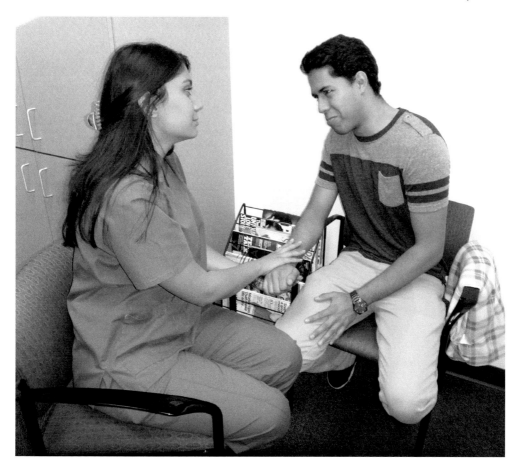

Figure 14.3 Acceptable touching of a patient.

Focus on non-verbal communication cues

Non-verbal communication cues are important in five ways. They can repeat a verbal message, contradict a verbal message, substitute for a verbal message, complement or add to a verbal message, or accent a verbal message. Therefore, it is very important to be aware at all times of which non-verbal cues you are sending out along with what you are saying.

Improving your communication skills

It is important to continually try to improve your communication skills, so that you will become an efficient communicator. Every day, we use listening, interpersonal, and assertiveness skills in order to hear, understand, interpret, and respond to others. Each of these skills has a variety of components that must be learned in order to facilitate positive communication.

Listening skills

To listen to others effectively, you not only hear their words, but interpret the messages they are conveying. It is crucial to pay attention to their words, but also to their non-verbal cues and body language. Listening can be active or passive, as follows:

- *Active listening* – Involves two-way communication. As you actively listen, you ask questions or offer feedback (see Figure 14.4). Active listening is used when interviewing a patient about his or her medical history, and therefore is a crucial skill in the health care facility.
- *Passive listening* – Involves listening to another's words without needing to reply. An example is listening to the weather or news on a radio.

Ways to improve your listening skills include assuming an open posture, sitting or standing on the same level as the person who is speaking, relaxing, and listening attentively. You should maintain the appropriate personal space and make eye contact. Before you respond, think about what you will say. Give the speaker feedback and restate what you heard in your own words. If you do not understand something that was said, ask the speaker to repeat it.

Interpersonal skills

The ability to offer good interpersonal skills is crucial in health care. This is demonstrated by being friendly to others, showing respect, having empathy, being genuine and open, and remaining considerate and sensitive to their needs.

- *Friendliness* – You should show warmth to patients, but remain professional. Greet them pleasantly and smile. This sincerity will help patients to relax and be more open with you about their needs.
- *Empathy* – This involves identification with another person's feelings, and showing sensitivity to their situation. When a patient is in pain, acknowledge its severity and show care while providing support.

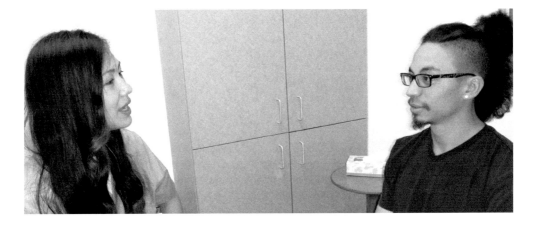

Figure 14.4 Active listening, between a health care professional and patient.

- *Respectfulness* – Use the proper title for each patient, such as "Mr." or "Mrs." Show each patient that you acknowledge his or her wishes or choices and are not passing judgment.
- *Genuineness* – Show patients that you really care about them and their individual needs. This is accomplished by giving them your full attention and treating them in a respectful manner. Your genuine attitude helps the patient to trust you and the information you supply.
- *Openness* – You should be receptive to each patient's needs, and show that you listen to and consider their concerns. When you are open, you accept others and have no bias for or against their viewpoints.
- *Sensitivity* – By showing consideration for each patient, thinking about their needs, and treating them kindly, you prove that you are sensitive to their needs and situations, and even what worries them about their health.

Assertiveness skills

It is important to be assertive with others, but not to show aggression while doing so. Assertiveness requires you to be open, direct, and emotionally honest, including in your body posture. Aggressiveness is shown by attempting to tell others what to do without taking into consideration their needs and feelings. Assertive professionals are firm, principled, and yet always respectful. If a patient looks worried about a procedure, ask him or her if you can do anything to increase comfort or reduce discomfort. This shows the patient that while you are sure about what needs to be done, you are still completely focused on his or her needs.

Assertiveness skills help you increase your own professional confidence and feelings of self-worth. These skills help to improve your abilities as a leader, while peacefully resolving or preventing conflicts. Most people respect assertive professionals and admire them. Assertive behaviors are expressive, self-enhancing, individually chosen, focused on achieving goals, and offer value to others.

Therapeutic communication

It is important when communicating with patients to keep your verbal and non-verbal communications consistent. You should ask the patient to provide feedback about what you have communicated, in order to facilitate his or her complete understanding. The patient should be encouraged to ask questions, to which you must provide positive and open information. If further explanation is needed, it should be given clearly. Once again, the patient must be asked for feedback to ensure understanding.

Therapeutic communication requires continual exchanges of information, questioning, explanations, and clarification. Remember that a patient who does not fully understand important information may experience a negative outcome to treatment. It is a great idea to follow-up verbal communication with written instructions, in order to reinforce what was discussed and increase understanding.

Positive communication

Positive communication is an essential component in the health care setting. It promotes the comfort and well-being of patients. Examples of positive communication include the following:

- Encouraging questions – Patients should feel comfortable to ask anything
- Having instructions repeated – Ask patients to repeat your instructions so that you know they understand them
- Smiling naturally – A natural smile encourages patients to be receptive
- Listening carefully – Don't talk while the patient is talking; just listen
- Good eye contact – Look directly at patients while speaking with them
- Being attentive, friendly, and warm
- Speaking clearly and slowly
- Focusing – Encourage the patient to stay on the topic
- Showing concern – Tell patients that you are concerned about them
- Summarizing – Organizing and restating the important discussion points gives the patient an awareness of progress that has been made toward better understanding of his or her health needs.

Negative communication

Negative communication gives the receiver impressions that impede the exchange of information. Examples include appearing bored, uninterested, impatient, or judgmental, speaking too quietly or indistinctly (*mumbling*), speaking too loudly or aggressively, interrupting, being discourteous, staring, or avoiding eye contact. Negative body language (closed posture) or frowning may convey the impression that communication is not being received well or, when performed by the sender, can show lack of respect or aggression. Anything that makes a patient feel as if he or she is being treated impersonally results in negative communication. The following should be refrained from in order to avoid negative communication:

- Showing approval or disapproval – Approving of a patient's behavior may cause the patient to receive praise instead of make progress; disapproving tells the patient that you are passing judgment – avoid appearing moralistic and stay focused on the patient's needs
- Reassuring – By indicating to the patient that there is no need to worry, you devalue his or her feelings, providing false hope if there is a negative outcome; you must show understanding and empathy instead
- Agreeing or disagreeing – Agreeing tells the patient that he or she is right, when this may not be correct – you should not provide opinions or make conclusions; disagreeing reduces your status as caregiver, provoking arguments that are counterproductive to good treatment
- Probing – Making a patient uncomfortable by discussing something he or she does not want to share
- Advising – Telling a patient what you think should be done is outside your scope of practice – do not advise patients
- Requesting explanations – By asking the patient to explain behaviors, you may provoke intimidation or confusion; often, the patient does not know why they behaved a certain way

- Defending – Do not protect yourself or your facility from verbal attack, because the patient may stop communicating
- Minimizing feelings – Avoid judging or making the patient feel like his or her discomfort is not that important; always perceive the situation from the patient's point of view, not yours
- Lack of explanation – Do not use statements that are meaningless to the patient, such as, "Just take the medication"; you must explain things in reasonable, thoughtful ways so that the patient feels that their treatment is individualized and focused.

Focus on health care "burnout"

A meaningful situation that may result in negative communication is "burnout." This is a direct result of the chronic stress many health care professionals experience in their daily work. When it occurs, the individual may feel exhausted, cynical, and unable to listen well or show compassion. Negative communication often results, along with more errors, in lower quality of care and reduced patient satisfaction.

Interprofessional communication

In the health care profession, there are communications between all types of workers, in many disciplines. It is very important to understand proper and effective communication techniques, regardless of whether you are communicating with coworkers or superiors.

Communicating with coworkers

It is extremely important to communicate effectively with your coworkers because this helps to develop positive working environments. When the working environment is positive instead of negative, everyone can function as a team, which supports good patient care.

Communicating with superiors

The same is true of positive communication with your superiors. There should always be an open line of communication between the people who supervise others and their subordinates. Workers must understand their job responsibilities, and this means that superiors must develop effective communication to explain what is required. Always keep superiors informed about what is being done, show initiative in your work, minimize interruptions so that you can focus on your work, and ask questions when you need more information to work effectively.

Methods of communication

Though much communication in the health care setting is face-to-face, it may also include communication that utilizes telephones, fax machines, computers and e-mail, telecommunication conferences and meetings, the Internet, voice mail, and pagers.

Computers

Computers are more prevalent than ever before in all industries, including health care. All health care professionals must be thoroughly proficient in their use, which may include Internet searches, e-mail, conferencing, and various types of software. E-mail is the exchange of information between computers, through Internet connections. For e-mails, you must ensure that your wording and grammar are clear and correct. It is wise to double-check all e-mails, including the recipient's name and e-mail address, before they are sent.

At the top of an e-mail, there should be an informative subject line. It is always suggested that you acknowledge receiving an e-mail, even if you have no immediate reply. All information must be verified, ensuring confidentiality and appropriateness. E-mails should be kept as short as possible so that they can be read and answered with efficiency. They should be written in the same manner as when you are writing professional correspondence with your facility's letterhead. At the bottom of every e-mail, it is good to include an e-mail signature with full contact information. E-mails must be used only for business communications when you are at work.

Clinical e-mail is sent between health care professionals using *electronic medical records (EMRs)*. This type of e-mail is more secure than regular e-mail, shares patient information between colleagues, and often has patient records attached. *Attachments* to e-mails allow documents, images, and other file types to be sent along with e-mails, but must be used carefully since they are commonly used to spread *computer viruses*. You should never click on an attachment to open it unless you know it is from a verified source.

Fax transmission

It is important to use cover letters when sending faxes so that the person receiving the fax is able to respond correctly if there are any problems or questions about the information sent. Though fax machines are used less today than in the past because of the advent of computers, they are still common. In previous years, fax machines could only be used by connecting to a telephone line. Today, fax machines are also able to interact with computers so that a fax machine is not required on both ends of a connection.

Telecommunication

Telecommunication involves telephones and/or computer systems. Examples of telecommunication in health care include conversations between medical facilities, pharmacies, researchers, insurers, and many others. They should be handled similarly to regular meetings, with scheduled times, etiquette, and a planned agenda.

Telephone skills are vital to health care, and require excellent tone of voice, a pleasant demeanor, and professionalism. When answering a phone call, you should identify the place of business, then give your name, and finally ask the caller what you can do to help them. When you are required to make a phone call, always introduce yourself, your place of business, and the reason for your call.

Photocopying

Copy machines are still routinely used in the health care setting to make *photocopies* of all types of documents. Before using a copy machine, make sure that your master documents are not stapled or clipped together, that the machine has enough paper to make all the copies you need, and that the pages are arranged in the correct order. Copiers can make multiple copies of all the pages that you require and *collate* them, which means to arrange all pages in each copy of the entire document in order. Some copiers can also sort, make double-sided copies, and even staple documents. It is important to avoid distractions when copying so that the final copies are in the correct order.

When making copies of patient medical records, it is essential to ensure that patient confidentiality is protected at all times. Never leave any copies of patient records in a copying machine, where another individual may have unauthorized access to them. Prior to copying patient records, verify that the patient has authorized this information to be released. For any copies that are printed incorrectly, make sure to shred them completely in a shredding machine.

> ## You should remember
>
> Patients must feel that all of their private health information will be handled with the strictest confidence by everyone participating in their health care. When a patient cannot trust a health care professional to treat information as confidential, they may withhold it. This means that vital information required for accurate assessment and treatment may not be shared, or the patient's health care may suffer as a result.

Barriers to communication

There are many types of barriers that reduce the effectiveness of communication. They can be very dangerous, since accurate and timely communication may reduce life-threatening errors. Barriers might include noise, excessive numbers of people in a facility, lack of privacy, compromised patient confidentiality, anger, violence, stress, and inadequate time to complete procedures. Of these barriers, the most significant barrier to communication is stress. Barriers to communication also include environmental barriers such as physical impairments, language difficulties, hearing impairments, and prejudice.

Environmental barriers (physical impairment)

Environmental barriers that involve physical impairments to communication may include poor acoustics, high levels of noise, and lack of confidentiality because of the design of the workspace. Poor acoustics can cause information to be interrupted or disrupted between health care professionals and patients, affecting the quality of patient care. High levels of noise, likewise, might impede the flow of communication and cause errors to occur. A patient who feels he or she is not receiving enough confidentiality about private information may be hesitant to communicate, or even become dishonest about information. Environmental barriers to communication must be reduced to a minimum so that patients will feel that they are being treated with confidentiality, care, concern, and courtesy.

Non-English-speaking people

English is the predominant language of the United States, but many people in the country are not able, or not fully able, to communicate effectively except in their native language. If English is not understood sufficiently, the health care professional may have to use simple and direct terms, visual aids, specific gestures, preprinted instructions in the patient's language, or interpreters. The non-English-speaking person must be treated with professionalism and concern until a suitable mode of communication can be established.

Hearing impairment

When an individual cannot hear sufficiently, the health care professional may be required to make special considerations to assist them in communicating. Sometimes, simply moving into a smaller, quieter room is sufficient for the individual to be able to hear your words. For others, it might be necessary to use written communication, sign language, lip reading, or an interpreter.

Prejudice

Prejudice is created when personal and social bias causes an individual to discriminate against another. Discrimination is unfair treatment of another, based on gender, race, handicap, religion, nationality, or other reasons. It is totally unacceptable, immoral, unethical, and socially wrong in all situations. Discrimination might also be illegal, and is a definite barrier to effective communication.

Written communication

Excellent written communication plays another important role in health care settings. Your writing must be accurate and clear, utilizing correct grammar, punctuation, and spelling, in order to avoid potential confusion. Written communications may include letters, memos, e-mails, supply orders, records, financial paperwork, labels, envelopes, packages, prescriptions, and many other forms. Often, written communication is used as a back-up to verbal communications, in order to reinforce instructions and other information.

Medical writing

Medical writing requires a higher level of accuracy and clarity than other types of correspondence, such as personal or business correspondence. Since medical writing may be incorporated into permanent medical records of patients, a great degree of careful attention must be utilized. Any mistake could potentially cause injury or death, and result in lawsuits or other negative outcomes for your employer and yourself. In medical writing, abbreviations and symbols, capitalization, numbers, and spelling all have strict rules governing their use.

- Abbreviations and symbols may be used to save time when taking notes, but words should be fully spelled out when typing the final version of a written medical document. The health care facility will probably have a list of approved abbreviations and symbols that it uses regularly. You must be familiar with this list and know how to use it correctly.

- Capitalization must also follow certain guidelines. When in doubt, you must verify that all capitalization is used correctly by checking with another individual who knows the correct usage.
- Numbering in medical writing is used as follows: the numbers *one* through *ten* are usually spelled out, while larger numbers are written using their numerals, such as *11*, *15*, *30*, *50*, or *100*. However, units of measurement, such as *10 g*, should be written as numbers regardless of their amount. Sentences that begin with a number should have the number spelled out.
- Ensuring correct spelling requires regular proofreading of all written communications. This should be done even if computer spell-checking is also used. The spell-check in a computer's word processing program is not able to find incorrect usages of words, even though they may be spelled correctly.

Focus on medical writing

Medical writing is an interdisciplinary field that attempts to articulate medical information in the most effective ways possible. Its goals are to accurately represent research, provide unique perceptions and insights, and to make complex material easier to share with people outside of the field of research.

Defense mechanisms

People often use defense mechanisms when dealing with situations that seem threatening or uncomfortable. These may be subconscious mechanisms used to protect an individual's emotions. Defense mechanisms help us cope with difficult events. Common defense mechanisms are listed in Table 14.1.

You should remember

There are three common defense mechanisms that, when used in moderation, are relatively healthy ways of dealing with difficult situations: humor, sublimation, and suppression. Humor helps patients to distance themselves from the pain of their conditions. Sublimation redirects negative emotions into positive actions, such as educating others about a disease or condition. Suppression allows the patient to deal with urgent matters while temporarily delaying acknowledgment of certain painful emotions.

Table 14.1 Defense mechanisms

Type	Explanation
Acting out	Performing extreme behaviors to express feelings or thoughts that the individual feels cannot be otherwise expressed
Apathy	Acting as if you do not care; this may develop after receiving repeated disappointments
Assertiveness	Emphasizing thoughts or needs in a way that is received as firm, direct, but respectful
Compartmentalization	A lesser type of *dissociation* in which some parts of the self are separated from others, resulting in behaviors that seem to come from different sets of values
Compensation	Trying to overcome something by developing another trait or ability
Denial	Refusing to accept a reality or fact, or pretending something painful or disagreeable did not exist
Depersonalization	Removing a feeling from something perceived as stressful
Displacement	Shifting behaviors or emotions from original objects to more acceptable objects
Dissociation	Losing track of time and/or person, and finding another self-representation in order to continue; often related to childhood abuse
Intellectualization	Overemphasis of thinking when confronting an unacceptable thought, behavior, or situation; it avoids the use of emotion
Projection	Misappropriation of one's own undesirable thoughts or feelings onto another person who does not have the same thoughts or feelings
Rationalization	Assigning logical excuses or reasons for actions that may have occurred because of emotions, such as self-interest, that a person does not want to acknowledge
Reaction formation	Converting dangerous or unwanted feelings or thoughts into their opposites
Regression	Returning to an earlier emotional stage of growth and development

Table 14.1 Continued

Type	Explanation
Repression	Unconscious exclusion of unacceptable thoughts or emotions from one's own awareness
Sarcasm	The expression of bitter, sharp remarks when experiencing an uncomfortable situation, feeling, or thought
Selective inattention	Not allowing oneself to hear or pay attention to information that causes anxiety
Sublimation	Channeling unacceptable emotions or thoughts into more acceptable ones
Suppression	Making the decision to put painful or uncomfortable thoughts out of one's own awareness
Undoing	Attempting to make up for behaviors or feelings that cause guilt

Dealing with conflict

Conflicts in the health care setting can occur when there are misunderstandings between members of the team, or when communications break down due to various types of interference. There must be mutual trust and respect between all team members. In order to deal with potential conflicts, there are several things you should and should not do on a continual basis. You should try to be supportive and personable to everyone, at all times. You should always act in a professional manner. Things to avoid include participating in the negative attitudes of other people, stereotyping, passing judgment on others, gossiping, and jumping to conclusions about others' actions or motives. Instead of concluding things incorrectly, it is important to ask them directly.

CASE STUDY

John had been working in a physician's office, as a medical assistant, for three years. In his last employee review, some of the constructive criticism John received included that he didn't seem to be overly interested in his job, did not really interact with the other employees, and seemed defensive about new areas of work with which he was not familiar.

1   What could John do to communicate more interest in his work?
2   What behavioral changes could John make to better interact and communicate with the other employees?
3   What should John try to do in regard to his attitude about new tasks at work?

Chapter highlights

This section answers the Objectives found at the beginning of the chapter.

1 Describe the communication process.

- The steps of the communication process involve two or more individuals, and the exchange of information between them. The five basic steps in communication include: a sender or source, a message, a channel or mode of communication, a receiver, and feedback. The channel may involve spoken words, written messages, and even non-verbal body language. Feedback involves body language or verbal expressions, and expresses an understanding from the receiver about the message that was received.

2 Briefly explain the five Cs of communication.

- Complete – the message contains complete information, which means everything that is necessary to be communicated
- Concise – the message does not contain any unnecessary information
- Clear – it should not be obscure or ambiguous
- Cohesive – it should be organized and logical
- Courteous – it should show respect and consideration to others.

3 Differentiate between open and closed feedback.

- Open (positive) feedback is encouraged to be used by the sender of a message – it is accepting, engaged, interactive, interested, non-interrupting, responsive, respectful, sincere, thoughtful, and involves active listening.
- Closed (negative) feedback must be avoided – it includes attacking, ignoring, defensive, denying, disrespectful, patronizing, rationalizing, and superficial actions, and involves inactive listening.

4 Compare verbal with non-verbal communication.

- In verbal communication, words are exchanged, as well as vocal quality and inflections, tone, pitch, body posture, facial expressions, and various behavioral responses. Phrasing refers to the style of speaking and the chosen words. Pronunciation, word presentation, diction, enunciation, accurate listening, comprehension, information sharing, feedback, and documentation also play important roles in verbal communication. Non-verbal communication is also called body language, and may convey true feelings better than words. Body language includes eye contact, facial expressions, grooming, hand gestures, clothing, personal space, posture, tone of voice, and touching.

5 Describe the importance of therapeutic communication.

- Therapeutic communication requires consistent verbal and non-verbal communication, and to be successful requires that the patient provide feedback about the information. The patient should be encouraged to ask questions and provide additional feedback to the responses to these questions to ensure further understanding. Continual exchanges of information are required for good patient communication. This will help avoid negative outcomes to treatment. Verbal communication should be followed up with written instructions to increase understanding.

6 Discuss examples of negative communication.

- Negative communication presents impressions to the receiver that become real barriers to the exchange of information. It may result from appearing bored, uninterested, impatient, or judgmental. Mumbling can be interpreted negatively, and interruption is considered negative. Avoiding courtesies, staring at another person, or avoiding eye contact are all negative. Aggressive forms of speaking and negative body language are also forms of poor communication. In general, anything that makes a patient feel as if he or she is being treated impersonally should be avoided.

7 Describe barriers to communication.

- Barriers to communication can cause life-threatening errors, and include noise, excessive numbers of people, lack of privacy, compromised patient confidentiality, anger, violence, stress, and inadequate time for procedures. Environmental barriers include physical impairments, language difficulties, hearing impairments, and prejudice.

8 Explain why defense mechanisms may be used.

- People often use defense mechanisms when dealing with situations that seem threatening or uncomfortable. These may be subconscious, in order to protect the emotions of the individual. They help us to cope with difficult events.

9 Define the terms compensation, displacement, dissociation, and rationalization.

- Compensation is trying to overcome something by developing another trait or ability. Displacement is shifting behaviors or emotions from original objects to more acceptable objects. Dissociation is losing track of time and/or person, and finding another self-representation in order to continue. It is often related to childhood abuse. Rationalization is assigning logical excuses or reasons for actions that may have occurred because of emotions (such as self-interest) that a person does not want to acknowledge.

10 Describe how to deal with conflict.

- In dealing with conflict, you should try to be supportive and personable, and remain professional. Avoid participating in negative attitudes, stereotyping, passing judgment, gossiping, and jumping to conclusions about others' actions or motives.

Summary

Communication is the sharing of thoughts, ideas, information, and feelings. It requires a sender (source), message, channel (mode of communication), receiver, and feedback. For effective communication, messages must be complete, concise, clear, cohesive, and courteous. Feedback involves non-verbal communication (body language) or verbal expressions that express an understanding of a message. Listening is crucial for effective communication, and may be active, passive, or evaluative.

In health care, written communication such as medical writing requires a high level of accuracy, clarity, and care in order to avoid mistakes that could cause patient harm. Aside from face-to-face communication, today's health care settings involve a great deal of communication via computers, telephone, and other methods. Communication may be interrupted by environmental barriers, language barriers, hearing impairment, prejudice, and defense mechanisms. Overall, positive, effective communication helps health care professionals to work as a respectful team, which in turn allows the delivery of excellent patient care.

Review questions

1 In the communication process, what is feedback?
2 What is the most important form of non-verbal communication?
3 What is personal space?
4 If you encourage a patient to ask questions, ask the patient to repeat your instructions, and tell the patient that you are concerned, what type of communication are you sharing?
5 What is clinical e-mail?
6 When photocopying, what must you ensure at all times?
7 What do the terms prejudice and discrimination mean?
8 When does negative communication occur in relation to a patient?
9 What do the defense mechanisms known as intellectualization and projection mean?
10 When can conflicts in the health care setting occur?

Bibliography

American Academy on Communication in Health Care. 2016. AACH Home Page. Available at: www.aachonline.org. Lexington, Kentucky: American Academy on Communication in Health Care.

American Hospital Association. 2016. Communicating with Patients. Available at: www.aha.org/advocacy-issues/communicatingpts/index.shtml. Chicago: American Hospital Association.

American Medical Writers Association. 2016. AMWA Home Page. Available at: www.amwa.org. Rockville: American Medical Writers Association.

Angelo, G. 2014. *The 7 Effective Communication Skills: How to Be a Better Communicator Now*. Seattle: SN & NS Publications. Electronic.

Back, A., Arnold, R., and Tulsky, J. 2009. *Mastering Communication with Seriously Ill Patients: Balancing Honesty with Empathy and Hope*. New York: Cambridge University Press. Print.

Burgo, J. 2012. *Why Do I Do That?: Psychological Defense Mechanisms and the Hidden Ways They Shape Our Lives*. New York: New Rise Press. Print.

BusinessBalls.com. 2016. How to Read Body Language Signs and Gestures – Non-Verbal Communications – Male and Female, for Work, Social, Dating, and Mating Relationships. Available at: www.businessballs.com/body-language.htm. Eynsford: BusinessBalls.com.

Christianson, J., et al. 2012. *Physician Communication with Patients: Research Findings and Challenges*. Ann Arbor: University of Michigan Press. Print.

Chron.com. 2016. Advantages of Teamwork in Today's Health Care Organizations. Available at: http://work.chron.com/advantages-teamwork-todays-health-care-organizations-5143.htm. Houston: Houston Chronicle.

Creativity in Care. 2011. Conflict in Care Settings. Available at: http://creativityincare.org/conflict-in-care-settings. London: Creativity in Care – Karrie Marshall.

Deepermind.com. 2016. Abraham Maslow – Hierarchy of Needs. Available at: www.deepermind.com/20maslow.htm. Newark: Deepermind.com.

Dinkin, S., Filner, B., and Maxwell, L. 2012. *The Exchange Strategy for Managing Conflict in Healthcare: How to Defuse Emotions and Create Solutions When the Stakes Are High*. New York: McGraw-Hill Education. Print.

Dutta, M.J., and Kreps, G.L. 2013. *Reducing Health Disparities: Communication Interventions*. New York: Peter Lang Publishing Inc. Print.

Employee Assistance Network, Inc. 2016. Tips for Communicating Effectively With Your Boss. Available at: www.eannc.com/employees/tips-for-communicating-effectively-with-your-boss. Asheville: Employee Assistance Network of North Carolina.

Fitzgerald, A. 2014. *Healing Conversations: Essential Communications for Healthcare Professionals*. Seattle: CreateSpace Independent Publishing Platform. Print.

Helpguide.org – Trusted Guide to Mental Health. 2016. Improving Your Non-Verbal Communication Skills. Available at: www.helpguide.org/articles/relationships/nonverbal-communication.htm. Santa Monica: Helpguide.org.

Hugman, B. 2009. *Healthcare Communication*. London: Pharmaceutical Press. Print.

Institute for Healthcare Communication. 2016. IHC Home Page. Available at: http://healthcarecomm.org. New Haven: Institute for Health Care Communication.

Johnson, K.S. 2016. Non-Confrontational Communication with Coworkers. Available at: http://work.chron.com/nonconfrontational-communication-coworkers-8667.html. Houston: Houston Chronicle.

Kelly-McCorry, L., and Mason, J. 2011. *Communication Skills for the Healthcare Professional*. New York: Lippincott, Williams, & Wilkins. Print.

LittleThingsMatter.com. 2010. Verbal Communication Skills Worth Mastering. Available at: www.littlethingsmatter.com/blog/2010/11/30/10-verbal-communication-skills-worth-mastering. Chicago: W. Todd Smith.

Matsumoto, D., Frank, M.G., and Hwang, H. 2012. *Nonverbal Communication: Science and Applications*. Thousand Oaks: SAGE Publications. Print.

Monarth, H. 2013. *Breakthrough Communication: A Powerful 4-Step Process for Overcoming Resistance and Getting Results*. New York: McGraw-Hill Education. Print.

PsychCentral. 2016. PsychCentral Home Page. Available at: http://psychcentral.com. Newburyport: PsychCentral.

Ragan's Health Care Communication News. 2016. Health Care Communication Home Page. Available at: http://healthcarecommunication.com. Chicago: Ragan's Health Care Communication News.

Safer Healthcare. 2016. Conflict Resolution in Hospitals and Healthcare Facilities. Available at: www.saferhealthcare.com/high-reliability-topics/conflict-management-in-healthcare. Centennial: Safer Healthcare.

Schreiner, E. 2016. 5 Steps to the Communication Process in the Workplace. Available at: http://smallbusiness.chron.com/5-steps-communication-process-workplace-16735.html. Houston: Houston Chronicle.

Scott-Conner, C. 2015. *Medical Writing: A Brief Guide for Beginners*. Seattle: CreateSpace Independent Publishing Platform. Print.

Silverman, J., Kurt, S., and Draper, J. 2013. *Skills for Communicating with Patients, 3rd Edition*. Boca Raton: CRC Press. Print.

Whitborne, S.K. 2016. Fulfillment at Any Age -. Available at: www.psychologytoday.com/blog/fulfillment-any-age/201110/the-essential-guide-defense-mechanisms. New York: Psychology Today.

Wolf, J. 2015. *Body Language: Master the Art of Reading Anyone Through Nonverbal Communication*. Seattle: CreateSpace Independent Publishing Platform. Print.

Chapter 15

Computers and technology in health care

After study of the chapter, readers should be able to:

1 Explain various types of computers used in health care.
2 Describe patient monitoring systems.
3 Explain the advantages of electronic medical records.
4 Identify the functions of spreadsheets used in health care.
5 Give examples of computerized diagnostic imaging methods.
6 Explain the basics of fiber optics in health care.
7 Describe the two techniques that are combined for all image-guided surgery, since they allow for three-dimensional accuracy.
8 As part of bioinformatics, explain the Human Genome Project.
9 Explain how telemedicine is revolutionizing health care.
10 List simple steps to protect computer data.

Overview

Computers and related technology are crucial for today's health care professions. Every health care professional has some interaction with computerized technology, and often the majority of a specific job centers on it. It is important to understand at least the basics of computers when entering the workforce. For each specific health care profession, training in the use of computers and technology is a component of college courses that prepares each student for how their work will utilize these devices. The final and perhaps most important component involving computers and related technology is security, since inadequate computer security affects patients, health care professionals, facilities, and society in general.

Types of computer

The health care professionals of today work with a variety of types of computer. Therefore, understanding of computer basics is an essential component of employment in the field. There are four basic types of computer in use today, each of which is designed for particular types of work and work facilities. The four basic types include supercomputers, mainframe computers, minicomputers, and personal computers.

Supercomputers

Supercomputers are the largest and most complicated computers used today. They offer extremely fast processing of information, and are mostly used in research medicine, such as for cancer or DNA research, or for genetic coding. The future of medicine is largely based on the advances made in the design of supercomputers.

Mainframe computers

Mainframe computers are able to process and store enormous amounts of information. They are mostly used by larger health care institutions, including hospitals and universities, as well as by the government. Medicare and Medicaid are examples of government programs that utilize mainframe computers.

Minicomputers

Minicomputers are larger than personal computers, yet smaller than mainframe computers. They are primarily used in *networks*, which link multiple computers together as part of a computer system. Most minicomputers function as *servers*, which are centralized storage locations for information that is shared between multiple computers. Personal computers are quickly becoming as powerful as minicomputers, and may replace them in the future.

Personal computers

Personal computers are also known as *microcomputers*, and are found nearly everywhere today. Since they are relatively small and self-contained, they are perfect for use in offices, schools, and homes. There are several different types of personal computer available, and their designs are based on the needs of different types of user.

Desktop
Desktop personal computers are designed to fit on desks and other flat surfaces (see Figure 15.1). Therefore, they are the most common type of personal computer used in medical facilities. Many desktop computers have a *tower case* that contains their operating components. This type of case is often placed on the floor near the workstation so that there is more surface area available for the user.

Laptop and notebook
Laptop personal computers are smaller than desktop computers, weighing only a few pounds (see Figure 15.2). Approximately the size of a magazine, they can operate via AC electrical power or by battery. Laptops and notebook computers allow health care

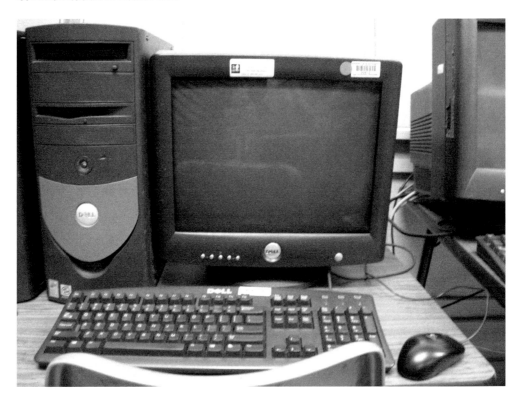

Figure 15.1 A desktop computer.

Figure 15.2 A laptop computer.

professionals to communicate easily with medical office computer systems, to access data and information from multiple locations. These types of computer are becoming extremely popular in medical offices, since they are mobile and easy to move between examination rooms and other areas. They easily exchange electronic health records with other computers.

Subnotebook and tablet PC

Subnotebook personal computers are smaller than laptops, with screens that measure 14 inches or less. They are being replaced by *tablet PCs*, which are small mobile computers that offer touchscreens and/or graphics tablets (see Figure 15.3). Users can operate them with their fingers, a stylus, or a digital pen, and do not have to use a keyboard or mouse. This type of computer is quickly becoming the preferred computer for many users.

Personal digital assistant (PDA)

Personal digital assistants are small computers that are common in health care facilities, since they allow physicians and other health care professionals to easily look up reference information and medications. The PDA allows users to easily enter data into the patient's chart. This is the most popular personal computer for use by many health care professionals.

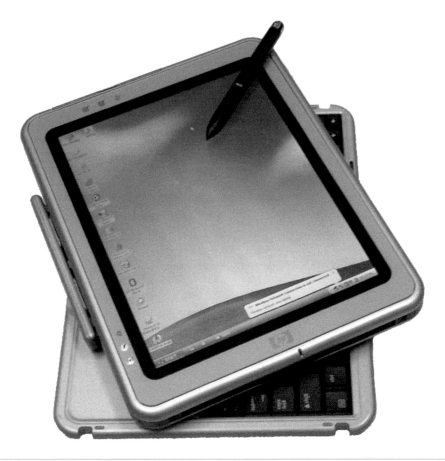

Figure 15.3 A tablet PC.

Computers in health care

In health care, computers are utilized on a daily basis. This means that all health care professionals need to be adept at using computers in order to function effectively in their careers. All departments of health care facilities utilize computerization. Computers are able to store massive amounts of information that can be manipulated with high accuracy and speed. This allows extremely high-speed communication of information, via computer networks, to occur. Computers reduce the need for workers to complete repetitive, time-consuming tasks such as mathematical calculations. The results of data manipulation and calculation become immediately available for others to use.

Examples of the use of computers in health care include electronic patient record systems, processing of information from patient monitoring devices, word processing of medical information, scheduling, electronic prescribing and prescription processing, medical coding, supply inventories, billing, and medical test processing. Table 15.1 summarizes some of the benefits of computer use in health care systems.

Therefore, health care professionals must be able to perform a variety of computer-related tasks. Often, employees in smaller facilities have to perform more varied computer tasks than those in larger facilities. Usually, larger facilities have information technology or *IT* departments that oversee the computer systems.

Focus on computers in health care

Survey of patients reveals that more than 74% feel that their quality of care has been increased by the use of computers in health care.
Source: www.ncbi.nlm.nih.gov/pmc/articles/pmc4554529/.

Patient monitoring

Today, patients are commonly monitored using computerized technology. For example, when heart or respiration is monitored, there are alarm systems running simultaneously to alert health care professionals to any problems. Data can be entered and tracked, which aids patient monitoring. Movable computer terminals allow the entering of all patient information needed. In *point-of-care charting systems*, this is done at the bedside in the hospital, or from the bedside of the patient in his or her own home. Patient monitoring systems keep track of vital signs, physical status, and other factors. In hospitals and similar facilities, monitoring systems are linked to central locations such as nursing stations, and are constantly recorded and observed.

Laptop computers have become very popular for patient monitoring, and offer benefits such as record-keeping and charting. Hospitals utilize laptops on movable carts. They are part of hospital-wide computer systems, which allow the exchange of patient data quickly and easily through all departments. Through internal hospital websites, health care professionals can access information from outside the hospital to improve patient care. Laptops are also commonly used by health care professionals who work in the home health care setting (see Figure 15.4). In these settings, the term telemonitoring is used, in which data are collected about the patient's health from his or her own home. Telemonitoring usually utilizes patient interaction about health status, the display of reminders concerning when medications should be administered, and wireless monitoring devices connected to the Internet or a phone line.

Table 15.1 Benefits of computer use in health care systems

Benefit	Comments
Improved quality of care	Computers improve order entry, data storage and analysis, billing, pharmacy needs, radiology needs, documentation, monitoring, medication dispensing and usage, clinical problem solving, diagnostic testing and imaging, and many other factors. They generate alerts, reminders, and integrated patient reports
Decreased costs	Computers link directly with electronic medical records, help to reduce needed testing, reduce paperwork, improve time management, offer streamlined communication, and organize schedules – all of which lower costs
Uniformity	Computers offer the potential for worldwide integration of healthcare systems, reference materials, database linking, automatic updating, better utilization of medical terminology, and many other factors
Patient knowledge	Computers help patients become more involved in their own healthcare options. They increase patient knowledge by offering visual images, educational databases of information, frequently asked questions and answers, and many other factors
Internet capability	Computers offer advanced telemedicine and telepharmacy to many people, including home-bound patients; they utilize sensory and input devices that alert health care professionals to emergencies
Patient accessibility	Computers allow patients to be more involved in their health care. They encourage social networking and offer a variety of applications that can be used and enjoyed by individuals to monitor daily health. Patient–provider interaction has become more convenient and more constant as a result of computers

Computers are also used in dispensing systems to supply patients with predetermined amounts of medication at the correct intervals. Some allow patients to control their own medication administration, such as bedside devices used for pain management. However, these are limited so that the patient cannot overuse them and exceed dosing allowances.

Information management

The managing of large amounts of information helps health care professionals to do their jobs with accuracy as well as speed. Information management involves a variety of functions. For example, a database utilizes software that structures information so that it is searchable in many different ways. Databases can be small or large, and are designed for all

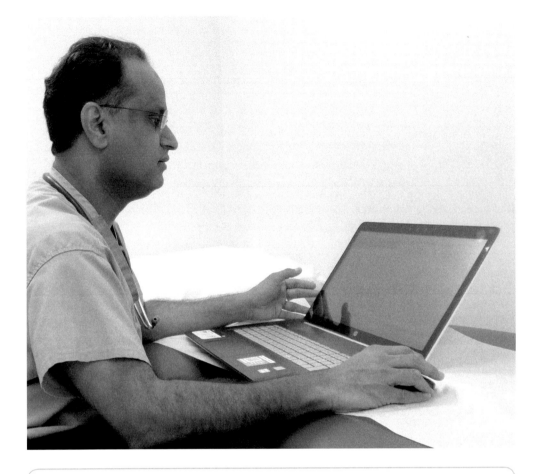

Figure 15.4 A health care professional using a laptop computer in a home care setting.

types of medical office. In a database, each group of related data is called a *record*, such as an individual patient record. To enter data into an individual record, the user types it into fields that are predefined. Common fields in a patient record include *name, telephone number, address, occupation,* and *insurance company.* A group of related fields makes up a file.

In health care management, computerized databases offer easy and fast retrieval of records, which can be accessed and sorted, or used to create reports. Records can be searched in many ways, such as by last name of the patient, address information, insurer, or dates. More than one individual can access information at the same time. Changes to records can be easily made. Also, quality improvement studies are able to be performed using computerized databases.

It is important to enter data accurately, since errors can affect patient outcomes in many different ways. Lawsuits may result when information is entered or managed incorrectly. Computerized databases must be correctly constructed in order to serve the needs of the facility and the customers.

Computerization of medical records

Today, electronic medical records *(EMRs)* are the most common forms of health care information utilized for patients. The computerization of medical records offers better efficiency, lower costs, and safer patient care. The federal government now requires that health care facilities computerize their record-keeping. This was enforced by the cutting of Medicare reimbursements to those who did not comply by 2015. The process of totally computerizing all areas of health care practice is ongoing, but it is becoming a reality for nearly all in the United States. The major impediments to this process have been resistance by physicians, lack of IT staff, expensive initial costs, and expensive maintenance costs.

The goal of EMRs is that they are shareable and useable by all types of health care facility. Different software packages currently may not be able to interface between them. Uniformity must happen so that patients can receive adequate care that utilizes accurate sharing of their health information no matter where they are when something occurs that requires medical treatment. Software used for EMR is being consistently improved, offering accuracy, speed, and compatibility while reducing all types of error. The basic information contained in an EMR includes the following:

- Patient identification information
- Emergency department visits
- Preventive care
- Clinic notes
- Inpatient notes
- Laboratory data
- Pharmacy data
- Radiology data
- Surgical procedures
- Billing information.

Spreadsheets

The primary use of electronic **spreadsheet** software **programs** is to calculate numerical data quickly and accurately. Each spreadsheet consists of rows and columns that are made up of individual blocks called *cells*. For calculations, numbers and calculation formulas are inserted into specific cells. Budgets may be easily constructed using spreadsheets. They are used widely in billing and accounting. Changes to only one section, several sections, or many can be easily made and then recalculations can be performed quickly.

Spreadsheets are also important since they easily link to electronic billing programs, including those related to Medicare and Medicaid. Medical coding can be matched to procedures for fee schedules and bills. Insurer codes can also be used when needed. Spreadsheets allow for calculations about future hiring needs and required financing over time. They allow the creation of charts and graphs so that information can be more readily understood. Accuracy is, of course, essential when using spreadsheets so that calculations are correct.

Diagnostics

Computerized diagnostics include diagnostic imaging, expert systems, fiber optics, and patient questionnaires. **Diagnostic imaging** allows images to be mathematically converted into measurements. This means that better viewing of soft tissues can now be done. These are much more detailed and clear than traditional X-rays. The ability of computers to convert mathematical measurements into images has vastly improved patient care.

Digital X-rays are also available, which allow patients to be examined with much less radiation exposure. This utilizes small electronic chips that are linked to computers and monitors, as well as directly to patient records. Other diagnostic methods involving computers include computed tomography (CT), magnetic resonance imaging (MRI), positron emission tomography (PET), and ultrasound (see Figures 15.5a and 15.5b).

CT utilizes X-rays taken from many angles, with tissue density measurements converted into cross-sectional views. MRI uses a magnetic field, in which hydrogen atom activity inside body tissues is measured, then converted into cross-sectional images. In PET, a radioactive substance is injected into the patient's body, which can be detected by a scanner and translated into three-dimensional images. In ultrasonography, high-frequency sound waves bounce off tissues and organs as echoes, from which signals are used to create images. A newer, experimental technology called electrical impedance tomography (EIT) uses skin electrodes that allow electrical currents to be measured, detecting tissue differences.

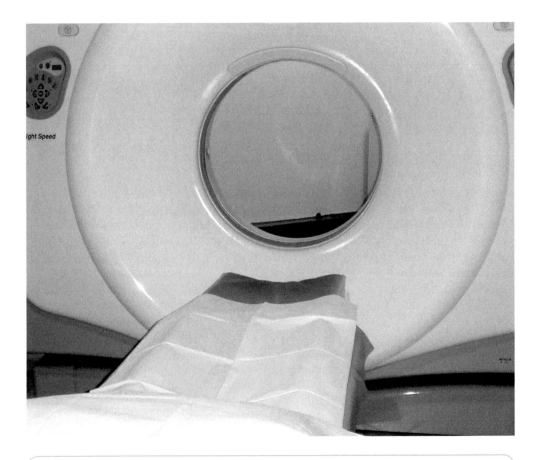

Figure 15.5a Computed tomography (CT) scan.

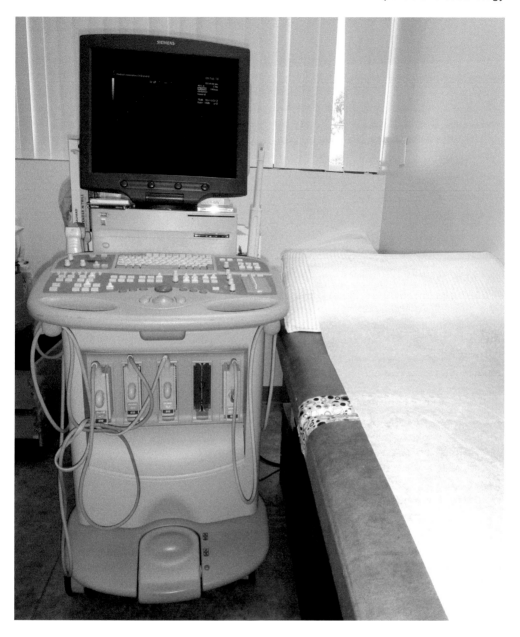

Figure 15.5b Ultrasound (ultrasonography).

Focus on diagnostic imaging

Magnetic resonance imaging (MRI) and ultrasound are safer than other types of diagnostic imaging, because they operate without *ionizing radiation*.

Expert systems

Expert systems help to diagnose and treat specific conditions. They utilize artificial intelligence, which is the ability of a computer to perform tasks that normally require human intelligence, including visual perception, speech recognition, decision-making, and language translation. Since the 1970s, expert systems have been used, but only in more recent years have they advanced to the point of offering enough accuracy to be widely useful. Artificial intelligence is intended to assist health care professionals in their decision-making, not to replace human interaction. Common examples of these expert systems include:

- *ATHENA* – used for hypertension and opioid therapy
- *CEMS* – used for psychiatric and mental conditions
- *GIDEON* – used for infectious diseases and epidemiology
- *TherapyEdge HIV* – used for patients with the HIV virus.

Fiber optics

An area of applied science, Fiber optics is the means by which an organ or cavity can be viewed by using plastic fibers to transmit light through a specially designed tube, reflecting a magnified image. It is used for diagnosis, treatment, and medical data transfer. Examples of fiber optics include the *fiberoptic colonoscope*, *fiberoptic duodenoscope*, and the *fiberoptic bronchoscope*. The science of fiber optics utilizes tiny cables, as thin as human hairs, to transmit data. Fiber optics has many applications in medicine, and is becoming more prevalent in most specialization areas. It allows better visualization during patient examinations, and also improves patient understanding of their own conditions by being able to be shown actual images. Fiber optics has greatly increased safety for many surgical procedures since it allows tiny cameras to be inserted through narrow tubes, which project images over cables onto screens. This allows tiny incisions to be made, usually of less than one half-inch, while physicians are able to view the procedure more clearly. Examples of surgeries that commonly utilize fiber optics include repair of hip fractures and spinal fusions. When a surgical procedure is needed, it is then done through tiny instruments inserted through other tubes. The screen images guide the surgical procedure with great accuracy.

Patient questionnaires

The use of *patient questionnaires* is also becoming more prevalent, in which patients use computer terminals to enter information into computerized forms. Related health assessment software helps to identify patient conditions. The patient can answer questions about their health, which are then used to identify risk factors and to perform health screening. Some individuals answer these types of question with more honesty and completeness than when they are interviewed face-to-face. There are also *health calculators* available that aid367in determining target heart rates, body mass index, energy expenditure, and other information.

Treatment

For patient treatment, there are many developments related to computerization. **Robotic surgery** allows the use of minimally invasive procedures that offer increased accuracy over traditional forms of surgery. The surgeon guides the robot during surgery, and must have extensive specialized training in robotic surgery. These robots interact with cameras offering three-dimensional imaging in extremely high resolution, and are able to respond to voice commands. The tiny tools used by the robots allow for minuscule incisions to be made, keeping the potential of infection to a minimum and reducing healing time. Robotic surgery is commonly used for cancers of the head and neck, in cardiac surgery, for gynecological cancer surgery, and in urological (prostate cancer) surgeries.

Another type of computer-linked technology includes laser surgery. Light rays that have been finely focused are used in these procedures, such as in corrective surgery of the eyes. For all image-guided surgery, CT is combined with infrared technology, which uses *invisible radiant energy* to allow for three-dimensional accuracy. When the two technologies are combined, it greatly helps in controlling surgical instruments. Image-guided surgery offers more accuracy as well as being less invasive. Computer modeling is also used in dentistry, and both cosmetic and reconstructive surgery.

You should remember

Most surgeons only need to make two or three small incisions in order to successfully perform robotic surgery. The average length of each incision is only 2 cm. The rate of robotic surgeries in the United States is increasing 25% annually.

Sources: www.allaboutroboticsurgery.com/surgicalrobots.html; www.beckersasc.com/asc-turnarounds-ideas-to-improve-performance/ 11-things-to-know-about-robotic-surgery.html.

Research

Health care research is easier today than ever before, via thousands of available computerized resources. Detailed searches for very precise data are possible, interacting with medical journals, electronic books, and research databases. On the Internet, however, only trusted sources for research should be used, in order to ensure the highest accuracy of information. Popular information databases include the National Library of Medicine (MEDLINE and PubMed), the Cumulative Index to Nursing and Allied Health Literature or CINAHL, PsychINFO, and the Educational Resources Information Center or ERIC.

Electronic research is much faster and more accurate than traditional research using only printed materials. The organization of biological data into electronic databases is called bioinformatics. With these resources, health care professionals can access data globally. Perhaps the best example of bioinformatics is the Human Genome Project, an international collaboration that collected all research information about human genes and heredity. The project organized all of the genes involved in human DNA, and became the basis for today's gene therapy.

Focus on the Human Genome Project

The total number of human genes is between 30,000 and 35,000. The functions are unknown for over 50% of them.

Gene therapy is a specialized area that uses normal genes, which are inserted into cells, replacing abnormal genes that are linked to disease. Drug therapy has also greatly benefited from computerized research, and the development of new drugs is able to occur more quickly than ever before as a result, helping many patients worldwide.

Telemedicine

Telemedicine uses telecommunication equipment and IT to provide clinical care to individuals at distant sites, as well as to transmit medical and surgical information and images needed to provide that care. It is revolutionizing health care. Telemedicine may involve primary care physicians, specialists, referral services, remote patient monitoring, medical education, consumer medical information, and consumer health information. It is now used by hospitals, clinics, home health agencies, private physicians, and all varieties of health care organization.

Telemedicine links emergency caregivers with physicians to provide better on-site care, allows vital signs of home-bound patients to be transmitted to health care facility monitoring systems, gives patients access to specialists who are located far away, allows long-distance physical examinations to be performed, allows monitoring of pacemakers, and even allows electrocardiograms to be performed between different locations.

Telemedicine is somewhat ahead of state licensing guidelines concerning a physician's ability to practice. Currently, a physician licensed in one state is not allowed to diagnose, suggest treatment, or otherwise work with patients in another state, but this is an area of contention that will likely be changing. Also, telemedicine over long distances will probably influence changes in regulations put forth by private insurers and government programs such as Medicare and Medicaid. Legal outcomes will undoubtedly result from cases involving telemedicine and the transmission of images and information.

Already, however, long-distance telemedicine has helped U.S. troops in other countries. Treatment has been performed successfully, guided by American specialists. Robotic systems have been used in this manner via telemedicine, to send data from robotic probes to physicians who can then direct what must be done to treat the wounded individual. Telemedicine will also offer vital assistance to people in areas of the world who do not otherwise have access to the latest imaging equipment.

> ### You should remember
>
> As of 2014, more than 90% of health care organizations had begun developing or implementing telemedicine programs.
> *Source:* www.wexhealthinc.com/healthcare-trends-institute/
> telemedicine-statistics-show-big-growth-potential/.

Telepharmacy

Telepharmacy is the delivery of pharmaceutical care via the use of telecommunications equipment, to patients in locations where there is not direct contact with a pharmacist. In telepharmacy, a drug can be dispensed at a location other than a pharmacy. Using telephone lines or other modes of communication, prescriptions are sent to computerized dispensing units that prepare and release the prescribed dosages. These systems have protections built in that do not allow incorrect dosages or types of medication to be dispensed. Telepharmacy is a good way to assist dispensing between commercial pharmacies located far away from medical facilities.

Central pharmacy sites also use telepharmacy to dispense medications to rural citizens in distant locations. Video conferences can occur between pharmacists, patients, and dispensaries. All of the same procedures that can be performed personally for a patient in a local pharmacy can be performed via telepharmacy, including patient counseling. With telepharmacy, a remote pharmacy can serve a patient without having to have a pharmacist on location, but instead communicating electronically.

Computer security

In the health care setting, computer security cannot be stressed enough. Private patient health information must be protected from those who do not have authorized access. There is a variety of laws related to computer security, the most important of which is the Health Insurance Portability and Accountability Act, or HIPAA, which is also discussed in Chapters 3 and 16.

For computer security, simple precautions that provide protection of data include the use of passwords that are unique to every user. In this way, the individual accessing data is identified by the computer system. Passwords should never be shared, under any circumstances. If an unauthorized user gains access to a facility's files, they may be able to delete or falsify information. Often, such activities are related to payments and other financial transactions. The best passwords are those assigned by the facility to each user, since many users choose personal passwords that are simple and relatively easy to guess.

Computer security also requires that users do not leave their workstations unattended, and that they close all open programs before leaving the computer terminal. Patients and other unauthorized individuals must be kept away from areas where they could view information. Printouts from the computer must be shredded before being discarded.

It is important not to create, change, or delete any records unless you are authorized to do so. This can compromise the accuracy and completeness of needed records. Files must be regularly backed up so that accidentally deleted information can be restored from backup copies.

A major concern affecting computer security is **computer viruses**, which are destructive programs that attempt to access information illegally. They are capable of slowing down or even destroying entire computer systems, and most commonly are spread from programs **downloaded** via the Internet, or from *infected* files loaded into the computer from a source such as a **CD-ROM**. All computers, regardless of their location or type, can be infected by viruses, making this a very important factor. To prevent viruses in the health care facility, you must follow all policies and procedures concerning the use of e-mail, the Internet, software, and antivirus programs. Basically, Internet usage should only involve work-related tasks. It is not appropriate to "**surf**" the Internet for personal reasons while at work. Avoiding this practice helps to reduce the possibility of visiting websites infected with viruses.

When using a laptop computer in a public setting, public Internet access points called *hot spots* are very popular. For example, a user can bring his or her laptop to lunch at a restaurant that offers this free Internet access, and easily "surf" the Internet. The problem is that other individuals are easily able to access your private information that is transmitted over the wireless technology offered in these locations.

CASE STUDY

Most physicians today feel that the use of electronic medical records has greatly improved their practices, and in some cases has saved lives. A physician specializing in cancer recently instituted an EMR system for his practice, which almost immediately helped him to better diagnose his patients. It helped identify cases of asymptomatic breast cancer in three patients.

1 What key component of EMR systems may have played a part in identifying asymptomatic breast cancer?
2 How can EMRs increase knowledge about breast cancer between health care providers?
3 Do statistics show that patients are more likely to participate in cancer screening because of EMR alerts?

Chapter highlights

This section answers the Objectives found at the beginning of the chapter.

1 Explain various types of computer used in health care.

- Supercomputers are the largest and most complicated type, offering extremely fast processing of information. They are mostly used in research medicine, such as for cancer or DNA research, or for genetic coding.
- Mainframe computers are able to process and store enormous amounts of information. They are widely used by larger health care institutions, including hospitals and universities, as well as by the government (including Medicare and Medicaid).
- Minicomputers are smaller than mainframe computers and are primarily used in computer networks, usually functioning as servers (centralized storage locations for shared information).
- Personal computers (microcomputers) are used nearly everywhere. They include desktops, laptops, notebooks, subnotebooks, tablet PCs, and personal digital assistants (PDAs).

2 Describe patient monitoring systems.

- Computers are used to monitor various body systems, including the cardiovascular and respiratory systems of patients. They allow for alarm systems that alert health care professionals, data entering and tracking, portability, point-of-care charting, and monitoring of vital signs, physical status, and other factors. Patient monitoring systems link patients at home or in facilities to a variety of health care professionals. Laptop computers have become very popular for patient monitoring. Telemonitoring is used in home health care settings, allowing data to be collected about a patient from his or her own home.

3 Explain the advantages of electronic medical records.

- Electronic medical records (EMRs) offer better efficiency, lower costs, and safer patient care. Since the federal government now requires the computerization of health records, there is increased sharing and use between all types of health care professional. Software used for EMRs is being consistently improved, offering accuracy, speed, and compatibility while reducing errors.

4 Identify the functions of spreadsheets used in health care.

- Calculation of numerical data
- Budgets, billing, and accounting
- Linking to Medicare, Medicaid, and other electronic billing programs
- Use of insurer codes
- Calculations about future hiring needs and required financing over time
- Creation of charts and graphs.

5 Give examples of computerized diagnostic imaging methods.

- Digital X-rays
- Computed tomography (CT)
- Magnetic resonance imaging (MRI)
- Positron emission tomography (PET)
- Ultrasound.

6 Explain the basics of fiber optics in health care.

- Fiber optics utilizes tiny cables to transmit data
- It is used for diagnosis, treatment, and medical data transfer
- It allows better visualization during examinations
- It improves patient understanding by showing actual images
- It increases safety in surgery, as well as accuracy, by using tiny cameras to project images, allowing smaller incisions to be made and clearer viewing.

7 Describe the two techniques that are combined for all image-guided surgery, since they allow for three-dimensional accuracy.

- Computed tomography (CT) – utilizes X-rays taken from many angles, with tissue density measurements converted into cross-sectional views.
- Infrared technology – which uses *invisible radiant energy*.

8 As part of bioinformatics, explain the Human Genome Project.

- The Human Genome Project is an international collaboration that collected all research information about human genes and heredity.
- It organized all of the genes involved in human DNA, and became the basis for today's gene therapy.

9 Explain how telemedicine is revolutionizing health care.

- Telemedicine involves medical practice that takes place over mobile devices and telephone lines.
- It allows transmission of important types of data such as digital images.
- It may involve many types of health care professional, and is used by all varieties of health care organization.
- Telemedicine links emergency caregivers with physicians, transmits vital signs to monitoring facilities, gives patients access to specialists over long distances, allows long-distance examinations to be performed, offers pacemaker monitoring, and allows long-distance electrocardiograms to be performed.

10 List simple steps to protect computer data.

- Assigning passwords that are unique to every user, and not shared
- Avoiding leaving workstations unattended
- Closing all open programs before leaving terminals
- Keeping unauthorized individuals away from private information
- Shredding computer printouts before discarding them
- Avoiding the alteration of computer records unless authorized to do so
- Regularly backing up files
- Avoiding computer viruses by strictly following your facility's procedures concerning e-mail, the Internet, software, and antivirus programs.

Summary

Health care professionals, at all levels, must be computer-literate in order to be effective in their careers. Computers are used for all types of functions in clinical, administrative, treatment, and diagnostic areas. Mobile devices such as laptop computers are becoming more popular every year, offering the ability to access and utilize data regardless of location. Computers are even involved in automated functions such as prescription dispensing and robotic surgery. Electronic medical records allow health care professionals to quickly access, alter, and share patient data with greater accuracy and efficiency than ever before. Patient diagnoses and treatments have been highly improved by the use of computerized imaging, fiber optics, and artificial intelligence. Advances in telemedicine and telepharmacy have made today's health care more effective than ever, since patients can now be treated over long distances. However, all of these advances require increased computer security to protect the private health information of patients.

Review questions

1 What do the terms "medical coding" and "information technology" mean?
2 How does telemonitoring work?
3 What were the major impediments to the process of totally computerizing all areas of health care practice in the United States?
4 What is artificial intelligence?
5 What is robotic surgery commonly used for?
6 How does gene therapy work?
7 How does telepharmacy work?
8 What is the most important law related to computer security?
9 What is a computer virus?
10 What is the danger of using a laptop computer in a public setting?

Bibliography

Agency for Healthcare Research and Quality. 2015. AHRQ Home Page. Available at: www.ahrq.gov. Rockville: Agency for Healthcare Research and Quality.

All About Robotic Surgery. 2015. The Official Medical Robotics News Center. Available at: www.allaboutroboticsurgery.com/surgicalrobots.html. New York: AVRA Surgical Robotics.

Becker's ASC Review. 2016. 11 Things to Know About Robotic Surgery. Available at: www.beckersasc.com/asc-turnarounds-ideas-to-improve-performance/11-things-to-know-about-robotic-surgery.html. Chicago: Becker's Healthcare.

Donovan, P., and Papay, J. 2012. *Pharmacists and Medication Adherence: Brief Interventions, Motivational Interviewing & Telepharmacy.* Wall Township: Healthcare Intelligence Network. Print.

Ehrenfeld, J.M., and Cannesson, M. 2014. *Monitoring Technologies in Acute Care Environments: A Comprehensive Guide to Patient Monitoring Technology.* New York: Springer. Print.

Fong, B., Fong, A.C.M., and Li, C.K. 2010. *Telemedicine Technologies: Information Technologies in Medicine.* Hoboken: Wiley. Print.

Forbes.com. 2013. The Different Ways that Technology is Transforming Health Care. Available at: www.forbes.com/sites/bmoharrisbank/2013/01/24/5. Jersey City: Forbes Media LLC.

Gartree, R. 2011. *Electronic Health Records: Understanding and Using Computerized Medical Records, 2nd Edition.* Upper Saddle River: Prentice Hall. Print.

Glandon, G.L., et al. 2013. *Information Systems for Healthcare Management, 8th Edition.* Arlington: Health Administration Press. Print.

Healthcare Information and Management Systems Society (HIMSS). 2015. *Preparing for Success in Healthcare Information and Management Systems: The CPHIMS Review Guide, 2nd Edition.* Chicago: HIMSS Publishing. Print.

Healthcare Information and Management Systems Society. 2015. HIMSS Home Page. Available at: www.himss.org. Chicago: HIMSS.

Hoyt, R.E., and Yoshihashi, A.K. 2014. *Health Informatics: Practical Guide for Healthcare and Information Technology Professionals, 6th Edition.* Raleigh: Lulu.com. Print.

Informatics and Nursing. 2015. Computer Development and Health Care Information Systems 1950 to Present. Available at: http://dlthede.net/Informatics/Chap01IntroNI/healthcare_computers.html. Philadelphia: Informatics and Nursing.

InformationWeek. 2013. Remote Patient Monitoring: 9 Promising Technologies. Available at: www.informationweek.com/mobile/remote-patient-monitoring-9-promising-technologies/d/d-id/1110968. San Francisco: InformationWeek / UBM.

Joos, I., Nelson, R., and Smith, M.J. 2013. *Introduction to Computers for Healthcare Professionals, 6th Edition.* Burlington: Jones & Bartlett Learning. Print.

Lambert, A.A. 2014. *Advanced Pharmacy Practice, 3rd Edition.* Boston: Delmar Cengage Learning. Print.

Lyuboslavsky, V. 2015. *Telemedicine and Telehealth 2.0: A Practical Guide for Medical Providers and Patients.* Seattle: CreateSpace Independent Publishing Platform. Print.

McCormick, K., and Gugerty, B. 2013. *Healthcare Information Technology Exam Guide for CompTIA Healthcare IT Technician and HIT Pro Certifications.* New York: McGraw-Hill Education. Print.

National Institutes of Health. 2016. NIH Home Page. Available at: www.nih.gov. Bethesda: National Institutes of Health.

Preim, B., and Botha, C.P. 2013. *Visual Computing for Medicine, 2nd Edition.* Burlington: Morgan Kaufmann. Print.

Sequelmed.com. 2015. Telemedicine Regulations. Available at: www.sequelmed.com/Articles/Future%20Healthcare_EMR%20Issue%20April%202009_Sequel%20Systems.pdf. Melville: SequelMed.

Sequelmed.com. 2016. Computerization of Health Records. Available at: www.sequelmed. com/Articles/Future%20Healthcare_EMR%20Issue%20April%202009_Sequel%20 Systems.pdf. Melville: SequelMed.

Shortliffe, E.H., and Cimino, J.J. 2013. *Biomedical Informatics: Computer Applications in Health Care and Biomedicine, 4th Edition.* New York: Springer. Print.

Tang, J., and Agaian, S.S. 2013. *Computer-Aided Cancer Detection and Diagnosis: Recent Advances.* Seattle: SPIE Press. Print.

Terry, K. 2012. Telepharmacy Really Does Make A Difference. Available at: www.information-week.com/healthcare/clinical-information-systems/telepharmacy-really-does-make-a-difference/d/d-id/1106265. San Francisco: Information Week / UBM.

Topol, E. 2015. *The Patient Will See You Now: The Future of Medicine Is in Your Hands.* New York: Basic Books. Print.

U.S. Health. 2016. How Technology is Transforming Health Care. Available at: http:// health.usnews.com/health-news/hospital-of-tomorrow/articles/2013/07/12/how-technology-is-transforming-health-care. New York: U.S. News and World Report.

U.S. National Library of Medicine. 2015. Ethnically Diverse Patients' Perceptions of Clinician Computer Use in a Safety-Net Clinic. Available at: www.ncbi.nlm.nih.gov/pmc/articles/pmc4554529/. Bethesda: National Center for Biotechnology Information.

Veney, J.E., Kros, J.F., and Rosenthal, D.A. 2009. *Statistics for Health Care Professionals: Working with Excel, 2nd Edition.* San Francisco: Jossey-Bass. Print.

Wachter, R. 2015. *The Digital Doctor: Hope, Hype, and Harm at the Dawn of Medicine's Computer Age.* New York: McGraw-Hill Education. Print.

Wager, K.A., Lee, F.W., and Glaser, J.P. 2013. *Health Care Information Systems: A Practical Approach for Health Care Management, 3rd Edition.* San Francisco: Jossey-Bass. Print.

WexHealthInc.com. 2016. Telemedicine Statistics Show Big Growth Potential. Available at: www.wexhealthinc.com/healthcare-trends-institute/telemedicine-statistics-show-big-growth-potential/. Simsbury: Wex Health Inc.

Williams, T., and Samarth, A. 2010. *Electronic Health Records for Dummies.* Hoboken: Wiley Publishing. Print.

Chapter 16

Record-keeping

Objectives

After study of the chapter, readers should be able to:

1 List the documents that are included in the medical record.
2 Differentiate between source-oriented and problem-oriented medical records.
3 Identify what the abbreviation "SOAP" signifies.
4 Describe what is included in the CHEDDAR format of medical records documentation.
5 Describe why electronic health records are superior to traditional paper records.
6 Identify basic suggestions for the usage of electronic medical records.
7 Identify the contents of a personal health record.
8 Describe the contents of an employee's medical record according to the requirements of OSHA.
9 Explain the primary concerns of HIPAA related to the medical record.
10 Describe the HIPAA Security Rule.

Overview

Medical records play an essential role in health care, and accurate record-keeping is an important administrative function. Maintaining a well-organized, easy-to-use records management system is essential in providing good patient care. No health care professional is able to remember every detail of care, such as the results of a physical examination or doses of certain medications. A variety of people in the primary care physician's office have contact with patients, as well consultants, laboratories, and hospitals. It is important that each interaction is recorded in the patient's medical record, which may be electronic or written. Regardless of their form, medical records must be handled safely and securely and adhere to the privacy rules of the Health Insurance Portability and Accountability Act, or HIPAA. Each patient's permanent health record is formed by medical records, which include health information, insurance forms, notes, physician orders, test reports, and other data. Patient records are considered legal documents, and may be used in court cases, meaning that they must contain accurate and correct information. The use of computers for electronic medical records has revolutionized all types of health care profession.

Contents of the medical record

The medical record is the only permanent legal document that includes everything about a patient's medical history, laboratory tests, and appointments with health care professionals. It consists of many different documents containing specific information, which are explained in the following sections.

Admission sheet

The admission sheet contains information from the patient prior to the first visit to the provider, including: name, address, phone number, birthdate, Social Security number, gender, marital status, race, and employer's name, address, and phone number. It may also include the primary health insurer, policy number, insurer address and phone number, co-payment or deductible information, and secondary insurer information. The admission sheet is usually updated every year so that all patient and other information is as current and up-to-date as possible. Copies of any insurance cards may be attached to the admission sheet. The initial visit of a patient to a provider should include information about the chief complaint, in the patient's own words.

Medical history

A patient's medical history contains previous medical information, including allergies, childhood diseases, current and past medications, hospitalizations, immunizations, previous illnesses, and surgeries. Family history, including causes of death, is important because of hereditary and familial components of certain diseases.

Social history

Social history reviews patient education, occupation, marital status, diet, sexual history, alcohol and tobacco use, and hobbies. It is important because lifestyle factors can affect illnesses, and vice versa. Social history is also used to educate the patient about changes that may improve health status.

Physical examination form

The physical examination form is used to ensure consistency of information and minimize the risk of incomplete documentation. It includes a review of the patient's body systems, results of the general physical examination, identification of any signs or symptoms, and the patient's responses to the provider's questions. The review of systems (ROS) and physical examination are usually performed by a physician, nurse practitioner, or physician's assistant, though vital signs are often documented by a medical assistant.

Physician orders

Medical orders for patient care include medications, tests, treatments, and follow-up care, in a precise, highly detailed format. Electronic medical orders allow information to be sent automatically between health care professionals, eliminating errors, loss, and misreading of information.

Progress notes

Progress notes document all contacts between patients and health care providers, regardless of their form. Findings are summarized chronologically, such as changes in conditions and effects of treatments. Progress notes provide a brief overview of the patient's health and always include entry dates, times, and provider names. In a hospital, this is very important since many different individuals may access the patient record. There is no standard format for progress notes, and in electronic form they are more organized and accurate.

Laboratory reports

Laboratory reports include results from tests, including blood tests, electrocardiographs, computed tomography (CT) scans, magnetic resonance imaging (MRI) scans, and X-rays. Tests may be conducted in the physician's office or elsewhere. The reports section includes consultations with other providers.

Diagnostic imaging information

Diagnostic imaging information must be recorded in the medical record. It includes X-rays, cardiac catheterizations, echocardiography, cerebral angiograms, fetal ultrasound, gastrointestinal studies with contrast media, MRI, and others. Today, diagnostic imaging information is often reproduced onto CDs or DVDs, which allows patients to carry their diagnostic images in a format that can be used by other health professionals, if needed.

Types of medical records

There are two ways in which personal health records are organized. These are the *source-oriented medical record (SOMR)* and the *problem-oriented medical record (POMR)*. In both formats, the most recent information always appears first, and older information follows. This is called a *reverse chronology*, in which data gets chronologically older as you move backwards, while the first page contains the latest information. Every entry requires a date and time stamp as well as the signature or initials of the professional who made the entry. Information must be entered only after an event occurs, never before.

Source-oriented medical records

In a source-oriented medical record (SOMR), information is organized based on type, such as various types of report, and who supplied each of them – the patient, the physician, specialists, hospitals, laboratories, radiologists, cardiologists, and others. When special forms are used to attach such documents to the medical record, there is usually space for the patient's or physician's comments to be added. The SOMR is also sometimes called the *conventional method* or *SOMR approach*.

The primary difficulty with the SOMR format is that tracking progress of a certain condition or illness is more difficult than in the POMR format. This is because the specific ailment will be listed chronologically with any other conditions or illnesses the patient experienced. Should a condition recur a few years later, it remains listed chronologically and is not "grouped" with its initial occurrence.

Problem-oriented medical records

In a problem-oriented medical record (POMR), information is organized based on the problem the patient is experiencing. Each individual problem appears on the first page, given a number and date of first occurrence, and all related documentation bears the same problem number. The problem list may include items affecting the patient's health, including family, social, or work-related problems. It is important to differentiate between *signs*, which are objective and measurable, and *symptoms*, which are subjective and experienced by the patient. When a problem does not exist anymore, that fact is recorded in the progress notes. An "X" is marked next to the problem on the *problem list*.

The next section is the *database*, which contains medical history, review of systems, information from the initial patient interview, physical examination results, lab reports, and other test results. The *educational, diagnostic, and treatment plan* indicates tests and treatments that are required, diagnostic workups, and patient instructions. The final section contains *progress notes*, which are grouped together and numbered according to the problem list. The chronological order of documents includes the patient's condition, problems, complaints, treatment, and responses to care. The POMR is generally preferred over the SOMR because it is easier to use in relation to tracking patient progress.

Focus on "charting by exception"

The *charting by exception* format documents significant or abnormal findings in a problem-oriented method. This method is commonly used with electronic medical records, allowing for shorter charting times and lower costs, greater emphasis on important data and communications between providers, easy data retrieval, faster bedside charting, better tracking of patient comments, and standardized assessment.

SOAP documentation

SOAP documentation, also known as *SOAP notes*, contains four components: *Subjective data*, *Objective data*, *Assessment*, and a *Plan*. This type of documentation originated from the problem-oriented medical record format, and is used by health care providers to communicate between various disciplines, since it clearly documents the patient's progress.

● Subjective data includes patient statements and symptoms in the patient's exact words. Examples of subjective data include statements such as "I have a headache," or "My heart feels like it is beating really fast."

- Objective data includes the health care provider's observations of the patient, such as things that can be seen, felt, heard, or measured. Test results and vital signs may be included. Examples of objective data include "The patient's temperature is 101 °F/38.3 °C," or "The heart rate is elevated at 122 beats per minute." Objective data also includes results of special procedures, diagnoses, X-ray reports, progress notes, and prescribed treatments.
- The assessment portion contains the diagnosis, based on the subjective and objective data. If no final diagnosis can be made, possible disorders that can be ruled out can be listed.
- The plan describes what will be performed, including testing, treatments, and follow-ups.

CHEDDAR format

A more detailed method of medical records documentation is known as the *CHEDDAR format*. This acronym stands for the following:

- *Chief complaint* – including the presenting problems and subjective statements
- *History* – including past medical, family, and social histories, the history of the presenting problems, and other contributing information
- *Examination* – including the extent of body systems examined
- *Details* – focusing on the problem and complaints
- *Drugs* and dosage – includes a list of current medications, dosages, and frequency of administration
- *Assessment* – focusing on the diagnostic process and the physician's diagnosis
- *Return* – concerns return visits or any applicable referrals.

Electronic health records

The majority of health care facilities today utilize electronic health records. These are defined by the National Alliance for Health Information Technology, or NAHIT. Written, printed records are becoming a thing of the past. *Electronic health records (EHRs)* or *electronic medical records (EMRs)* contain an individual's health information that has been created and gathered by more than one health care organization. These records are managed by clinical health care professionals, as well as those directly involved in the individual's treatment. Computerization provides better accuracy, file management, and accessibility of records. EHRs can be transferred quickly and easily between facilities, and can be accessed simultaneously by many health care professionals. Aside from computers in the health care facility, electronic information can also be accessed by laptops, smartphones, tablets, and other hand-held devices.

Large selections of software and file formats are available for electronic medical record management. Electronic records are easier to store, retrieve, securely back up, edit, and read. There is nearly unlimited file space available for use. Computers also allow for many related functions, such as ordering services and supplies, and for financial data activities.

Like all changes, increased usage of EMRs requires policies and procedures about patient information privacy and confidentiality. The type of information that can be accessed, for what reasons, and by which individuals must be spelled out in the policies and procedures of each facility. Patients must give consent for the use and release of their EMRs.

Guidelines for this usage are set out by the American Health Information Management Association (AHIMA) and other associations. Basic suggestions include the following:

- Only authorized personnel should be allowed to change, create, or delete electronic medical records.
- Correct protocols must always be followed when making corrections, such as listing mistaken entries, adding in corrected information, and initialing the new information.
- Computer terminals should never be left unattended once an individual has logged on.
- Personal passwords or computer signatures should never be shared.
- Sensitive material may require additional confidentiality procedures – this includes patients with HIV/AIDS.
- Protected health information should never be e-mailed unless it has been encrypted.
- Electronic copies of computerized files should be documented in a log or other similar type of record.
- Patient information should never be left displayed on a monitor that might be seen by unauthorized personnel.
- Records must be backed up regularly according to accepted protocols.

Advantages of electronic health records are summarized in Table 16.1.

You should remember

The patient's ethical right to confidentiality and privacy is protected by law. Only the patient can waive this right regarding his or her own health information.

Personal health records

Personal health records must always be accurate, complete, and legible. They create a clear record of each patient's personal health care. All documentation related to the patient must remain part of his or her permanent medical record. Entries must be accurate and non-repetitive, yet thorough, in order to ensure effective patient care. Factual entries that include correct acronyms, abbreviations, medical terminology, and spelling are essential. In electronic form, errors should not be deleted, but listed as "mistaken entries" and corrected. In paper form, they should not be erased, but listed as "errors" and corrected. It is also important to make sure that the correct patient file is being worked with prior to entering or correcting any information.

Personal health records also include e-mails, phone messages, and other correspondence between patients and providers. Dates and times are essential to include, along with any supporting documentation about reports or tests. Entries should be brief, including only relevant information. The patient's name does not need to be used in his or her record for each entry – the word "patient" is sufficient. Only universal abbreviations and acronyms are acceptable. These are often listed in each medical facility. Any abbreviation or acronym that may cause confusion should be avoided. The full term should be written out instead.

In a paper record, legibility is crucial, since many individuals may access the record to read what it contains. Illegible writing increases the chance of errors. Certain electronic systems allow personnel to enter information by using a stylus instead of a keyboard. This

> ## Table 16.1 Advantages of electronic health records

Component	Comments
Chart notes	Immediately available information that helps with referrals or consultations with other providers
Coding	CPT or ICD codes can be assigned when a patient visit occurs, helping to simplify the insurance filing process
Coordination	Streamlining the efforts of multiple providers; elimination of duplicate or incompatible tests and treatments
Database	Searchable information containing allergies, demographics, better accessibility to providers, and lab results
Ease of transmission	Sharing of information between providers and other departments, reducing treatment times and notifications concerning critical values
Electronic prescriptions	These reduce errors caused by poor handwriting and reduce time to process prescriptions; this software also screens for allergies and interactions, decreasing adverse reactions
Photographs	When the individual patient appears in the electronic record, this helps to avoid mistakes in identification
Reminders	Electronic alerts concerning when tests, vaccinations, or procedures are due
Trending of information	Analysis of information over time to identify potential problems earlier
Voice recognition	Software that reduces costs by eliminating the need for transcription, and improves availability of printed records

means that poor handwriting can cause the software to interpret the characters incorrectly, and transform them into an incorrect word or phrase.

Medical documentation

Accurate medical documentation allows health care professionals to communicate with each other, utilizing up-to-date patient information. For a single patient, an annual check-up may result in the need for different medications. This means that a number of health care professionals can access the patient's record to verify the patient's previous or current medications, in order to determine which medications can be safely prescribed. Dosages can be verified based on patient vital signs, weight, and other factors.

If any tests have shown results that might impact the use of certain medications, this will be listed in the patient's record. Also, testing technicians access the patient's record to interpret certain substances that may be in the patient's bloodstream. Changes in test results over time are also noted, which may impact future medication decisions by the prescriber. Pharmacists also check the patient's record to determine any allergies or the use of other prescription medications that may conflict with a newly prescribed medication. Therefore, it is easy to see that accurate medical records are of crucial importance to the health management of every patient.

Patient assessments also form part of the medical record. As mentioned previously, they include vital signs such as blood pressure, pulse, respiration rate, and temperature. Other assessments include the patient's medical history, the reason for the current visit to the medical office, and the present symptoms. Assessments of different visits can be compared, which helps physicians to determine correct diagnoses and treatments.

The quality of care given to a patient over time is also documented in the medical record. This information proves whether the physician and other health care professionals have met the expected standard of care. When determining whether a medical facility is meeting its standards, an accrediting agency uses quality of care documented in the medical record. This is also linked to reimbursement by insurers and government plans. These entities review why patients sought medical care and what they received, as well as diagnoses, tests, and treatments. Reimbursement decisions are made based on these types of information. Specific codes are used for each type of service, which are then submitted to insurers and government plans. The billing codes are reviewed with the medical record to make sure everything is correct before reimbursements are issued.

Moral, legal, and ethical standards must be met by all health care professionals in order to avoid a breach of contract between providers and patients. These situations may result in patient harm or embarrassment, and result in fines or lawsuits to the health care professionals involved. Patient records may be admissible as evidence in court cases, such as in those concerning malpractice or negligence. They are also used in injury or accident claims.

The medical record can be used to train new medical professionals. Health educators often use actual patient records during their clinical portions. Records also help for research. By examining similar cases in health records, researchers may accurately determine conditions and make determinations about treatments. In research, medical record data aid in determining how effective a therapy might be, contributing factors to disease states, and important similarities between disease types.

OSHA requires that employers maintain accurate records of every health care employee who may be at risk of occupational exposures. These records must be kept confidential, except for review by OSHA officials and as required by law. The records must include each employee's name, social security number, hepatitis B vaccination status including dates of vaccination, results of any post-exposure examinations, medical testing, and follow-up procedures. A written evaluation of exposure incidents, along with copies of exposure incident reports, must also be included. Employers are required to maintain records for the duration of employment, and for 30 years thereafter.

HIPAA and the medical record

The Health Insurance Portability and Accountability Act, or HIPAA, was passed in 1996, to improve portability and continuity of health insurance coverage; reduce waste, fraud, and abuse; promote medical savings accounts; improve access to long-term care; and simplify health insurance administration. Regarding medical records, HIPAA has resulted in many changes in how they are managed and protected. Patients must sign a HIPAA notice of privacy practices, and if they refuse, this must be correctly documented in the medical record. The primary concerns of HIPAA concerning the medical record include:

- Protecting the privacy of each patient's health information
- The establishment of electronic transmission standards concerning this information as well as claims
- Making sure that all electronic health information is secure.

The *HIPAA Privacy Rule* requires providers to notify patients of their privacy rights and about the usage of their health information. It also requires providers to develop privacy procedures and train employees about them. Providers are encouraged to designate certain individuals that can oversee proper adherence to privacy procedures. They must also secure patient records containing Individually Identifiable Health Information to prevent them from becoming available to unauthorized personnel.

The *HIPAA Notice of Privacy Practices* must be written in plain language, describing uses and disclosures of private health information, patient rights and duties, and how complaints may be registered if privacy violations are suspected. A header must be included that reads, "This notice describes how medical information about you may be used and disclosed, and how you can get access to this information. Please read carefully." These notices must also specify effective dates and points of contact. They must state that the entity or provider reserves the right to change privacy practices.

Patients have many rights, including the right to access, copy, and inspect their own information, to request amendments to their information, to obtain accountings of specific disclosures of their information, to receive different types of communications from their providers, and to complain about violations of regulations and provider policies. A privacy violation complaint form is shown in Appendix B.

HIPAA allows providers to use health care information concerning treatment, payment, and operations. If use of patient information does not fit into one of these categories, written authorization must be obtained before the information can be shared. Also, the *HIPAA Security Rule* describes how patient information is protected on the Internet, computer networks, computer disks and other storage media, and also on *extranets*, which are private networks using similar technology to the Internet.

For electronic medical records, HIPAA mandates that each facility assign a security officer, also known as a privacy officer. The HIPAA Security Rule requires all health care providers to demonstrate compliance in four areas, which are explained in Table 16.2.

Table 16.2 The four areas of compliance under the HIPAA Security Rule

---

1. Confidentiality, integrity, and availability of all electronic protected health information (PHI) that is composed, received, maintained, or sent out
2. Policies and procedures must be in place that protect against use or disclosures of this information that the Privacy Ruling does not allow
3. Other policies and procedures must protect against hazards or threats to this information
4. There must be compliance within the workplace to the Security Ruling

---

It is important to adhere to these four areas, so that when an audit occurs, documentation requested by the Centers for Medicare and Medicaid Services (CMS) can be supplied. Documentation will be needed for administrative, physical, and technical safeguards, and organizational requirements. Training must be given to employees concerning the maintenance of records security.

Focus on protected health information

When a patient requests his or her health information not to be disclosed to anyone, the health care provider must follow through on this request.

CASE STUDY

Accurate medical record-keeping is an essential component of today's health care, since inaccuracies have the potential to cause severe patient harm. A young woman named Frances went to see her family physician, who had just installed a new electronic health records system. Some of the employees at the physician's office were still getting used to the new system at the time of Frances' appointment. Though the EHR system can greatly improve patient care, errors can be copied between sections of a patient's file and result in additional errors. In Frances' case, a clerk in the office clicked on the wrong area in the "allergies" section of her file, when in fact she had an allergy to penicillin. Her gender was selected as "male" instead of "female," and her birthdate was entered as "4/19/1986" instead of the correct date, "4/19/1996."

1 What could the incorrect allergy information have caused?
2 Could the incorrect gender have influenced any incorrect medication choices being made?
3 Could the incorrect birthdate have affected any future testing?

Chapter highlights

This section answers the Objectives found at the beginning of the chapter.

1 List the documents that are included in the medical record.

- Admission sheet
- Medical history
- Social history
- Physical examination form
- Physician orders
- Progress notes
- Laboratory reports
- Diagnostic imaging information.

2 **Differentiate between source-oriented and problem-oriented medical records.**

- Source-oriented medical records organize information based on their type, such as various types of report, and who supplied each of them.
- Problem-oriented medical records organize information based on the problem the patient is experiencing.

3 **Identify what the acronym "SOAP" signifies.**

- Subjective data – patient statements and symptoms in his or her exact words.
- Objective data – the health care provider's observations of the patient, such as things that can be seen, felt, heard, or measured; test results and vital signs may be included, as well as results of special procedures, diagnoses, X-ray reports, progress notes, and prescribed treatments.
- Assessment – the diagnosis, based on the subjective and objective data; if no final diagnosis is made, possible disorders that can be ruled out can be listed.
- Plan – what will be performed, including testing, treatments, and follow-ups.

4 **Describe what is included in the CHEDDAR format of medical records documentation.**

- Chief complaint – the presenting problems and subjective statements.
- History – past medical, family, and social histories, history of the presenting problems, and other contributing information.
- Examination – the extent of body systems examined.
- Details – focused on the problem and complaints.
- Drugs and dosage – list of current medications, dosages, and frequency of administration.
- Assessment – the diagnostic process and the physician's diagnosis.
- Return visits – also, any applicable referrals.

5 **Describe why electronic health records are superior to traditional paper records.**

- Computerization provides better accuracy, file management, and accessibility of records.
- EHRs are easily transferred quickly between facilities, and can be accessed simultaneously by many health care professionals.
- They can also be accessed by laptops, smart phones, tablets, and other hand-held devices.
- EHRs are easier to store, retrieve, securely back up, edit, and read.
- There is nearly unlimited file space available for use.

6 **Identify basic suggestions for the usage of electronic medical records.**

- Only authorized personnel should be allowed to change, create, or delete them.
- Correct protocols must be followed when making corrections.
- Computer terminals should never be left unattended.
- Personal passwords or computer signatures should never be shared.
- Sensitive materials may require additional confidentiality procedures.
- Protected health information should never be e-mailed unless encrypted.
- Electronic copies of computerized files should be documented in a log or other type of record.
- Patient information should never be left displayed on a monitor that might be seen by unauthorized personnel.
- Records must be backed up regularly according to accepted protocols.

7 **Identify the contents of a personal health record.**

- Personal health records contain all documentation related to the patient, which must remain part of his or her permanent medical record.
- They also include e-mails, phone messages, and other correspondence between patients and providers.
- Dates and times are essential to include, along with any supporting documentation about reports or tests.

8 **Describe the contents of an employee's medical record according to the requirements of OSHA.**

- Employee names
- Social security numbers
- Hepatitis B vaccination status including dates of vaccination
- Results of any post-exposure examinations, medical testing, and follow-up procedures
- Written evaluation of exposure incidents
- Copies of exposure incident reports.

9 **Explain the primary concerns of HIPAA concerning the medical record.**

- Protecting the privacy of each patient's health information
- The establishment of electronic transmission standards concerning this information as well as claims
- Making sure that all electronic health information is secure

10 **Describe the HIPAA Security Rule.**

- The HIPAA Security Rule describes how patient information is protected on the Internet, computer networks, computer disks and other storage media, and also on extranets, which are private networks using similar technology to the Internet.

Summary

In health care, accurate record-keeping is essential to providing good patient care. The medical record is a permanent legal document containing everything about a patient's medical history. The medical record may be organized in two different ways: as a source-oriented medical record (SOMR) or as a problem-oriented medical record (POMR). Documentation may take the form of "SOAP" – which stands for subjective data, objective data, assessment, and a plan – as well as a more detailed "CHEDDAR format" system. EHRs have almost entirely replaced traditional paper records, and offer faster, easier, and more accurate records management. Every patient's personal health records become part of his or her permanent medical record. Quality in medical documentation helps health care professionals to meet all moral, legal, and ethical standards. Medical records are largely governed by the regulations set forth in the Health Insurance Portability and Accountability Act (HIPAA). The major goal of this Act was to protect the privacy and security of health information of all people.

Review questions

1 Which government Act established the privacy rules that govern the safe and secure handling of medical records?
2 Why is a patient's family history an important part of his or her medical history?
3 In a hospital, why are progress notes important?
4 Is a SOMR or a POMR preferred as a type of medical record, and why?
5 What type of data is provided by a patient's description of his or her symptoms?
6 What do electronic health records (or electronic medical records) contain?
7 How should errors in personal health records, whether electronic or written, be corrected?
8 What is included in a "patient assessment"?
9 How does documentation of quality of care affect accreditation and reimbursement?
10 What document must feature the header that reads, "This notice describes how medical information about you may be used and disclosed, and how you can get access to this information"?

Bibliography

Al-Ubaydli, M. 2011. *Personal Health Records: A Guide for Clinicians*. Hoboken: Wiley-Blackwell. Print.

Amatayakul, M.K. 2013. *Electronic Health Records: A Practical Guide for Professionals and Organizations, 5th Edition*. Chicago: AHIMA. Print.

AmeriHealth. 2015. Medical Record Keeping Standards. Available at: www.amerihealth.com/members/quality_management/medical_record_standards.html. New York: AmeriHealth.

Buck, C.J. 2016. *Step-by-Step Medical Coding*. Philadelphia: Saunders. Print.

Carlton, M.E. 2011. *My Doctor Book: A Personal Medical Records Organizer*. London: Notebook Publishing Company. Print.

CME Resource/NetCE, and Jackson, L. 2014. *Beyond Therapy: The Basics of Clinical Documentation*. Seattle: CME Resource/NetCE. Digital.

EHealthInsurance.com. 2016. Keeping a Personal Health Record. Available at: www.ehealthinsurance.com/ehealthinsurance/aboutuscopy/keepingapersonalhealthrecord.html. Washington, D.C.: EHealthInsurance.com.

Freudenheim, M. 2012. The Ups and Downs of Electronic Medical Records – The Digital Doctor. Available at: www.nytimes.com/2012/10/09/health/the-ups-and-downs-of-electronic-medical-records-the-digital-doctor.html?pagewanted=all&_r=0. New York: The New York Times.

Gartee, R. 2011. *Electronic Health Records: Understanding and Using Computerized Medical Records, 2nd Edition*. Upper Saddle River: Prentice Hall. Print.

GroupHealth. 2016. Medical Records and Documentation Standards. Available at: https://provider.ghc.org/open/render.jhtml?item=/open/workingwithgrouphealth/records-standards.xml. Seattle: GroupHealth.

Hamilton, B. 2012. *Electronic Health Records, 3rd Edition*. New York: McGraw-Hill Education. Print.

HealthIT.gov. 2013. How is My Health Information or Medical Record Protected by HIPAA?. Available at: www.healthit.gov/patients-families/faqs/how-my-health-information-or-medical-record-protected-hipaa. Washington, D.C.: HealthIT.gov.

Herold, R., and Beaver, K. 2014. *The Practical Guide to HIPAA Privacy and Security Compliance, 2nd Edition.* Boca Raton: Auerbach Publications/CRC Press. Print.

HHS.gov. 2016. For Individuals: Your Medical Records. Available at: www.hhs.gov/hipaa/for-individuals/medical-records/index.html. Washington, D.C.: U.S. Department of Health and Human Services.

Hipaa.com. 2016. HIPAA Compliance Made Easy. Available at: www.hipaa.com. Washington, D.C.: Hipaa.com.

Kettenbach, G. 2009. *Writing Patient/Client Notes: Ensuring Accuracy in Documentation, 4th Edition.* Philadelphia: F.A. Davis Company. Print.

Krager, C., and Krager, D. 2008. *HIPAA for Health Care Professionals (Safety and Regulatory for Health Science).* Boston: Delmar Cengage Learning. Print.

Louisiana State University Health Services Center – Shreveport. 2012. Medical Records Content/Documentation. Available at: www.sh.lsuhsc.edu/policies/policy_manuals_via_ms_word/hospital_policy/h_6.5.0.pdf. Shreveport: Louisiana State University.

MedicalRecords.com. 2015. HIPAA Requirements. Available at: www.medicalrecords.com/physicians/hipaa-and-medical-records. Cambridge, Massachusetts: MedicalRecords.com.

MyPHR / AHIMA Foundation. 2016. What Is A Personal Health Record? (PHR). Available at: www.myphr.com/startaphr/what_is_a_phr.aspx. Chicago: AHIMA Foundation.

Nagle, J. 2014. *Jump-Starting a Career in Health Information, Communication & Record Keeping (Health Care Careers in 2 Years: Book 7).* New York: Rosen Classroom. Print.

Peter Pauper Press. 2015. *My Personal Health Record Keeper.* White Plains: Peter Pauper Press. Print.

Schanhals, R. 2012. *Electronic Health Records: Understanding the Medical Office Workflow.* Philadelphia: Saunders. Print.

Sullivan, D.D. 2011. *Guide to Clinical Documentation, 2nd Edition.* Philadelphia: F.A. Davis Company. Print.

U.S. Department of Health and Human Services. 2015. Electronic Health Records. Available at: www.cms.gov/medicare/e-health/ehealthrecords/index.htm. Baltimore: U.S. Centers for Medicare and Medicaid Services.

Unit VII

Predictions for health care in the United States

Contents

17 Research and advancements in health care 393

Overview	393
Types of research	394
Research ethics and conflicts of interest	401
Patient satisfaction	403
Future challenges	403
Case study	405
Chapter highlights	405
Summary	407
Review questions	407
Bibliography	408

18 The future of health care 409

Overview	409
Essentials of reform	410
Clinical advancements	410
Increasing ambulatory, outpatient, and home care	412
Predictions for long-term care	413
Increasing populations	414
Increasing obesity	415
Case study	417
Chapter highlights	418
Summary	419
Review questions	420
Bibliography	421

Chapter 17

Research and advancements in health care

Objectives

After study of the chapter, readers should be able to:

1. Describe the various types of research regarding today's health care.
2. Explain double-blind studies.
3. Describe cohort studies.
4. Identify advantages of descriptive studies.
5. Describe the goal of the National Institutes of Health (NIH).
6. Explain the role of the Agency for Health Care Policy and Research (AHCPR).
7. Explain what *outcomes research* provides, evaluates, and investigates.
8. Identify how comparative effectiveness research improves health care treatment choices.
9. Describe conflicts of interest concerning research.
10. Identify some of the future challenges regarding health care.

Overview

Many of the advancements in today's health care begin with research. Health services research is a newer field, beginning in the last half of the 20th century, that focuses on how our health care system actually works. This research is primarily funded by the federal Agency for Healthcare Research and Quality. One of the most important advances has come from using statistical probabilities based on the accurate findings of carefully controlled clinical studies. Additional research that is advancing U.S. health care focuses on the quality of care and how problems are solved. Professional journals of today are reviewed by many health care professionals and monitor the progress of discoveries and advancements.

The data they contain are based on rigorous scientific studies with extremely accurate statistical results. Therefore, they are much more accurate than information published in the general media, which are often incomplete and lacking in accuracy. Inaccurate reporting often results in consumers being disappointed or deceived. Though the future will present unique research challenges, our growing understanding will probably be able to provide many unforeseen advancements in health care.

Types of research

There are many different types of research being conducted regarding today's health care. Regardless of the type, each new discovery is improving the effectiveness and efficiency of our health care system. Different types of research include:

- Biomedical – focusing on organisms
- Clinical – focusing on patients
- Disciplinary – focusing on medical theory
- Health services – focusing on the health care system
- Public health – focusing on communities.

Professionals who conduct research in basic science include biochemists, biologists, pharmacologists, physicians, and others. These individuals focus on the areas of science that help us to understand the human body's anatomy and physiology, as well as how it responds to external stimuli. They are often concerned with research into body cells, and usually work in extremely high-level laboratories. Additional research into basic science involves human and animal studies. All clinical medical advances are based upon basic science research.

Biomedical research

Biomedical research is also known as *experimental medicine*. It consists of basic medical research, which supports the increase of medical knowledge. Biomedical research is a rapidly evolving area. It includes a new paradigm known as *translational research*, which focuses on feedback between basic and clinical research that helps to increase the speed of knowledge sharing. Biomedical research incorporates a large variety of disciplines, which include biochemistry, microbiology, physiology, oncology, surgery, and research into many non-communicable diseases.

The major benefits of biomedical research have included vaccines for polio and measles, insulin used to treat diabetes, many different antibiotics, high blood pressure medications, improved AIDS medications, a variety of treatments for atherosclerosis, microsurgery and other newer surgical techniques, and improving treatments for various types of cancer. The Human Genome Project has resulted in new types of testing and treatments that are continually improving.

The majority of this type of research is performed by biomedical scientists. Additional contributions are made by other types of biologists, along with chemists and physicists. When biomedical research involves human studies, it strictly follows codes of medical ethics. In the United States, biomedical research is mostly funded through the National Institutes of Health and private pharmaceutical companies, followed by biotechnology companies, medical device manufacturers, other federal sources, state and local governments, and private foundations and charities.

Clinical research

Clinical research is mostly focused on early detection, diagnosis, and treatment. It is also concerned with maintaining mental, physical, and social functions, as well as limiting and rehabilitating patients with disabilities and palliative care of the terminally ill. Clinical research is conducted by medical, nursing, allied health, and related specialists. These individuals often work with people conducting basic science research. Clinical research is often experimental. Controlled studies of technological developments, new drugs, and diagnostic or therapeutic procedures are common. A brief overview of advances due to medical research is outlined in Table 17.1.

New drugs or treatments are often tested against currently used drugs or treatments. When there is no "standard" drug available, or if such a drug is too easily identified, a *control group* of individuals will receive a placebo in order to minimize *subject bias*, which is when participants believe they know the purpose of the study and react in ways that support or discredit the study. Another way to reduce bias is to use *random selection* for the selection of members in the experimental and control groups. *Double-blind studies* are defined as those in which neither the "patients" nor the researchers know who is receiving the actual drug or treatment being tested, and who is not. The identities of the participants and what they received are revealed only when the study is completed.

In research studies, a variety of *safeguards* are used to protect each volunteer participant's rights and safety. *Peer-review committees* are used to judge whether each government-funded clinical study has scientific value in how it is designed, and in whether its findings will be valid. After this, *institutional review boards (IRBs)* or *hospital-based boards* verify that participants were protected adequately and that ethics were followed properly. Every volunteer participant must sign an *informed consent form* that clearly explains the expected benefits of the study, as well as potential risks or adverse effects. Therefore, participants are able to determine that they will receive the most up-to-date care and close monitoring of their conditions, to help advance science. The potential risks can be compared to these positive outcomes.

Table 17.1 Overview of advances due to medical research

Date	Advancement
1901	Blood typing
1903	Electrocardioscope (electrocardiograph)
1921	Insulin
1927	Tuberculosis and tetanus vaccines
1928	Penicillin
1952	Polio vaccine
1985	Robotic surgery
2003	Human genome

> ## Focus on double-blind studies
>
> When both participants and researchers do not know who is receiving a treatment that is being tested, it is called a double-blind study. An example of a double-blind study is one performed for sildenafil, a drug used for erectile dysfunction. This particular study focused on men who had type 2 diabetes, to see whether the drug was safe and well tolerated. By using this technique, the placebo effect could also be understood since no one involved knew who actually received sildenafil.

Disciplinary research

Disciplinary research utilizes a holistic approach to research because it combines various medical disciplines or areas. Research focuses on subjects that affect several disciplines, an example of which is the use of information systems as part of biomedical research. Methods that were often developed as part of one area are utilized by other areas involved in the research.

The term *transdisciplinarity* is used to explain the use of various types of knowledge within disciplinary research. These include system, target, and transformation knowledge. *System knowledge* focuses on the cause of a problem and future developments. *Target knowledge* concerns values and normalcies used to form goals to solve the problem. *Transformation knowledge* is related to transforming and improving the situations surrounding the problem.

The individuals conducting disciplinary studies interact openly and relate different perspectives and sets of information to each other. Researchers combine their own individual depth of knowledge with the abilities to moderate and mediate the knowledge of others. Disciplinary research works with four central questions: causation, ontogeny (development of organisms), adaptation, and phylogeny (relationships with other organisms) – all of which are essential in medical research.

Health services research

Health services research is also known as *health systems research* and *health policy and systems research*. It involves many different disciplines and focuses on several areas:

- How patients get access to health care practitioners and services
- The costs of health care
- Patient outcomes as a result of health care.

Health services research takes into account health policy, social factors, financing, health care organization, medical technology, quality of care, quality of life, and the effects of personal behaviors upon health care.

Health services research is a newer area of study that combines social science with contributions from the health care system. Its primary goals are to identify the best ways to improve health care services, reduce medical errors, and improve patient safety. Researchers in this area may include pharmacists, physicians, epidemiologists, nurses, psychologists, economists, and health care administrators. Additional support is sometimes given by geographers, political scientists, public health professionals, biostatisticians, engineers, and even patients.

The two major approaches to health services research are as follows:

- Implementation research – analysis of public policies; effectiveness evaluations concerning specific health interventions
- Impact evaluation – emphasis on health care practice effectiveness and how care is organized; uses more narrow methods of study, including systematic reviews of health interventions.

Health services research is generally divided into three areas in the United States. These include government-sponsored, university-sponsored, and "think tanks" formed by professional organizations. Government-sponsored health services research is conducted by the U.S. Department of Veterans Affairs as well as the Institute of Medicine. University-sponsored health services research includes the Center for Surgery and Public Health (affiliate of Harvard University) and the Institute for Healthcare Policy and Innovation (affiliate of the University of Michigan). Think tanks concerning health services research include the Society of General Internal Medicine and the Rand Corporation Health Division.

Public health research

Public health research focuses on preventing disease and improving health and mortality via the combined efforts of public and private communities, individuals, organizations, and society in general. It is concerned with health threats based on analysis of population health. It takes into account not only diseases, but also mental and social wellness. Public health research includes many different areas, including epidemiology, biostatistics, health services, environmental health, behavioral health, economics, public policy, insurance medicine, mental health, and occupational safety and health.

Surveillance is conducted of disease cases and health indicators. The effects of preventive measures such as breastfeeding, hand washing, vaccinations, and condom distribution are studied. Comparison studies are conducted that assess the differences in public health between developed and developing populations. Many intercontinental studies are conducted with the support of the World Health Organization (WHO). Within the United States, public health research is conducted through the United States Public Health Service and the Centers for Disease Control and Prevention (CDC).

Unfortunately, public health research receives less government funding than other research areas. Still, this type of research has been instrumental in developing many effective treatments for HIV/AIDS, diabetes, water-borne diseases, antibiotic resistance, and diseases that affect both humans and animals. Public health research covers a variety of areas, including assessment of the health care system in regard to various populations, cost-effectiveness, and determining long-term outcomes of various public health programs – including their successes and failures.

Ongoing public health research includes studies on such diverse subjects as use of seat belts in automobiles, maternal and child health problems, malnutrition, poverty, food security, improving water and sanitation, malaria, SARS, obesity and resultant diabetes, the effects of disasters, and the development of new diseases such as Zika. Public health research is highly concerned with preventive medicine. Topic areas that are being studied today include opioid dependence, mental illness in relation to substance abuse, drug addiction, differences in disease prevalence between minority groups, gene variants related to changes in bone mineralization, and glaucoma links to genetic transcription factors.

Expenditures for research and development

The American Recovery and Reinvestment Act (ARRA) allocated $10.4 billion to fund the National Institutes of Health (NIH), primarily for research and development. However, funding was ended by the Budget Control Act in 2011, since funding for biomedical research had totaled $136.2 billion. This represented a 35% increase since 2007. Most spending on research and development goes to the private biotechnology, private pharmaceutical, and medical device industries. In 2011, these three areas made up 57% of all research and development spending. The United States spends the most of all other countries, yet does not have the best health care system.

Epidemiology

The study and analysis of disease patterns, causes, and effects of health and disease conditions in defined populations is called epidemiology. It is focused on human health and factors that affect health or cause diseases and injuries. In general, epidemiological research is *observational*. This means that it collects data about human behaviors and characteristics, naturally occurring phenomena, effects of environment and locations, and exposures to various events and circumstances. Observational studies are of two types:

- Analytical studies – often explore differences between human populations that have different behaviors or characteristics, such as smokers versus non-smokers. Cohort studies are analytical studies of a specific population over a certain time period, focusing on factors such as diet, exercise, weight, and other data related to heart disease or similar conditions. Analytical studies help to explain disease patterns and processes. They also document data concerning the effects of certain agents or activities upon health. Analytical studies often follow descriptive studies, in which they attempt to find associations between causes of disease and outcomes.
- Descriptive studies – identify conditions and factors determining distribution of disease and health in specific populations. Descriptive studies use interview surveys, databases, patient records, and other sources. These studies document biological or disease characteristics and details, as well as how often or how significantly they occur. Descriptive studies are usually quicker to complete than analytical studies, as well as less expensive. They commonly find questions that need to be answered, or hypotheses requiring testing.

Experimental epidemiological studies usually follow observational studies. In these experimental studies, a variable being tested is manipulated by an investigator to see how it affects another variable. These studies are technically difficult to perform, and often are considered unethical. However, they are the best way to test *causes and effects*. To ensure that non-experimental variables will not affect the outcome, control populations are used. Ethical issues may be raised when a clinical procedure is used that could expose test subjects to unknown or meaningful risks. Additional ethical problems might occur when an experimental study withholds a potentially beneficial medication or procedure from individuals in the control group, in order to test whether an experimental drug or procedure is effective.

In epidemiological studies, methods and principles are used that can be applied to many different problems, in several fields. This requires the use of data from large-scale populations. Quantitative methods have been used to increase understanding of health and disease, as well as to evaluate health care services. These methods are also used to anticipate health needs of specific populations, determine the number of health professionals needed, and to determine outcomes of treatments in different clinical settings. As epidemiology and statistical theories have advanced, today's researchers can utilize data from large insurance-oriented databases such as Medicare. Often, findings from diverse areas of the world, in relation to various treatment procedures and costs, have been influenced by analysis of these databases.

> ## You should remember
>
> Observational studies, used in epidemiology, are qualitative when they do not use control or comparison groups. In this type, they can be compared to the techniques used by newspaper reporters, in that they attempt to simply describe what has been naturally observed. A less complicated form of observational study is one that is analytical or quantitative, and has a control or comparison group.

Health services research

Health services research developed out of needed improvements in health care system effectiveness and efficiency. It also came about because of the need to determine which treatment options for specific conditions would produce the best outcomes. Earlier in history, research was focused on increasing understanding of health and disease. It attempted to find better ways to diagnose and treat disease, and ultimately to improve life quality and increase lifespans of the population. In the 1950s and 1960s, federal health care policy was dominated by supply-side *subsidy programs* such as Medicare, Medicaid, and others. These programs were based more on politics than on research, and were the primary forces that eventually would result in health services research.

Over time, data collected from Medicare and other government programs showed important deficiencies of the U.S. health care system to deliver essential knowledge and skills either efficiently or effectively. Evidence continued to grow showing huge variations in amounts and types of care delivered for *the same* health conditions. This meant that, quite often, treatments were being selected that were based on conflicting data. Health care that was provided often was inappropriate or questionable, and the best methods of treating the condition were often confusing and unclear to clinical personnel.

Important advances in health services research began in the late 1960s, when John Wennberg documented vast differences in how medical and surgical procedures were utilized by physicians in small geographical areas. Additional studies showed exceedingly costly health care practices that resulted from such differences. Rates of surgeries performed related directly to the number of surgeons in a specific area. Also, numbers of available hospital beds related directly to rates of hospitalization in a given population – instead of being related to differences among patients. For example, in Boston, per capita expenditures for hospitalization were almost always *double* those of New Haven, which is a nearby city. Many clinical procedures were performed differently by physicians, without consistency. There was also a lack of measurement concerning desired outcomes for specific health care interventions.

The federal government would react to these findings over the following years. For example, the NIH was created, in part, because of variances in diagnoses and treatments that resulted in unacceptable fluctuations in health care outcomes. Over time, federal legislation addressed the development of strict clinical guidelines. In 1989, the Agency for Health Care Policy and Research (AHCPR) was established to replace the National Center for Health Services Research and Health Care Technology and become one of the eight agencies of the Public Health Service, a part of the Department of Health and Human Services.

The AHCPR focused on development and review of clinical guidelines that assisted health care professionals in disease prevention, diagnosis, treatment, and management. The agency was authorized to establish panels of qualified experts to review findings of many clinical studies, and then recommend guidelines to assist practitioners and patients about making appropriate decisions on health care.

Two types of research project were funded by the AHCPR: large patient-outcome research teams and smaller **meta-analysis** (or literature synthesis) projects. Both projects compared patient outcomes with alternative practices, and then recommended changes when they were required. The AHCPR was important for about ten years, supporting studies that created many publications about quality and costs of health care, clinical decisions, assessments of technology, and outcomes of treatment. The agency still exists, but today supplies private, non-government groups with evidence used to develop their own guidelines.

In 1996, the AHCPR had difficulties with national organizations of surgeons because of its guidelines concerning the discouragement of surgical procedures for back conditions. Congress was convinced by lobbyists for the surgical organizations that the AHCPR was exceeding its authority and not considering the expertise of the surgeons themselves.

Outcomes research

Outcomes research provides information that helps governments, insurers, employers, and consumers make better health care decisions. It evaluates health care procedures in medical facilities, which is a much more realistic way to study related factors than in traditional controlled environment studies. *Effectiveness research*, utilizing actual practice settings, is more accurate than *efficacy research* conducted via controlled clinical trials. Outcomes research investigates the well-being and functional status of patients, and takes into account the patient's satisfaction with his or her care. The functional status of a patient involves three factors:

- Physical functioning within the patient's regular environment
- Role functioning, or how health status disrupts normal daily activities
- Social functioning, or whether health status alters normal social activities.

A patient's mental health, mood, personal view of overall health status, and the sense of having quality of life are collectively referred to as *personal well-being*. This includes both mental and physical components. The way each patient feels about health care access, communication, convenience, financial coverage, and technical quality make up *patient satisfaction* with health care.

Outcomes research assesses the treatments that work best in different circumstances, in relation to certain clinical problems. It utilizes meta-analyses, which summarizes comparable findings from multiple studies. In order to determine the procedures that should or should not be performed in various circumstances, *appropriateness studies* are conducted. Not every procedure is appropriate for a patient in all circumstances, even though it may be proven otherwise effective.

Our health care system has a significant quality of care problem that is related to the number of inappropriate clinical interventions that occur. Research is continuing to develop methods of identifying patient preferences when given various options for treatment. Outcomes research can potentially reveal *underuse* of appropriate services as well as *overuse*. However, potential cost savings, achieved by reductions in unnecessary care and service overuse, are usually at the core of most debates related to appropriate services.

The only way to measure the real value of outcomes research is according to how its results will affect actual care. Ideally, outcomes research must result in changes of behavior for health care institutions, providers, payers, and patients. Clinical practice guidelines must be promoted in ways that will be accepted, and that will result in change regarding the choice of the most appropriate type of care for each situation. The United States cannot continue to spend nearly $3 trillion every year for the relatively poor overall results being achieved.

In 2009, ARRA expanded *comparative effectiveness research* by the NIH as well as the Agency for Healthcare Research and Quality (AHRQ). A Federal Coordinating Council was created, to produce research activity guidelines and to recommend research priorities. The Institute of Medicine (IOM) recommended many areas needing funding to support priority research, which resulted in better direction of research funds. Comparative effectiveness research improves health care treatment choices by increasing available information that is based on benefits, effectiveness, and harms of available health care options. Related research compares drugs, medical devices, surgeries, tests, and health care delivery methods.

Comparative effectiveness research is better than traditional research methods, since it compares two or more options for health care. It uses analyses of insurance claims, computer modeling, practical clinical trials, and systemic reviews of literature. Findings are produced quickly in a form that is easily usable. The identification of the best health care interventions available can reduce unnecessary treatments and lower costs. In 2010, the Affordable Care Act created the Patient-Centered Outcomes Research Institute (PCORI), which is dedicated to comparative effectiveness research, and funded it with more than $1 billion.

Focus on outcomes research

Outcomes research studies the end results of health care. Over time, it has been used to measure health status or outcomes in terms of physiological measurements, through test results, complications of disease, or death.

Research ethics and conflicts of interest

Research ethics requires fundamental ethical principles to be applied during research studies. There must be a foundation of trust between researchers, the people involved in research studies, and those who interpret study results. There cannot be any bias in research or conflicts of interest. The basic principles of ethical research include avoiding unnecessary harm, deceit, extensive rewards, plagiarism, and fraud. Researchers must always obtain informed consent, preserve privacy and confidentiality, and take all needed precautions to ensure safety. Conclusions of research must be accurate and truthful, based on the results, and not altered because of the opinions of individuals who funded the research.

Biomedical research has been supported by the U.S. federal government since the 1950s. Outstanding medical research has occurred as a result of this, and the United States has made many research advancements. However, many new technologies have focused on curative methods for ongoing conditions or diseases, instead of preventive medicine. Adequate research into public health problems such as AIDS has only occurred because of the epidemic proportions. Funding for medical research must benefit society and not only the practice of medicine. The goal of the PCORI is to include health care consumers in research activities by allowing them input into the studies that are conducted. The institute also wants to identify the best ways to translate findings into clinical practice that will educate people in a clear manner.

However, there are conflicts of interest that occur. This is, in part, due to increased research funding that comes from medical device and pharmaceutical manufacturers. For example, pharmaceutical companies have been accused of misstating the results of their studies or keeping unfavorable results from reaching public awareness. With more and more commercial research firms conducting studies instead of academic institutions, conflicts are increasing with respect to tests of new drugs and medical devices. Conflicts of interest have arisen between physicians conducting research for large medical device manufacturers, such as when certain physicians were financially compensated with company stock certificates in exchange for reporting findings as requested.

Another area of concern is the FDA, which regulates nearly one-fourth of the U.S. economy, since the administration is now heavily funded by the pharmaceutical companies it monitors, instead of only by the federal government. Obviously, political pressure from these companies has influenced FDA decisions, such as the famous case of inadequate monitoring concerning risks of common arthritis drugs. The administration has mishandled clinical trial data after product approvals by not giving the public complete reports on the safety and effectiveness of drug products. The FDA attempted to defend its position by stating that research data is protected under *proprietary information* legislation. Examples of drugs approved by the FDA that were later found to have significant health risks include:

- Acne medication (Accutane®)
- Antidepressants (Effexor®, Paxil®, Prozac®, Lexapro®, Zoloft®)
- Birth control medications (Yasmin®, Yaz®)
- Anticoagulants (Pradaxa®, Xarelto®)
- Diabetes medications (Actos®, Avandia®)
- Dialysis medications (GranuFlo®, NaturaLyte®)
- Hair loss medication (Propecia®)
- Mood stabilizer (Depakote®)
- Osteoporosis medication (Fosamax®).

Another violation of ethics includes pharmaceutical employees who write scientific articles, then compensate respected physicians to take credit for what was written in an attempt to defraud the public by increasing product sales. These physicians worked for major U.S. medical schools, and the NIH has suggested that these schools should reprimand the physicians involved. However, most college administrators will not comply, and publication of fraudulent biomedical literature continues today.

Patient satisfaction

Patient satisfaction is very important as part of quality of care. Patients' subjective ratings of their health care involve criteria that are very different from what providers believe to be important. However, patient preferences involve areas of perceived quality that are still extremely important. Today, providers must monitor their facilities' organization, management systems, and characteristics that will be perceived by patients. Patients list many things that satisfy or do not satisfy them concerning health care, including interpersonal and technical skills of providers, appointment waiting times, responses to emergencies, staff members' helpfulness and communication, and pleasing appearances of facilities.

Health care facilities and insurers work to monitor patient satisfaction on a regular basis. They may use patient satisfaction survey forms or questionnaires, as well as follow-up phone surveys. Regardless of the method used, asking patients about recent experiences at the health care facility can effectively determine both good and bad perceptions and attitudes. These results give providers the ability to correct problem areas and improve overall quality of care.

Future challenges

Today's research into health care focuses more on societal demographics, as well as patient health factors. More attention is paid to how the patient population as a whole perceives quality of care, rather than how individuals feel. Substantial challenges will involve changing provider behaviors, rejecting new information due to cognitive bias, differing payment incentives, and lack of resources to promote research findings. Basic research continues to discover more about genetics, immunology, microbiology, neuroendocrinology, aging, cell growth, and age-related mental degradation. Advances in gene manipulation will result in clinical, ethical, and legal issues requiring more research and court cases.

Deoxyribonucleic acid (DNA) research is an ongoing area of study and is being used for a number of applications. In Denmark, scientists are testing a new technique to "flush" the AIDS virus from reservoirs that exist in human DNA. The virus can then be destroyed naturally by the immune system. In the United Kingdom, scientists have identified chemical "tags" on DNA in tumors that could help physicians decide the type of chemotherapy women with advanced ovarian cancer should receive. The tags are known as *epigenetic markers*. For Alzheimer's disease, researchers have identified a number of genes that might increase risks for the late-onset form of the disease. Discovering these genetic risk factors helps us to better understand how the disease develops, and increases the chances of identifying possible treatments to study.

Another DNA study in the United Kingdom is focused on using *circulating tumor DNA* in the blood to predict metastatic relapse of early-stage breast cancer. In the United States, it has been discovered that genetic changes can predict cancer up to 13 years in the future. Protective caps on the ends of chromosomes, known as telomeres, function to prevent DNA damage. Telomeres appear more "worn" in people who eventually develop cancer. Understanding this pattern of telomere growth may prove to be an accurate biomarker in the prediction of cancer.

Research into two different obesity vaccines involves the targeting of somatostatin, a hormone that can promote weight gain. The vaccines work by creating antibodies against somatostatin. However, these vaccines are still being studied since their effects are very short, lasting less than two weeks. It is known that by reducing the effects of neuropeptides that control appetite, obesity can be controlled.

Bioinformatics utilizes large computer databases to study health, disease, and medications. Considered the future of biotechnology, bioinformatics has already provided enormous amounts of information about human body structures, functions, and the sequences of genes and proteins. *Genomics* is the study of genetic material within chromosomes. This area of study resulted in the sequencing of the human genome, which will help to improve disease diagnoses and produce more effective medications. Several drug companies are researching how to make medications more effective, with fewer side effects.

Future challenges will occur in relation to maintaining life in people who are considered terminal or unresponsive, as well as with respect to organ transplantation. For example, if recipients for a heart transplant must be chosen, who is to determine this? Complicated personal, professional, ethical, religious, and economic issues arise. Previous clinical research creates new problems for future studies as knowledge progresses.

With the increased occurrence of antibiotic-resistant microorganisms, many people are worried that eventually, there will be bacterial infections that cannot be treated by any available medications. Common antimicrobials are already unable to kill certain strains of staphylococcus or streptococcus bacteria. Since staphylococcus bacteria cause many hospital infections, this is an enormous concern. Slightly fewer than 99,000 hospitalized patients in the United States die every year because of bacterial infections.

It has been known for decades that antibiotic misuse or overuse would eventually cause drug-resistant pathogens with the potential to kill. Warnings were not heeded, and new antimicrobials continued to be developed. There have been some measures taken, involving limiting use of antibiotics or the creation of added fees designed to pay for estimated costs of antibiotic resistance. One encouraging factor is bacterial genetics, which might be able to combat the problem. Many authorities suggest that the U.S. drug approval process be reorganized so that new antibiotics can be brought to market and offer more alternatives to treat pathogens.

Continued health services research will monitor our health care system to determine what changes are required. Multi-disciplinary, value-focused efforts are essential. Finances, socioeconomics, training, health care team management, and the interaction of these factors all contribute to quality of care. A better health care system can be achieved only by understanding what health care is best for every unique situation, and then applying changes to the system to make them happen.

Epidemiology and public health research must find ways to solve differences in health behaviors, care, and the effectiveness of our system. As the cornerstone of public health research, epidemiology can determine the needs of the total population. Health policies can be designed, organized, and paid for by assessing health conditions and effects of care. Epidemiologists play an important role in identifying disease outbreaks, transmission patterns, and outcomes of treatment as well as prevention. The future of health care in the United States depends upon continued research and improvement in quality for everyone.

You should remember

The top antibiotic-resistant microorganisms in the United States include three that are ranked as having an "urgent" hazard level by the CDC. The three microorganisms are *Clostridium difficile* (which causes life-threatening diarrhea), *Carbapenem-resistant Enterobacteriaceae* (which causes systemic infection that is fatal in nearly half of affected patients), and *Neisseria gonorrhoeae*, the causative organism of gonorrhea.

Source: www.cdc.gov/drugresistance/biggest_threats.html.

CASE STUDY

Cohort studies begin with a group of people who do not have a certain disease, and the participants are grouped by whether or not they are exposed to a potential cause of the disease. A *case-control study* begins with the selection of people with a certain disease and a control group of people without the disease. In this case study, the disease being examined is gastroenteritis, which may or may not be linked to contaminated drinking water.

1 Which type of study provides the best information about the cause of the disease, since you follow the individuals from exposure to drinking water and then the occurrence of gastroenteritis?
2 Which type of study is easier to conduct, and usually takes less time?
3 Which type of study is usually about the life histories of people in a certain population segment?

Chapter highlights

This section answers the Objectives found at the beginning of the chapter.

1 Describe the various types of research regarding today's health care.

- Biomedical – focusing on organisms
- Clinical – focusing on patients
- Disciplinary – focusing on medical theory
- Health services – focusing on the health care system
- Public health – focusing on communities.

2 Explain double-blind studies.

- Double-blind studies are those in which neither the patients nor the researchers know who is receiving the actual drug or treatment being tested, and who is not. The identities of the participants and what they received are only revealed when the study is completed.

3 Describe cohort studies.

- Cohort studies are analytical studies of a specific population over a certain time period, focusing on factors such as diet, exercise, weight, and other data related to heart disease or similar conditions. They are a type of analytical study, which is a study that helps to explain disease patterns and processes, and document data concerning the effects of certain agents or activities upon health. Several variables can be studied at once.

4 Identify advantages of descriptive studies.

- Advantages of descriptive studies include that they are quicker to complete than analytical studies, as well as less expensive.

5 **Describe the goal of the National Institutes of Health (NIH).**

- The NIH was created, in part, because of variances in diagnoses and treatments that resulted in unacceptable variations in health care outcomes.

6 **Explain the role of the Agency for Health Care Policy and Research (AHCPR).**

- The AHCPR focused on development and review of clinical guidelines that assisted health care professionals in clinically significant disease prevention, diagnosis, treatment, and management. It was authorized to establish panels of qualified experts to review clinical study findings, then recommend guidelines to assist in making appropriate health care decisions.
- The AHCPR funded both large patient-outcome research teams and smaller meta-analysis (literature synthesis) projects, both of which compared outcomes with alternative practices, then recommended changes if required.
- Today, the AHCPR supplies private, non-government groups with evidence used to develop their own guidelines.

7 **Explain what *outcomes research* provides, evaluates, and investigates.**

- Outcomes research provides information that helps governments, insurers, employers, and consumers make better health care decisions.
- It evaluates health care processes in medical facilities, and investigates the well-being and functional status of patients, taking into account the patient's satisfaction with his or her care.

8 **Identify how comparative effectiveness research improves health care treatment choices.**

- Comparative effectiveness research increases available information that is based on benefits, effectiveness, and harms of available health care options.
- It compares drugs, medical devices, surgeries, tests, and health care delivery methods.
- It is better than traditional research since it compares two or more options for health care, using analyses of insurance claims, computer modeling, practical clinical trials, and systemic reviews of literature.

9 **Describe conflicts of interest concerning research.**

- Conflicts of interest concerning research are partly due to increased research funding that comes from medical device and pharmaceutical companies, which have been accused of misstating study results or keeping unfavorable results from reaching the public. Also, more commercial research collectives are conducting studies instead of academic institutions, causing conflicts of interest about tests of new drugs and medical devices. Other conflicts have occurred between physicians conducting research for manufacturers who were then compensated by those manufacturers.

10 **Identify some of the future challenges regarding health care.**

- Future challenges will occur related to maintaining life in terminal or unresponsive patients, organ transplantation, new research that uses older research, and antibiotic-resistant microorganisms.

Summary

Today's health care is being advanced by research into biomedical, clinical, disciplinary, health service, public health, and other areas. The majority of research is conducted by private biotechnology or pharmaceutical companies, as well as by the medical device industry. Epidemiology is the area of medicine that focuses on human health and the factors that affect it or cause diseases and injuries. Outcomes research is highly effective because it studies health care processes in actual medical facilities. Another good method is comparative effectiveness research, which improves health care treatment by increasing information that is available concerning treatment options. However, there are concerns about ethics and conflicts of interest related to research funded by companies that have a direct interest in outcomes. The Food and Drug Administration is also implicated since it is partially funded by pharmaceutical companies. Regardless of difficulties, health care advancements continue to be made into genetics, immunology, microbiology, neuroendocrinology, aging, cell growth, age-related mental degradation, DNA, cancer, obesity, and antibiotic resistance.

Review questions

1 What does clinical research focus on?
2 What do the terms *control group* and *subject bias* mean?
3 What is the focus of epidemiology?
4 How did health services research develop?
5 What three factors are involved in the functional status of a patient?
6 How is outcomes research measured, and what must it achieve?
7 How has the FDA mishandled clinical trial data?
8 What items are listed by patients in regard to their satisfaction with health care?
9 What does today's research into health care focus on?
10 How is DNA research progressing regarding various types of cancer?

Bibliography

Agency for Healthcare Research and Quality. 2016. Outcomes Research: Fact Sheet. Available at: www.ahrq.gov/research/findings/factsheets/outcomes/outfact/index.html. Rockville: Agency for Healthcare Research and Quality.

Bidwell, A. 2014. U.S. Medical Research Spending Drops while Asia Makes Gains. Available at: www.usnews.com/news/articles/2014/01/02/us-medical-research-spending-drops-while-asia-makes-gains. New York: U.S. News and World Report.

CDC. 2016. Biggest Threats involving Antibiotic / Antimicrobial Resistance. Available at: www.cdc.gov/drugresistance/biggest_threats.html. Atlanta: U.S. Centers for Disease Control and Prevention.

CDC. 2016. What is Epidemiology?. Available at: www.cdc.gov/EXCITE/epidemiology. html. Atlanta: U.S. Centers for Disease Control and Prevention.

Chen, A., Zhang, R., and Chen, J. 2016. *Challenges of Big Data Analytics Applications in Healthcare: The Future of Healthcare*. Seattle: Amazon Digital Services LLC. Digital.

Cherry, K. 2016. What is a Double-Blind Study?. Available at: http://psychology.about.com/ od/dindex/g/naturalobserv.htm. Loma Linda: American College of Lifestyle Medicine/ VeryWell.

Diering, S.L. 2004. *Love Your Patients! Improving Patient Satisfaction with Essential Behaviors That Enrich the Lives of Patients & Professionals*. Nevada City: Blue Dolphin Publishing. Print.

Education and Practice Committee on Conflict of Interest in Medical Research/Board on Health Sciences Policy. 2009. *Conflict of Interest in Medical Research, Education, and Practice*. Washington, D.C.: National Academies Press. Print.

Esteitie, R. 2013. *Medical Research Essentials*. New York: McGraw-Hill Education. Print.

Gordis, L. 2013. *Epidemiology, 5th Edition*. Philadelphia: Saunders. Print.

Graboyes, M. 2015. *The Experiment Must Continue: Medical Research and Ethics in East Africa, 1940–2014*. Athens: Ohio University Press. Print.

Grove, S.K. 2007. *Statistics for Health Care Research: A Practical Workbook*. Philadelphia: Saunders. Print.

Health Services Research. 2016. HSR Home Page. Available at: www.hsr.org. Chicago: Health Services Research.

Kane, R.L., and Radosevich, D.M. 2010. *Conducting Health Outcomes Research*. Burlington: Jones & Bartlett Learning. Print.

MedicalResearch.com. 2014. Patient Satisfaction and Quality of Care May Not Be Directly Associated. Available at: http://medicalresearch.com/author-interviews/patient_satisfaction_ and_quality_of_care_may_not_be_directly_associated/7052. Baltimore: MedicalResearch. com.

Merlino, J. 2014. *Service Fanatics: How to Build Superior Patient Experience the Cleveland Clinic Way*. New York: McGraw-Hill Education. Print.

The National Academies of Sciences Engineering Medicine. 2016. Conflict of Interest in Medical Research, Education, and Practice. Available at: http://iom.nationalacademies. org/Activities/Workforce/ConflictOfInterest.aspx. Washington, D.C.: National Academy of Sciences.

NIH Clinical Center. 2016. Patient Recruitment: Ethics in Clinical Research. Available at: http://clinicalcenter.nih.gov/recruit/ethics.html. Bethesda: National Institutes of Health.

Policy and Medicine. 2011. The Difficulties and Challenges of Biomedical Research and Health Advances. Available at: www.policymed.com/2011/02/the-difficulties-and-challenges-of-biomedical-research-and-health-advances.html. Washington, D.C.: Policy and Medicine.

Privacy and Confidentiality. 2016. Current Issues in Research Ethics. Available at: http:// ccnmtl.columbia.edu/projects/cire/pac/foundation. New York: Columbia University.

Schimpff, S. 2012. *The Future of Health-Care Delivery: Why It Must Change and How It Will Affect You*. Lincoln: Potomac Books. Print.

Topol, E. 2015. *The Patient Will See You Now: The Future of Medicine Is in Your Hands*. New York: Basic Books. Print.

U.S. Department of Health and Human Services. 2016. Research Design. Available at: http://ori.hhs.gov/education/products/sdsu/res_des1.htm. Washington, D.C.: U.S. Department of Health and Human Services.

U.S. Food and Drug Administration. 2015. Antibiotic-Resistant Bacteria: Consumer Update. Available at: www.fda.gov/ForConsumers/ConsumerUpdates/ucm349953.htm. Washington, D.C.: U.S. Food and Drug Administration.

Walker, D.M. 2014. *An Introduction to Health Services Research: A Practical Guide*. New York: Sage Publications Ltd. Print.

Chapter 18

The future of health care

After study of the chapter, readers should be able to:

1 Describe why health care reform is a complicated issue.
2 Describe the groups of Americans who do not have health insurance due to the cost of premiums.
3 Identify recent clinical advancements and technologies linked to improving health.
4 Identify the types of service now being offered in ambulatory and outpatient facilities.
5 Explain the problems concerning the future of long-term care.
6 Explain the terms "old-old population" and "young-old population" and their health care needs.
7 Describe the reason behind the upward shift in the elderly U.S. population and what it will cause.
8 Identify the amount of U.S. adults who are considered obese, related annual medical costs, and future predictions.
9 Explain factors related to the obesity epidemic in the United States.
10 Discuss how the U.S. government is trying to combat obesity.

Overview

The need for health care services will increase greatly over future decades, mostly because of the dramatic increase in the elderly population. It is projected that the future of health care in the United States will involve increased job opportunities but also increased costs, changes in quality of care, and legislative changes. There will be a much higher need for geriatric-specific training of all future health professionals. It is predicted that large health care organizations will increase in size and dominate more of the health care market. Physicians will be more likely to be employed by these organizations than by smaller companies. Overall, patients will be required to become more involved in their own health care.

Essentials of reform

Health care reform is a complicated issue that requires cooperation between primary health care providers, private insurance companies, and both state and federal governments. It will directly impact the availability of health insurance to the uninsured, and also increase access to health care. While most Americans currently obtain health insurance through employers, many smaller employers do not offer health insurance. Due to the cost of premiums, the self-employed, underemployed, and unemployed simply go without health insurance. Often, full-time employees avoid signing up for health insurance because their "employee share" of premiums is too high. Another important issue facing some individuals is when the cost of care reaches the insurer's lifetime limit due to serious illnesses or accidents. When this happens, the individual is often dropped by the health insurer.

The Affordable Care Act was modeled after the Massachusetts health care program, which is considered to be successful since more than 97% of residents of that state now have health insurance. However, health care costs in Massachusetts are still rising. Out-of-pocket expenses have been lowered, however, for people with chronic diseases and low income. The quality of care is rated as very good to excellent. Partly because of the increased numbers of people with health insurance, there is a shortage of primary care providers.

Clinical advancements

As the elderly population of the United States ages and increases in numbers, new clinical advancements will be required. Technology must increase, and new health care professionals must be continually recruited to address the needs of the population. It is estimated that between one-third and two-thirds of the workloads of future health care personnel will focus on the elderly. Training of health care professionals must be expanded to prepare them for a large variety of needed services. Funding will be required to support study and research into the psychological and physiological needs of the elderly.

Special clinical skills will be required to address future needs. This means that educational institutions must change and update their programs. Continuing education will also need to be revised. Health professionals of all disciplines will need to better interact and coordinate their efforts. More focus on geriatrics will be required. Beginning with future physicians, all students should receive geriatric medicine training, which includes care for chronically ill, elderly people. Clinical pharmacology must address the needs of many of these patients who require multiple medications, as well as how overall declining health and mental capacity influences medicine regimens.

Technology is offering clinical advancements for the future at an extremely fast rate. Technologies that are being tested and developed for regular use in the future are extremely diverse. They include the growing of organs, artificial organs, tumor testing, immune therapies for cancer, cellphone applications for better health, odor-sensing devices used to diagnose cancer, and saliva testing to determine the presence of cancer.

By using the body's ability to develop and heal, surgeons have directed blood flow to malformed left ventricles of infant hearts. This has triggered biological processes that promote heart growth. In the state of Virginia, pioneering steps were made toward being able to grow entire organs and tissues from stem cells, via manipulating the appropriate signaling of these cells. For cancer patients, tumor samples can be tested for more than 280 genetic mutations that are suspected of controlling tumor growth, resulting in genetic therapies that can reverse malignancies. Immune therapies for cancer involve experimental drugs that encourage the immune system to target and attack tumor cells. New *smartphone apps* are available for performing remote electrocardiograms, reading medical images, and tracking moles for signs of skin cancer.

The artificial pancreas, developed at colleges in Virginia and Massachusetts, is an automated insulin-delivery system that replicates the action of the human pancreas by mimicking healthy glucose regulation. It consists of an insulin pump, a continuous blood glucose monitor placed under the patient's skin, and advanced software embedded into the patient's smartphone that detects how much insulin must be provided, based on physical activity, stress, sleep, and metabolism. It works by predicting blood glucose levels in advance. Trials are ongoing in the United States and Europe.

A new implantable artificial kidney, approximately the size of a coffee cup, is able to perform functions that current dialysis machines cannot. It has been selected for a special fast-track approval process by the FDA, with human trials beginning in 2017. The artificial kidney will be powered from the patient's blood pressure, and utilize silicon nanotechnology in order to filter the blood. It passes blood through the filter to remove toxins, sugars, salts, and water – creating an *ultrafiltrate*. This moves to the opposite side of the device, where real kidney cells reabsorb the water, sugars, and salts back into the bloodstream. The kidney cells are obtained from organs rejected for transplantation. It is believed that the device would not trigger a rejection since the kidney cells are separated from the immune components of the patient's blood.

Newer clinical advancements, announced in 2016, include the *Odoreader*, which can analyze the odor of men to determine if prostate cancer is present. This new technology seems to be far more accurate than testing prostate-specific antigen (PSA) levels, which often gives false positives that lead to unnecessary biopsies. The new device uses a gas chromatography sensor system and was developed in the United Kingdom. It has also been proven useful in diagnosing bladder cancer and hematuria. Another new advancement, from California, is a saliva test that quickly and accurately identifies biomarkers of lung cancer. The test takes only ten minutes, can be performed in a physician's office, and began being used with patients in 2016. It is referred to as a "liquid biopsy," and detects circulating tumor DNA in saliva, but can be used in other body fluids as well. The biomarkers are detected by using an "electric field-induced release and measurement" process. It detects mutations in a cancer-linked gene called epidermal growth factor receptor, which provides instructions for making a receptor protein of the same name. Further trials are being conducted in collaboration with China. The next step is a saliva test for detecting mutations linked to cancers of the mouth and throat.

> ## Focus on clinical advancements
>
> Because of increased technology and information sharing, it is predicted that the speed of clinical advancements in the future will be faster than ever. It may become possible to predict disease outbreaks before they happen because of high-speed information processing and analysis. Advanced information technologies play a critical role in assessments of clinical practice, physician report cards, clinical guidelines, patient education, and many other areas.

Increasing ambulatory, outpatient, and home care

There has been a rapid growth in ambulatory, outpatient, and home care in the United States, based on the aging population and changes in hospital care. There has been large growth in the number of medical and surgical procedures performed in ambulatory and outpatient settings. Same-day surgery is possible for procedures that used to require hospital inpatient admission. This is partially due to advances in anesthesiology, diagnostic technology, and surgery. The large potential cost savings of ambulatory surgery was quickly recognized by third-party payers. As a result, many diagnostic and surgical procedures became non-reimbursable if patients were admitted to hospitals, unless extenuating circumstances existed. Therefore, these procedures increasingly came to be performed in ambulatory and outpatient facilities.

Federal and state incentives encouraged more ambulatory and outpatient facilities to be developed. Consumers came to accept these facilities for their needed services. As a result, nearly every type of service is now being offered in these on an ambulatory or outpatient basis. These facilities will continue to grow since they can offer comparable care to hospitals, much lower costs, and high patient satisfaction. Types of services now being offered in ambulatory and outpatient facilities include:

- Cancer treatment
- Diagnostic imaging
- Kidney dialysis
- Rehabilitative services
- Urgent care
- Sports medicine
- Certain surgeries
- Wellness and preventive medicine services.

Between 2001 and 2012, home health care episodes increased by nearly three million. By 2012, the number of home health care agencies had reached 12,200. Continued growth is expected as the population of older Americans continues to grow.

Predictions for long-term care

The U.S. population that is older than age 65 is dramatically increasing in size. As a result, the need for long-term care and its associated costs is increasing. For the future, dramatic methods of controlling costs must occur. There is also the possibility that there will be an inadequate number of people who can provide long-term care. Elderly people who are also disabled often have no one to help care for them with regard to their daily needs. Community-based services are helping to take the place of institutional care, but cannot administer to all of the people who need help. Other people requiring long-term care include those with chronic diseases, the mentally ill, those who have permanent disabilities, and impaired children.

Nursing homes make up approximately 70% of all long-term facilities. The remainder of these facilities include chronic disease hospitals, psychiatric and mental illness hospitals, and rehabilitation hospitals. Other forms of long-term care facilities include assisted living, shelter homes, workshops, home health services, and hospice.

Regarding the elderly and their needs for long-term care, it must be considered that predictions estimate the elderly population of the United States will have tripled by the year 2050. Therefore, the need for long-term care and its costs could be about ten times higher than they are currently. The "old-old" population, basically those over age 80, is increasing most rapidly, meaning that long-term care for the elderly with poorest health will be essential. For the "young-old" group, which is people between 65 and 80, there will be increased needs for preventive, primary, and acute care.

There will be increased need for community-based services for the elderly population. New areas of health care will be required, including evolving residential and living facilities, institutions, case management, rehabilitation facilities, self-care programs, and cost-sharing programs. Table 18.1 lists basic facts about long-term care.

Table 18.1 Long-term care statistics

Statistic	Comments
Most popular forms of long-term care	Home health agencies, followed by nursing homes, hospices, residential care communities, and adult day service centers
Who uses long-term care	About 63% are aged 65 and older
How much of the 65+ population are below the poverty level	14.8%
What are the percentages of long-term care types of service	66% of the disabled elderly are cared for by their families, 26% by family members along with paid help, and 9% from only paid help

Source: www.caregiver.org/selected-long-term-care-statistics.

> ### You should remember
>
> The elderly population of the United States in 2030 is projected to be twice as large as it was in the year 2000. This means it will be approximately 71.5 million people.
> *Sources:* www.ncbi.nlm.nih.gov/pmc/articles/pmc1464018; www.aarp.org/livable-communities/info-2014/livable-communities-facts-and-figures.html.

Increasing populations

Currently, about 25% of the U.S. population is made up of racial and ethnic minority groups. The Latino and Asian populations have doubled in recent decades, increasing populations that will also play a part in increased health care needs. This fact does not take into account the growth in other segments of the population. Changes in these and other populations will be reflected in the older adult population eventually. Minority groups – especially Latinos – will make up larger proportions of elderly people. Health care facilities will need to be culturally competent to treat all of the diverse populations of the country. Health literacy must be improved so that all populations receive adequate treatment. Limited health literacy is linked to worse health outcomes and higher costs.

Large differences exist between racial and ethnic groups and their individual occurrences of chronic conditions, mortality rates, preferred services, utilized services, and attitudes toward care. For example,

- Blacks in the U.S. have higher mortality rates than whites, and need more treatment for cerebrovascular disease, diabetes, hypertension, and diabetes
- Latinos also have higher rates of diabetes than the white population, yet they have lower rates of arthritis and hypertension.

The current total population of the United States is approximately 327 million people. The shift in the elderly portion of the population is mostly due to aging *baby boomers*. Because of advances in health care and medical technology, Americans are living longer than ever before. Since the elderly population is growing, this means there will be greater impact upon the health care system in regard to chronic diseases, which occur more often in the elderly.

Therefore, the increasing population, in all of its subgroups, means that more medical personnel will be required. Regardless of the Affordable Care Act's intentions, the shortage of health care professionals is a persistent and ongoing problem that appears likely to continue well into the future. There is an ever-increasing demand for nurses, nursing aids, and various therapists in what is termed the *acute-care sector*. Long-term facilities are not considered as attractive with respect to employment. As a result, many of them are highly understaffed. Funds are deficient both to meet the needs of older Americans who are dependent on Medicaid and to attract personnel into long-term care.

Our current health care system does not deal well with chronically ill, elderly people with multiple conditions and disabilities. Effective chronic illness care requires major changes. Since the U.S. health care system is still focused on acute care, the future does not look bright unless serious changes occur soon. Clinical and value-based attitudes and perceptions of health care professionals need to be revised. Geriatric practice is less multi-disciplinary and not as "exciting" as other areas of health care. The change that needs to occur requires

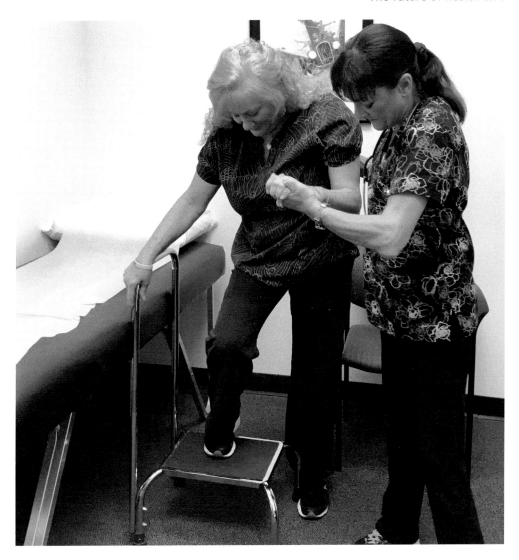

Figure 18.1 Assisting an elderly patient.

a refocus on maintaining optimal lifestyles for the chronically ill. The fee-for-service care model needs to be replaced by a more holistic approach.

Increasing obesity

According to the Centers for Disease Control and Prevention, more than one-third of U.S. adults are obese (see Figure 18.2). Obesity-related conditions include heart disease, stroke, type 2 diabetes, osteoarthritis, and cancer. Annual medical costs of obesity are more than $150 billion in the United States alone. Non-Hispanic blacks have the highest age-adjusted rates of obesity (47.8%). The age group, across all ethnicities, with the highest rates of obesity is 40–59 years (39.5%).

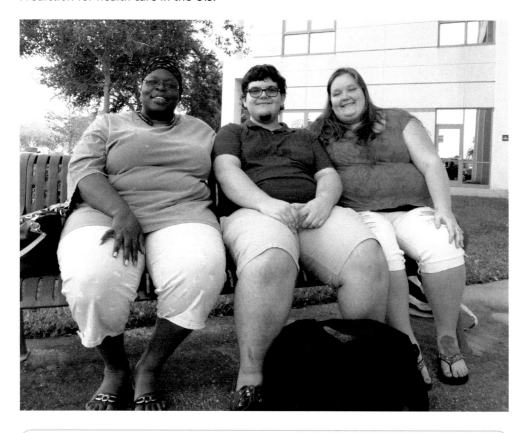

Figure 18.2 Obese patients.

Obesity is most prevalent in three states: Arkansas, Mississippi, and West Virginia, where 35% of more of citizens are obese. According to Johns Hopkins University, if current trends concerning obese and overweight Americans continue, it is possible that 86% of the population will be either obese or overweight by the year 2048. Most physicians believe that with increased education, the trend will be reversed. Healthier diets and exercise regimens are already improving the lives of many Americans.

To better understand why obesity has progressed over the years, consider the fact that in 1940s America, when fast food was just beginning, there were few obese people. Over the next 20 years, obesity rates began to rise, along with the proliferation of fast food chains and processed foods being sold in stores. Studies have shown that people who frequently eat fast food gain ten pounds more than those who do so less often.

Processed foods affect every type of dietary source, including carbohydrates, fats, and proteins. Along with Americans becoming less active and more sedentary, obesity rates have risen rapidly. Televisions, computers, and computer games have made many people accustomed to remaining relatively inactive for many hours of the day. When regular exercise is not part of a person's lifestyle, weight is likely to be gained, and future negative health outcomes are likely to occur. The health outcomes linked to obesity include the following:

- Heart disease
- Diabetes

- Cancer
- Liver disease
- Gallbladder disease
- Anxiety
- Depression.

The U.S. government has taken steps to try to combat the obesity epidemic. Obesity legislation is designed similarly to tobacco legislation: to reduce the number of diseases and deaths caused by obesity, and to reduce the huge impact of treatment costs upon the health care system. Legislation is designed to give manufacturers incentives to produce quality foods and drinks, as well as to educate the public.

Though future predictions about obesity are usually not encouraging, the most important thing to remember is that obesity is a reversible, treatable condition. As long as adequate education about healthy behaviors is provided, people have the ability to solve this problem and improve their health. Steps to reverse obesity include the following:

- *Reduce or stop eating sugar* – empty calories, quickly absorbed sugar, liquid sugar calories, and refined carbohydrates are all converted to sugar. This creates high insulin levels, leading to Type 2 diabetes. Chronically high insulin levels are also linked to hypertension, inflammation, cancer, depression, and poor sex drive.
- *Eat whole, unprocessed foods* – fruits, vegetables, omega-3 fats, coconut butter, olive oil, legumes, nuts, and seeds.
- *Take the right nutrient supplements* – if needed, high-quality multivitamins with minerals, omega-3 fatty acids, vitamin D3, alpha lipoic acid, chromium polynicotinate, and fiber.
- *Exercise* – walk up to 60 minutes per day, *vigorously*, getting the heart rate up to between 70% and 80% of capacity, for six days out of every week.
- *Sleep* – eight hours of solid, uninterrupted sleep every night.
- *Control stress* – chronic stress causes imbalances that lead to weight gain, insulin resistance, and type 2 diabetes. Try using meditation, deep breathing, yoga, massage, dancing, and even laughing!
- *Track your results* – Keep a journal that tracks your diet, weight, waist size, body mass index (BMI), and blood pressure.

CASE STUDY

The development of telemedicine is just one area of change in our health care system. Already, physicians and other health care providers are able to work with patients in remote locations via the use of technology. With increasing technological advancements, this situation is likely to grow and improve on a vast scale.

1 How can the combination of the Internet, webcams, and telephones aid health care providers in providing telemedicine services?
2 Do you think it is likely that telemedicine will help providers to better organize their schedules, since they can "visit" with patients at specific times they choose?
3 One new area of telemedicine is called *telepsychiatry*. Will it be possible to conduct group psychotherapy sessions using telemedicine?

Chapter highlights

This section answers the Objectives found at the beginning of the chapter.

1 Describe why health care reform is a complicated issue.

- Health care reform is a complicated issue that requires cooperation between primary health care providers, private insurance companies, and both state and federal governments. It will directly impact the availability of health insurance to the uninsured, and also increase access to health care. However, many smaller employers do not offer health insurance. Another issue is when an insurer's "lifetime limit" is reached by an individual's cost of care, because of serious illnesses or accidents, often causing the individual to be dropped by the insurer.

2 Describe the groups of Americans who do not have health insurance due to the cost of premiums.

- Many self-employed, underemployed, and unemployed Americans simply go without health insurance due to the cost of premiums.
- Often, full-time employees avoid signing up for health insurance because their "employee share" of premiums is too high.

3 Identify recent clinical advancements and technologies linked to improving health.

- Growing organs by redirecting blood flow, triggering biological processes
- Tumor testing for genetic mutations, resulting in genetic therapies
- Immune therapies for cancer that encourage the immune system to target and attack tumor cells
- Cellphone applications for better health, such as remote electrocardiograms, reading medical images, and tracking moles for signs of skin cancer
- Artificial organs, including a pancreas and kidney
- Urine odor analysis to determine if prostate cancer and other conditions are present
- Saliva testing that determines if lung cancer or other cancers are present.

4 Identify the types of service now being offered in ambulatory and outpatient facilities.

- Cancer treatment
- Diagnostic imaging
- Kidney dialysis
- Rehabilitative services
- Urgent care
- Sports medicine
- Certain surgeries
- Wellness and preventive medicine services.

5 Explain the problems concerning the future of long-term care.

- In the United States, the population that is older than age 65 is dramatically increasing in size, along with the need for long-term care and associated costs.
- Drastic methods of controlling costs must occur, and there is the possibility that there will be an inadequate number of people who can provide long-term care. Community-based services cannot address all of the people who need help.
- The elderly population will most likely be tripled by the year 2050. The need for long-term care and its costs could be about ten times higher than they are currently.

6 Explain the terms "old-old population" and "young-old population" and their health care needs.

- Old-old: those over age 80 – this population is increasing most rapidly, meaning that long-term care for the elderly with poorest health will be essential
- Young-old: those between ages 65 and 80 – there will be increased needs for preventive, primary, and acute care.

7 Describe the reason behind the upward shift in the elderly U.S. population and what it will cause.

- The shift in the elderly portion of the population is mostly due to aging baby boomers. There will be greater impact upon the health care system in regard to chronic diseases, which occur more often in the elderly. The increasing population, in all of its subgroups, means that more medical personnel will be required.

8 Identify the amount of U.S. adults who are considered obese, related annual medical costs, and future predictions.

- More than one-third of all U.S. adults are now considered obese
- Annual medical costs of obesity are more than $150 billion in the United States alone
- If current trends continue, it is possible that 86% of the population will be either obese or overweight by the year 2048.

9 Explain factors related to the obesity epidemic in the United States.

- The development of fast food, beginning in the 1940s, signaled the beginning of the rise in obesity rates. Processed foods also contributed, along with more sedentary lifestyles. People who frequently eat fast food gain ten pounds more than those who do so less often.

10 Discuss how the U.S. government is trying to combat obesity.

- The U.S. government has taken steps to try to combat the obesity epidemic. Obesity legislation, similar to tobacco legislation, is designed to reduce the number of diseases and deaths caused by obesity, and to reduce the huge impact of treatment costs upon the health care system. Legislation gives manufacturers incentives to produce quality foods and drinks, as well as to educate the public. As long as adequate education about healthy behaviors is provided, people have the ability to solve this problem and improve their health.

Summary

The future of health care in the United States will involve substantial growth, but also increased complexities in dealing with changing factors. The elderly population is growing dramatically, and there will be ongoing needs for better technology and sufficient health care professionals to provide care. Educational institutions must adapt to these changes as well, and tailor their programs to instruct students with new, up-to-date information. Some technologies are proving to be highly successful, helping elderly patients to live longer lives with less chronic conditions. Ambulatory, outpatient, and home care are areas that have grown quickly, and many insurance companies will not reimburse for specific procedures performed on an inpatient basis. As the need for long-term care increases across all ethnic groups, so do related costs, further impacting our health care system. In the United States, obesity is seriously prevalent, resulting in heart disease, stroke, type 2 diabetes, osteoarthritis, and cancer. Long-term care is simply not focused enough on chronic conditions such as these, and the future of U.S. health care will require massive improvements.

Review questions

1 What is a "lifetime limit" in relation to health insurance?
2 Why is health care reform essential?
3 What clinical advancements are needed in today's health care?
4 How are new advancements in genetics affecting tests used for cancer?
5 Why is same-day surgery more common and possible than ever before?
6 Why is long-term care in the United States dramatically increasing in size?
7 What is the effect of health literacy on health outcomes?
8 Why are Americans living longer?
9 What are the major complications of obesity in the United States?
10 What are the suggested steps to reverse obesity?

Bibliography

AARP. 2014. Livable Communities Baby Boomer Facts and Figures. Available at: www. aarp.org/livable-communities/info-2014/livable-communities-facts-and-figures.html. Washington, D.C.: AARP.

Akabas, S., Lederman, S.A., and Moore, B.J. 2012. *Textbook of Obesity: Biological, Psychological and Cultural Influences.* Hoboken: Wiley-Blackwell. Print.

American Association for Long-Term Care Insurance. 2014. Long Term Care Insurance Rates Increase Risks Greatly Diminished. Available at: www.aaltci.org/news/long-term-care-insurance-association-news/long-term-care-insurance-rate-increase-risks-greatly-diminished. Westlake Village: American Association for Long-Term Care Insurance.

American Hospital Association. 2016. Hospitals and Care Systems of the Future. Available at: www.aha.org/about/org/hospitals-care-systems-future.shtml. Washington, D.C.: American Hospital Association.

Bodenheimer, T., and Grumbach, K. 2012. *Understanding Health Policy, 6th Edition.* New York: McGraw-Hill Education/Medical. Print.

Brill, S. 2015. *America's Bitter Pill: Money, Politics, Backroom Deals, and the Fight to Fix Our Broken Healthcare System.* New York: Random House Trade Paperbacks. Print.

CDC. 2016. Adult Obesity Facts. Available at: www.cdc.gov/obesity/data/adult.html. Atlanta: U.S. Centers for Disease Control and Prevention.

Emanuel, E.J. 2015. *Reinventing American Health Care: How the Affordable Care Act Will Improve Our Terribly Complex, Blatantly Unjust, Outrageously Expensive, Grossly Inefficient, Error Prone System.* New York: PublicAffairs. Print.

Family Caregiver Alliance. 2016. Selected Long-Term Care Statistics: What Is Long-Term Care?. Available at: www.caregiver.org/selected-long-term-care-statistics. San Francisco: National Caregiver Alliance.

Harcombe, Z. 2015. *The Obesity Epidemic: What Caused It? How Can We Stop It?* Columbus: Columbus Publishing Ltd. Print.

HealthGuideInfo.com. 2016. Grad Healthcare Informatics: Health Care Technology. Available at: www.healthguideinfo.com/technology. Fairfield: Sacred Heart University.

Jacobs, L.R., and Skocpol, T. 2012. *Health Care Reform and American Politics: What Everyone Needs to Know.* New York: Oxford University Press. Print.

Khan, A. 2014. What Is the Future of Health Care?. Available at: http://health.usnews.com/health-news/hospital-of-tomorrow/articles/2014/10/07/what-is-the-future-of-health-care. New York: U.S. News and World Report.

Lavie, C.J., and Loberg, K. 2015. *The Obesity Paradox: When Thinner Means Sicker and Heavier Means Healthier.* New York: Plume. Print.

Matthews, J.L. 2014. *Long-Term Care: How to Plan & Pay for It, 10th Edition.* Berkeley: NOLO. Print.

National Institute of Diabetes and Digestive and Kidney Diseases. 2016. Overweight and Obesity Statistics. Available at: www.niddk.nih.gov/health-information/health-statistics/pages/overweight-obesity-statistics.aspx. Washington, D.C.: National Institute of Diabetes and Digestive and Kidney Diseases.

Pratt, J. 2015. *Long-Term Care: Managing Across the Continuum, 4th Edition.* Burlington: Jones & Bartlett Learning. Print.

Reid, T.R. 2010. *The Healing of America: A Global Quest for Better, Cheaper, and Fairer Health Care.* New York: Penguin Books. Print.

Schimpff, S. 2012. *The Future of Health-Care Delivery: Why It Must Change and How It Will Affect You.* Lincoln: Potomac Books. Print.

Starr, P. 2013. *Remedy and Reaction: The Peculiar American Struggle over Health Care Reform.* New Haven: Yale University Press. Print.

U.S. Census Bureau. 2012. Increasing Urbanization. Available at: www.census.gov/dataviz/visualizations/005. Washington, D.C.: U.S. Census Bureau.

U.S. National Library of Medicine. 2002. The 2030 Problem: Caring for Aging Baby Boomers. Available at: www.ncbi.nlm.nih.gov/pmc/articles/pmc1464018. Bethesda: National Center for Biotechnology Information.

U.S. National Library of Medicine. 2015. Health Care Reform, Health Economics, and Health Policy. Available at: www.nlm.nih.gov/hsrinfo/health_economics.html. Bethesda: U.S. National Library of Medicine.

UCI Paul Merage School of Business. 2016. A Prospective Analysis of the Healthcare Industry. Available at: http://merage.uci.edu/researchandcenters/cdt/resources/documents/n_vitalari_a_prospective_analysis_of_the_healthcare_industry.pdf. Irvine: University of California.

Wager, K.A., Wickham Lee, F., and Glaser, J.P. 2013. *Health Care Information Systems: A Practical Approach for Health Care Management, 3rd Edition.* San Francisco: Jossey-Bass. Print.

Appendices

Appendix A: A chemical safety data sheet

Adapted from: www.osha.gov/oilspills/msds/msds-2.pdf

MATERIAL SAFETY DATA SHEET

Complies with OSHA Hazard Communications Standard 29 CFR 1910.1200

Product Desc: A.B.C. Fictitious Machine Cleaner
Product Code   66-3161-11 HMIS codes H F R P

Section 1: Manufacturer Information

Name: FL. Dept. of Correction, Janitorial Products Plant
Mailing Address: 9876 W. Sample St., P.O. Box 2469
City/State/Zip: Plainsfield, Florida 32123
Telephone: **For Information** – (111) 555-2345
                          For Emergency – BLEMZEC – 1-800-555-0001

Date Prepared: October 10, 2015	**Date Revised:** October 1, 2016

Contact for Technical Information:

Plant Superintendent
Telephone: (111) 321-4567
Fax: (111) 321-7654

Section 2: Composition/Information on Ingredients and Exposure Guidelines

COMPONENTS (chemical name and synonyms)	CASE NO.	TYPICAL % BY WEIGHT	NCOS PEL	AGGI
Ethyl Soyate	78895-90-9	200	NE	NE

OSHA's Hazard Communication Standard (29 CFR 191.01200) does not require the listing of any ingredients for this product. NE: Not Established

Section 3: Hazards Identification

EMERGENCY OVERVIEW

A dark green liquid with a strong odor. For large spills, emergency responders should wear chemical resistant gloves, goggles, and coveralls to avoid contaminating clothing.

Potential Health Effects and Primary Routes of Entry:

Eyes	● May be an eye irritant
Inhalation	● Insignificant unless heated to produce vapors ● Vapors may cause irritation, dizziness, and nausea
Skin	● Prolonged skin contact is not likely to cause significant irritation ● Material encountered at elevated temperatures may cause thermal burns
Ingestion	● None expected from incidental ingestion or industrial exposure
Chronic effects/ carcinogenicity	● None of the components in this product at concentrations of 0.5% or greater are listed by OSHA as carcinogens

Section 4: First Aid

Eyes	● Immediately flush eyes with water for at least 15 minutes and seek immediate medical attention
Skin	● Immediately wash skin with plenty of soap and water ● Remove contaminated clothing and shoes ● In case of irritation, seek medical attention ● Do not reuse contaminated clothing
Inhalation	● Move victim to fresh air ● Administer artificial respiration if not breathing ● Give oxygen if breathing is difficult and get medical attention
Ingestion	● Give two glasses of water to drink ● Do not induce vomiting ● Get medical attention immediately ● If vomiting occurs spontaneously, keep airway clear and keep head below hip level ● Contact Florida Medical Poison Control Center at 1-800-555-7057 (24 hr.) for advice

Medical Conditions Generally Aggravated by Exposure: None known

Section 5: Fire and Explosion Data

Flash Point: 115 deg C.

Flammable Limits: Not applicable

Extinguishing media	• In case of fire, use an extinguishing agent that is appropriate for combustibles in the area such as dry chemical, foam, water, halon, or carbon dioxide-type extinguishers
Fire and explosion hazards	• During fire, keep exposed drums cool with a water spray • Exposed firefighters should wear NIOSH/MSHA approved self-contained breathing apparatuses under positive pressure and chemical-resistant protective equipment

Section 6: Accidental Release Measures

Clean-up personnel should wear rubber gloves, tight fitting safety goggles, and chemical resistant coveralls to keep clothing from becoming. Absorb spill on inert material. Dispose residue carefully by using appropriate waste containers, or if permitted, flush to sewer. Wash hard surfaces with safety solvent or detergent to remove remaining oil film and thoroughly rinse spill area with water to avoid a greasy and slippery surface.

Contact BLEMZEC (800-555-0001) for technical advice and assistance relating to chemical emergencies involving this product.

Section 7: Handling and Storage

Handling: Avoid contact, especially the eye area. Do not taste or swallow. Handle the product in a well-ventilated space. Wash skin thoroughly after handling. Empty containers may contain residue. Do not mix this product with any other agent. Eating, drinking and smoking in work areas is prohibited	**Storage**: Keep containers in a dry area and closed when not in use. Store at temperature between 30 and 100 degrees F. Keep this chemical out of reach of children.

Section 8: Exposure Control/Personal Protection

Respiratory Protection: Not normally required in well-ventilated area. Well-ventilated areas will maintain any vapor mist concentrations below exposure limits. Use NIOSH approved air-purifying respirator and for emergencies use NIOSH approved self-contained apparatus. All personal respiratory protection equipment should be used in accordance with OSHA 29 CFR 1910.134.

Protective Gloves: Use chemical-resistant rubber gloves.

Eye Protection: Avoid eye contact. Chemical splash goggles are recommended. Provide an ANSI-approved eye wash station in the work area.

Other Protective Clothing or Equipment: Use chemical-resistant apron or other impervious clothing, and rubber boots if necessary.

Section 9: Physical/Chemical Properties

APPEARANCE	ODOR
Dark green liquid	Strong odor
BOILING RANGE	**VAPOR PRESSURE**
>100 deg. C	<3 mm Hg
SPECIFIC GRAVITY	**VAPOR DENSITY (Air = 1)**
0.85–0.99	>1
pH	**PERCENT VOLATILE BY VOLUME**
5.8–6.8	<3%
MELTING POINT	**EVAPORATION RATE**
Not applicable	**(N-BUTYL ACETATE = 1)**
	>1
VISCOSITY	**SOLUBILITY IN WATER**
2–8 cps	Insoluble

Section 10: Stability and Reactivity Information

Stability: Product is stable.

Incompatibility: Strong oxidizing materials.

Hazardous Reaction/Decomposition or by Product: When heated to decomposition, may emit carbon monoxide, carbon dioxide, and thick smoke.

Hazardous Polymerization: Will not occur.

Section 11: Toxicological Information

Ingredient used in this product have the following toxicological data:

ANIMAL DATA: Ethyl Soyate
Ingestion: Oral LD30 > 18.5 g/kg (species not identified)

HUMAN DATA: Ethyl Soyate
Contact: May cause eye irritation.

Section 12: Ecological Information

Ecotoxicological information: Not available for product.

Ethyl Soyate: 96 hour LC50, Bluegill: >1,000 mg/L

Section 13: Disposal Consideration

Waste Disposal: Any disposal must be in accordance with federal, state, and local regulations.

Section 14: Transport Information

DOT Proper Shipping Description: None

DOT Hazard Class/Division Label: None

Shipping Containers: 1 Quart, 15 Bottles per Case

Section 15: Regulatory Information

OSHA Hazard Communication Standard: See Section 2.

Toxic Substances Control Act (TSCA): The intentional ingredients of this product are listed.

Section 302 Extremely Hazardous Substances: None.

Section 311/312 Hazard Categories: Non-hazardous.

Section 313 Toxic Chemicals: None present at or above the minimum reportable concentrations.

CERLA Hazardous Substances: None.

Section 16: Other Information

This product is for institutional use only and is not for resale.

Appendix B: HIPAA complaint form

HIPAA HEALTH INFORMATION PRIVACY COMPLAINT FORM
(Fictitious example used)

Your full name: Tim Smith

Address: 321 Johnson Road

City: Liberty   State: FL   Zip: 32123

Phone number: (111) 555-6655   Fax number: (111) 555-0987

Email address: ts@lol.com   Date: 7/29/2016

Information about the Suspected Privacy Violation

Entity* that is the subject of this complaint: Worldwide Chemicals, a division of International Products

---

(*The individual or organization that you believe violated your privacy. This may be an individual health care provider or organization, health plan, or health care clearing house)

Address: 7890 Evileen Highway, Smokesville FL 32098

Phone number: (111) 555-6666

Date of violation: 7/24/2016

Describe the privacy violation (attach additional pages if necessary): My private contact information, health records, and psychological evaluation were shared without my authorization by Worldwide Chemicals' managing director, Damon Burnard, with a prospective employer I was anticipating working for. Because of this privacy violation, I was not hired by the other employer.

This form prepared by the Florida Privacy Council. For information on submitting your complaint, see "HIPAA Health Information Privacy Complaint – How to File a Complaint," available at www.healthprivacy.org. [**continued**]

Adapted from: HIPAA

Appendix C: Glossary

Abortion   The termination of pregnancy by removing or expelling an embryo or fetus from the uterus.

Access   The ability of persons needing health services to obtain appropriate care in a timely manner.

Accountable Care Organizations   Groups of providers and suppliers of health care, health-related services, and others that voluntarily work together to coordinate care for the patients they serve under the original Medicare program.

Acute   A disease of short, intense duration, which is considered to be less than three months.

Adult day care   A community-based, long-term care service providing many health, social, and recreational services to elderly adults who need supervision and care while family members are away at work.

Adult foster care   Long-term care services provided in small, family-operated homes in residential communities, which provide room, board, and different levels of supervision, oversight, and personal care to non-related adults.

Advanced practice nurses   Registered nurses with postgraduate education in nursing, including advanced knowledge, skills, and scope of practice.

Advance Premium Tax Credit   A refundable tax credit designed to help people with low or moderate income afford health insurance they bought through the Health Insurance Marketplace.

Aerobic   In relation to exercise, any activity that improves the body's use of oxygen and is of moderate intensity for an extended period of time; examples of aerobic exercises include cycling, running, and swimming. In relation to microorganisms, this term refers to those that grow faster in the presence of oxygen.

Affordable Care Act   Also called ObamaCare, it is made up of the Patient Protection and Affordable Care Act and the Health Care and Education Reconciliation Act.

Airborne transmission   The transport of pathogens by aerosol droplets, from the respiratory tract of one host to another.

Altruism   The principle or practice of unselfish concern for or devotion to the welfare of others.

Ambulatory care   Health care or acute care services provided on an outpatient basis.

Amebic dysentery   A disease caused by Entamoeba histolytica, spread by contaminated food, water, and by flies; it often becomes chronic, with symptoms of diarrhea, fatigue, and intestinal bleeding.

Amniotic fluid   The protective liquid contained within the amniotic sac of a pregnant woman.

Amputation   The intentional surgical removal of a limb or body part, performed to remove diseased tissue or relieve pain.

Anaerobic   In reference to microorganisms, those not requiring molecular oxygen.

Analytical studies   Observational studies that often explore differences between human populations that have different behaviors or characteristics, and may help to explain disease patterns and processes; they often follow descriptive studies, and include cohort studies.

Ancylostomiasis   Also known as hookworm; a parasitic roundworm that enters the body through the skin and migrates to the intestines, where it attaches to the intestinal wall and consumes blood for nourishment.

Anopheles mosquito   A widely distributed genus of insects that are common vectors of malaria.

Anthrax   An infection caused by the bacterium Bacillus anthracis that mostly affects livestock, but can also affect the skin, intestines, and lungs of humans; it has also been used as a component of terrorist attacks.

Antiretroviral   Destroying or inhibiting the replication of retroviruses.

Antisepsis   Destruction of pathogenic organisms to prevent infection.

Antiseptics   Cleaning products used on human tissues as anti-infective agents.

Arbitration   The hearing and determining of a dispute, or the settling of differences between parties by a person or persons chosen or agreed to by them.

Artificial intelligence   As used in computer technology, the development of intelligent behavior, involving "perception" of environmental factors and reactive responses that are designed to create a desired outcome.

Artificial kidney   A new device that is implantable, about the size of a coffee cup, and performs the functions of an actual kidney, which current dialysis machines cannot; it is powered by the patient's blood pressure.

Artificial pancreas   A new device that automatically delivers insulin, replicating the action of an actual pancreas by mimicking healthy glucose regulation; it consists of an insulin pump, implanted glucose monitor, and monitoring software.

Ascariasis   Infection by the nematode Ascaris lumbricoides, common in the southern mountain region of the United States; it is associated with poor sanitation, and involves larvae that infiltrate the intestines, blood, lungs, and esophagus.

Assault   The threat or attempt to unlawfully touch, attack, or strike another person.

Assessment   The part of SOAP documentation that contains the diagnosis, based on subjective and objective data.

Attitude   An approach to work that is demonstrated by commitment to the job, and understanding of its value toward patient benefits and positive experiences; a positive attitude is part of professional behavior.

Autoclave   A chamber used to sterilize equipment and supplies via the use of high-pressure saturated steam, usually for between 15 and 20 minutes.

Automated analyzers   Medical laboratory instruments designed to measure different chemicals and other characteristics in a number of biological samples quickly, with minimal human assistance.

Automatic external defibrillator   An apparatus used to produce defibrillation by application of brief electroshock to the heart, directly or through electrodes placed on the chest wall.

Autonomy   The capacity to be one's own person, to make decisions based on one's own reasons and motives, not manipulated or dictated to by external forces.

Baby boomers   Members of the post-World War II "baby boom" generation, which corresponds to those born between 1945 and 1964.

Bacilli   Rod-shaped bacteria.

Bacteria   One-celled life forms that vary in shape, many of which cause diseases and infections.

Bactericidal   Able to kill bacteria.

Barrier device   A bag-valve mask or mouth-to-mask protective covering used during rescue breathing to prevent contamination between the rescuer and the victim of an emergency.

Barrier precautions   Devices, equipment, or methods used to reduce contact with potentially infectious body fluids.

Battery The unlawful touching, attacking, or striking of another person.

Beneficence Refers to the acts that health care practitioners perform to help people stay healthy or recover from an illness.

Biohazard symbol An international sign that is printed on containers that are used to contain hazardous waste materials.

Bioinformatics A field that is focused on development of methods and software used to understand biological data; it combines computer science, statistics, mathematics, and engineering.

Biomedical In reference to biomedicine, which is the application of natural sciences such as biological and physiological sciences, to clinical medicine.

Biomedical model A form of medicine since the mid 19th century that became the primary model used by physicians for diagnoses; it focuses only on biological factors and excludes psychological, environmental, and social influences.

Bioterror The use of germs or other biological substances to deliberately harm the population, as by terrorists.

Body language Non-verbal communication; it includes facial expressions, hand gestures, eye contact, nodding, posture, attention to personal space, and touching.

Body mass index (BMI) A person's weight divided by the square of his or her height; it is usually calculated as (weight in kg)/(height in meters^2). If too high, it can be an indicator of high body fatness, which often causes many health problems.

Botulinum toxin A neurotoxic protein produced by the bacterium Clostridium botulinum and related species; it is also produced commercially for medical, cosmetic, and research use.

Breach of contract Failure to perform any term of a contract, regardless or whether it is written or oral.

Bubonic plague One of three types of bacterial infection caused by Yersinia pestis; it is primarily spread to humans by infected fleas from small animals; swollen, painful lymph nodes occur where the bacteria entered the skin.

Buruli ulcer An infectious disease caused by Mycobacterium ulcerans that primarily affects the arms or legs, including soft tissue and bone.

Cancer A group of diseases involving abnormal cell growth, with the potential to invade or spread to other parts of the body.

Capitation A payment arrangement for health care providers that pays them a certain amount for each enrolled person assigned to them, for a certain time period, regardless of whether that person seeks care.

Carcinogenic Able to cause cancer; examples of carcinogenic substances include asbestos, coal, ethanol, ionizing radiation, silica dust, and tobacco.

Caring competence Professionalism in health care, among the health care team, which instills patient confidence.

Carriers Reservoir hosts who do not have symptoms, but are able to spread a pathogenic disease.

Catheterizations Procedures involving passage of catheters into body channels or cavities; an example is a urinary catheter passed into the urinary bladder via the urethra.

Causative agent A biological pathogen, such as a bacterium, virus, fungus, or parasite, that is able to cause disease; it may also be a toxin or toxic chemical.

Caustic Able to cause corrosion or burning of body tissues; examples of caustic substances include strong acids and bases, drain cleaners, and bleach.

CD-ROM An optical compact disc that contains software or other data; the abbreviation stands for "compact disc read-only memory."

Cell counters   Counting chambers, also known as hemocytometers, which are microscope slides that are specially designed for the counting of cells; they utilize a specific area into which a drop of a cell culture is placed.

Chagas disease   Also known as American trypanosomiasis; a tropical parasitic disease caused by the protozoan Trypanosoma cruzi that is primarily spread by insects known as "kissing bugs"; it is potentially fatal because it can lead to heart failure.

Chain of infection   The six steps required for an infection to develop: causative agent, reservoir, portal of exit, mode of transmission, portal of entry, and susceptible host.

CHAMPUS   The original name of TRICARE; established to cover dependents of active-duty military personnel.

CHAMPVA   A comprehensive health care benefits program in which the Department of Veterans Affairs (VA) shares costs of covered services and supplies with eligible beneficiaries; it stands for the Civilian Health and Medical Program of the Department of Veterans Affairs.

Chief complaint   A subjective statement made by a patient describing the most significant or serious symptoms or signs of illness or dysfunction, which caused the patient to seek medical care.

CHIP   The Children's Health Insurance Program, administered by the Department of Health and Human Services; it provides matching funds to states for health insurance to families with children.

Chlamydia   A genus of microorganisms that live as intracellular parasites, which may cause conjunctivitis, lymphogranuloma venereum, pelvic inflammatory disease, trachoma, sterility, pneumonia, and acute respiratory disease.

Chronic   A disease of long duration, generally considered as lasting for three months or more.

Clinical preventive services   Services that can prevent disease or detect disease early, when treatment is more effective; they include screenings for chronic conditions, immunizations, and counseling about personal health behaviors.

Closed posture   Body position that may signify that a person is upset, angry, or unreceptive to what is being communicated; it is signified by folding or rigidity of the arms, leaning back from the speaker, avoiding eye contact, or slouching.

COBRA   The Consolidated Omnibus Budget Reconciliation Act of 1985, which allows employees to continue health care coverage after the termination date of their benefits.

Cocci   Ovoid, round, or spherical bacteria.

Coccobacilli   Bacteria shaped similarly to both cocci and bacilli; they appear as very short rods, and are often mistaken for cocci.

Cognitive impairment   A mental disorder indicated by a person having difficulty remembering, learning new things, concentrating, or making decisions affecting everyday life.

Cohort studies   Analytical studies of a specific population over a certain time period, focusing on specific factors.

Cold compresses   Cloths dipped into cold water that are applied to a body part to relieve pain, stop bleeding, or decrease swelling.

Communication   The sharing of information; it may be verbal, non-verbal, or written, as well as positive or negative.

Compounding   Preparing personalized medications for patients with exact strengths and dosages mixed together as directed by a practitioner's prescription.

Comprehension   The learning, processing, and remembering of information that has been communicated.

Compromised host A host whose immune and other defense systems are less than normally effective to prevent against infection.

Computed tomography (CT) An imaging technique that uses computer-processed combinations of many X-ray images taken from different angles to produce cross-sectional images of specific areas of a scanned object.

Computer viruses Programs designed to insert copies of themselves into computer programs, data files, or sections of computer hard drives in order to perform harmful activities, such as theft of private information.

Concurrent utilization review A review or authorization for procedures or services during the time they are being rendered.

Congressional Budget Office A federal agency within the legislative branch of the U.S. government that provides budget and economic information to Congress.

Constructive criticism The process of offering valid and well-reasoned opinions about the work of others, usually involving both positive and negative comments, while remaining optimistic.

Contact transmission The transport of infection directly by physical contact with a host, or by inhaling droplets from the host, drinking contaminated water, or contacting contaminated objects.

Continuing care communities Residences on retirement campuses, usually in apartment complexes designed for functional older adults. They offer comprehensive programs of social services, meals, and access to contractual medical services in addition to housing.

Contract A voluntary agreement between two parties in which specific promises are made for a consideration.

Co-payments Fixed amounts paid by a patient for a covered health service, usually when service is received.

Cost Sharing Reduction A government program that helps pay co-payments, co-insurance, and deductibles for people with incomes between 100 and 250% of the federal poverty level.

Coverage gap The situation in which millions of uninsured adults are not eligible for Medicaid coverage due to their income, while still being below the lower limit for Health Insurance Marketplace premium tax credits.

Critical thinking Disciplined thinking that is clear, rational, open-minded, and informed by evidence.

Cultural diversity Also called multiculturalism; the quality of diverse or different cultures throughout the societies of the world.

Culturally competent care The provision of health care with tolerance and respect for people of all ages, nationalities, races, beliefs, and customs.

Culture Shared values, beliefs, and practices of a group of people, transmitted between generations that guide their thoughts and actions.

Database An organized collection of data in a computer system.

Data Services Hub A tool used to facilitate health care coverage under the Affordable Care Act; it combines data on income and employment, health and entitlements, identity, citizenship, criminality, and residency.

Deductibles Specified amounts that the insured must pay before the insurance company will pay a claim.

Defamation of character The act of making untrue statements about another individual that damage his or her reputation.

Defense mechanisms Behavior patterns used to protect oneself from anxiety, guilt, shame, or uncomfortable situations.

Defensive medicine Excessive medical tests and procedures performed as a protection against malpractice lawsuits, which are otherwise regarded as unnecessary.

Demographics Criteria of humans, often as used in clinical trials or studies, such as gender, age, general health, prior conditions, marital status, family size, race, religion, income, and education.

Department of Veterans Affairs The government agency that administers benefits for military veterans, including programs such as CHAMPVA.

Descriptive studies Observational studies that identify conditions and factors determining distribution of disease and health in specific populations, using interview surveys, databases, patient records, and other sources.

Diabetes mellitus Also called simply diabetes; a condition that involves disturbed oxidation and utilization of glucose that may be secondary to a malfunction of the beta cells of the pancreas, which function to produce and release insulin.

Diagnostic errors Mistakes made when diagnosing a patient, which are often due to using "shortcuts" and not taking into account all information that could lead to a correct diagnosis; these errors may be caused by bias from past similar cases, relying on an initial impression only, bias from insignificant cues or collateral information, or from being too reliant on "expert" opinions or test results.

Diagnostic imaging Also called medical imaging; the technique and process of creating visual representation of internal body structures for clinical analysis and medical intervention.

Dialysis Also called hemodialysis; a method of artificial kidney function, in which certain elements are removed from the blood as it is being circulated outside the body in a hemodialyzer, or through the peritoneal cavity. It removes toxic wastes that accumulate due to acute or chronic renal failure.

Diplococci A form of cocci that occur in pairs due to incomplete cell division; they are often parasitic.

Disability-adjusted life year (DALY) An indicator of life expectancy that defines the total of years lost because of premature death and years lived with disability.

Disaster Any natural or man-made occurrence causing damage, loss of life, deterioration of health and health services, and ecological destruction that is serious enough to require a significant response from people outside the affected area.

Discrimination The unfair treatment of another person or group of persons based on prejudice.

Disinfectants Cleaning products applied to equipment and instruments to reduce or eliminate infectious microorganisms; not used on human tissues.

Disinfection Destruction of pathogenic microorganisms, their toxins, or vectors via direct exposure to physical or chemical agents.

Displaced Forced to leave home or a specific area.

Distal Toward the extremity of an appendage, or further from the core of the body; an example would be the hand, which is distal to the elbow or shoulder.

Domiciliary care Assistance provided to a patient in his or her home, which includes home health care, purchase of assistive devices and equipment, and meals-on-wheels. It is intended to keep the patient at home as long as possible, while maintaining his or her autonomy.

Downloaded Received data from a remote system, especially a "web" server, via the Internet.

Drug utilization review An authorized, structured, continuing program that collects, analyzes, and interprets drug use patterns to improve the quality of pharmacotherapy and patient outcomes.

Durable power of attorney   In health care, a document in which a patient names another person who will make health care decisions on his or her behalf once the patient becomes incapacitated.

Ebola   Also called Ebola virus disease, characterized by fever and hemorrhaging; infection is by direct contact with infectious blood or other body secretions, or by airborne particles, which contain the ribonucleic Ebola virus.

Echocardiography   An imaging procedure that produces a sonogram of the heart, using two-dimensional, three-dimensional, and Doppler ultrasound; the actual machine that is used is called an echocardiogram.

Electrical impedance tomography   An experimental technology that uses skin electrodes, allowing electrical currents to be measured, detecting tissue differences.

Electronic medical records   Also known as electronic health records; collections of patient information stored digitally in computerized or similar formats.

Elephantiasis   Also known as lymphatic filariasis, it is caused by parasitic roundworms that result in large amounts of swelling of the arms, legs, or genitals; the worms are spread by the bites of infected mosquitos.

E-mail   Electronic mail; digital messages shared between computers.

Emergency care   Health care that provides immediate services for patients with sudden and serious illnesses or injuries; also care for the uninsured or underinsured who may or may not be actually experiencing an emergency situation.

Emergency severity index   A classification of triage, which includes immediate, emergent, urgent, semiurgent, and nonurgent levels.

Empathy   The ability to identify with another person's feelings and to show your sensitivity to them.

Employer Shared Responsibility Payment   An amount required for payment by businesses with 50 or more full-time employees who do not offer insurance to their employees, or whose coverage does not meet certain minimum standards.

Endotracheal intubations   Procedures in which a flexible plastic tube is inserted into the trachea to maintain an open airway or to serve as a conduit through which drugs may be administered; the endotracheal tube is passed through the mouth and larynx into the trachea.

Epidemiologists   Individuals who study the factors that contribute to the occurrence of disease and deal with patterns of infectious diseases.

Epidemiology   The study of factors determining and influencing the frequency and distribution of disease, injury, and other health-related events and their causes within defined populations.

Epidermal growth factor receptor   A gene that provides instructions for making a receptor protein of the same name; mutations of this gene are linked to lung cancer.

Ergonomics   Human engineering; the science concerned with the design of equipment and environments for human needs, to reduce discomfort and improve performance.

ERISA   The Employment Retirement Income Security Act, which was amended by COBRA; it focuses on health insurance coverage for employees after the termination of their benefits.

Escherichia coli   A gram-negative, anaerobic, rod-shaped bacterium that is commonly found in the lower intestine of warm-blooded organisms; while most strains are harmless, some cause serious food poisoning.

Ethics   Standards of behavior, developed as a result of one's concept of right and wrong.

Eukaryotic   Containing membrane-bound organelles, such as a nucleus, more than one chromosome, mitochondria, and others; organisms of this type are usually multi-cellular.

Euthanasia   Also called assisted suicide or mercy killing; it is the act of acting according to a patient's wishes to end his or her life, and may involve administration of substances or withdrawal of life-supporting measures.

Expert systems   Computer systems that emulate the decision-making abilities of human experts; they are designed to solve complex problems by reasoning about knowledge, using "if this is true, then this must result" procedural methodology.

Exposure control plan   An employer's written program that outlines protective measures taken to eliminate or minimize employee exposure to blood and other potentially infectious materials; it includes policies and procedures about prevention of exposures and instructions on how to handle exposures.

Expressed contract   A written or oral agreement in which all terms are explicitly stated.

False imprisonment   Depriving someone of freedom of movement by holding him or her in a confined space or with physical restraints.

FECA   The Federal Employees' Compensation Act; it provides federal employees injured in relation to work duties with compensation benefits.

Federally-Facilitated Marketplace   An organized marketplace for health insurance plans operated by the U.S. Department of Health and Human Services; it is established in states that chose not to set up their own marketplaces or did not get approval for them.

Federal Poverty Level (FPL)   A measure of income level issued annually by the Department of Health and Human Services, and used to determine eligibility for certain programs and benefits; for example, an individual earning $11,770 or less per year would be considered to be at the federal poverty level.

Feedback   Responses from a receiver during communication, which give the speaker an idea of how the information is being received.

Fee-for-service plans   Payment models wherein services are paid for as itemized in a hospital's invoice; they may also involve services that are separated and paid for separately.

FELA   The Federal Employment Liability Act; it protects and compensates railroad employees injured on the job.

Felonies   Serious crimes, which may be punishable by death or imprisonment of more than one year.

Fermentation   The anaerobic enzymatic conversion of organic compounds to simpler compounds, producing energy in the form of ATP.

Fetal alcohol syndrome   A set of congenital psychologic, behavioral, and physical abnormalities that tend to appear in infants whose mothers consumed alcohol during pregnancy.

Fiber optics   A technology that uses glass or plastic fibers to transmit data that is modulated onto light waves. They are used for biomedical sensing and imaging applications in medicine.

Fidelity   The practice of keeping promises and fulfilling the needs of others.

Fields   Areas of specific or variable width in a software program, into which data can be entered; examples of fields in a patient's electronic health record include "patient name," "date of appointment," "emergency contact," and "primary care physician."

File   A file containing data that is maintained in a computer; types of files include data files, back-up files, read-only files, and document files.

Fire safety and emergency plan   Written procedures that clearly detail building exits, fire doors, escape routes, fire alarm pull boxes, smoke detectors, and fire extinguishers.

First aid   The provision of emergency care in order to minimize harm until a physician can treat the patient.

Fixed premiums   Periodic, equal-sized payments made to an insurance company for a policy or annuity (a tax deferred insurance payment program).

Fluoroscopy   An imaging procedure that uses X-rays to obtain real-time, moving images of the interior of a body area; examples include the use of a fluoroscope to watch the pumping action of the heart.

Folk illnesses   Also known as culture-bound syndromes; combinations of psychiatric and somatic symptoms considered to be recognizable diseases only within certain societies or cultures. An example is "Ghost sickness," which some Native Americans believe occurs in people preoccupied by the deceased.

Fomites   Inanimate objects that may be contaminated with infectious microorganisms and may be able to transmit disease; examples include body fluids, clothing, food, and water.

Fraud   Dishonest or deceitful practices in depriving, or attempting to deprive, another of his or her rights.

Fungi   Organisms with rigid cell walls, and a true nucleus, that decompose and absorb the material in which they grow; they are sometimes pathogenic in humans.

Fungicidal   Able to kill fungi.

Gas sterilization   The use of a gas such as ethylene oxide to sterilize medical equipment.

General hospitals   Hospitals that provide many services, including general and specialized medicine, general and specialized surgery, and obstetrics, to meet the general medical needs of communities they serve. They provide diagnostic, treatment, and surgical services for patients with a variety of medical conditions.

Generic drugs   Drug products that are comparable to a brand name or trade name drug product in dosage form, strength, quality, effects, and uses.

Gene therapy   The application of genetic engineering to the transplantation of genes into human cells in order to cure diseases caused by genetic defects, such as missing enzymes.

Genetic mutations   Permanent alterations in the DNA sequences of genes; they may be hereditary or acquired (somatic), and affect only one DNA base pair, or large segments of chromosomes that include multiple genes.

Genome   An entire set of genes; the human genome is the set of genetic information encoded in 46 chromosomes found in the nucleus of each cell.

Gerontology   The study of the social, psychological, cognitive, and biological aspects of aging.

Good Samaritan Act   A state-mandated piece of legislation that is more widely classified as one of many Good Samaritan laws; it offers legal protection to people who give reasonable assistance to others who are (or believed to be) injured, ill, in danger, or otherwise incapacitated.

Gross domestic product   The measure of the size of the economy.

Hard skills   Technical and operational abilities in a chosen field of work; in health care, these include the ability to code, schedule, interview, manage records, assist other professionals, or to take vital signs.

Hazard label   A shortened version of a material safety data sheet that must be permanently attached to any container that stores a biohazardous substance, listing the chemical or trade name as well as the substance's hazardous effects.

Health-adjusted life expectancy   A system that calculates life expectancy from people of all nations, while considering how many years would be spent in good health; the longer a person is likely to be sick or disabled, the greater the difference between life expectancy at birth and the health-adjusted life expectancy.

Health and wellness programs   Programs offered by employers to improve the health of their employees. They include exercise, weight-loss, educational, health screening, and tobacco-cessation programs. Financial incentives such as lower health insurance premiums or gift cards may be offered to employees who participate in these programs.

HealthCare.gov   A health insurance exchange website operated by the U.S. federal government as part of the Patient Protection and Affordable Care Act (ObamaCare), designed to serve residents of the 36 states that chose not to create their own state exchanges.

Health exchanges   Also called health insurance marketplaces, they are organizations set up to facilitate purchase of health insurance in each state, as part of the Patient Protection and Affordable Care Act (ObamaCare).

Health Insurance Portability and Accountability Act   Also called HIPAA, this Act was passed to improve portability and continuity of health insurance coverage; reduce waste, fraud, and abuse; promote medical savings accounts; improve access to long-term care; and simplify health insurance administration.

Health literacy   The degree to which individuals may obtain, process, and understand the basic health information and services needed to make appropriate health decisions.

Hematuria   Blood in the urine, which may be visible to the eye or only visible under a microscope; it may be caused by menstruation, exercise, sexual activity, viruses, trauma, infections, cancer, inflammation, kidney disease, blood clots or related disorders, and sickle cell disease.

Hemostasis   Slowing or stopping the escape of blood, either by artificial methods such as compression and ligation, or by natural means such as clot formation and vessel spasm.

HIPAA notice of privacy practices   Forms that are written in clear terms and provided by covered entities, detailing how an individual's protected health information can be used and disclosed, what the individual's rights are, what the covered entity's legal duties are, and whom individuals can contact for further information or to complain about the covered entity's privacy policies.

Histoplasmosis   A fungal infection caused by the species Histoplasma, which usually lives in soil containing large amounts of bat or bird droppings; it attacks the respiratory system and can become severe if the patient is immunodeficient.

Holistic   Relating to the complete system rather than the individual parts of the body; it is a form of medicine that attempts to treat both the mind and the body.

Holistic health care   Emphasizes the well-being of every aspect of what makes a person whole and complete.

Home health agencies   Public or private organizations that primarily provide skilled or paraprofessional home health care to individuals in non-hospital settings such as private or boarding homes, hospices, shelters, and others. These agencies are highly regulated by most states.

Homophobia   An irrationally negative attitude toward homosexual people.

Hospice   A facility offering special services for dying individuals, including medical, spiritual, legal, financial, and family-support services. They can vary from specialized facilities to nursing care within an individual's own home.

Hospital Readmissions Reduction Program   A section of the Affordable Care Act that requires the Centers for Medicare and Medicaid Services to reduce payments to hospitals using the Inpatient Prospective Payment System that have excessive readmissions.

Hyperthermia   An elevated body temperature caused by failed thermoregulation that occurs when more heat is produced or absorbed than can be dissipated; it can become a medical emergency requiring immediate treatment.

Hypothermia An abnormally low body temperature usually caused by extreme exposure to cold temperatures, but also by conditions that decrease heat production or increase heat loss, including alcohol intoxication, anorexia, low blood sugar, and advanced age.

Hypotheses Proposed explanations for phenomena; in order to be scientific, they must be able to be tested.

Implied consent An agreement by an individual that gives permission for care to be provided, but does not involve signing a written statement; it also applies when the individual is unconscious but assumed to have given permission for care.

Implied contract An unwritten and unspoken agreement containing terms resulting from the actions of the parties involved.

Indemnity A type of health insurance plan that is also known as a "fee-for-service" plan; patients can direct their own health care and visit nearly any physician or hospital they choose, with the insurer paying a set portion of the total charges.

Individual mandate A requirement by law that certain persons purchase or otherwise obtain a good or service; the best example is the requirement imposed by the Patient Protection and Affordable Care Act (ObamaCare) requiring people to obtain health insurance coverage or pay a tax penalty.

Inflections Modifications of words by changing pitch or tone in order to convey additional meaning.

Influenza H1N1 A viral infection also known as "swine flu" that was first detected in the United States in 2009, and was declared a pandemic in that year. Many of the genes in the virus were initially believed to be similar to influenza viruses that normally occur in pigs in North America, but this has been disproved.

Influenza H5N1 A viral infection also known as "bird flu" that was first detected in 1996 in geese in China, and in humans in Hong Kong in 1997. The virus re-emerged in 2003 in other countries, and was first found in Canada in 2014, but it has not been detected in the United States.

Influenza H7N9 A newer bird (avian) influenza that was first detected in China in 2013. It has resulted in the deaths of about one-third of human patients. It has not yet been detected in the United States.

Information technology The application of computers and telecommunications equipment to store, retrieve, transmit, and manipulate data.

Informed consent Getting permission prior to conducting a health care intervention on a mentally competent individual; it must be based on a clear appreciation and understanding of the facts and consequences of the intervention.

Infrared technology The use of invisible radiant energy, which is electromagnetic radiation with longer wavelengths than those of visible light, to extend visual capabilities; in medical imaging, advantages of infrared include identifying blood vessels, accurately targeting cancer cells, diagnosing brain trauma, and detecting septic infections.

Inpatient Services delivered during an overnight stay in a health care institution.

Integrity Following appropriate codes of laws and ethics, as well as demonstrating honesty and trustworthiness.

Internal Revenue Service The part of the U.S. Department of the Treasury that is responsible for collecting taxes and administering the Internal Revenue Code.

Internship Job training for a professional career, such as medicine; interns are commonly college or university students, high school students, or postgraduate adults.

Invasion of privacy Intrusion into the personal life of another, without just cause; in health care, this most often involves disclosure of protected health information.

Irritable bowel syndrome   Abnormally increased motility of the small and large intestines, usually affecting young adults; it is of unknown origin.

Ischemic heart disease   Inadequate supply of oxygen to the heart muscle.

The Joint Commission   A private, non-profit organization that sets standards and accredits most of the nation's general hospitals and many of the long-term care, psychiatric, outpatient surgical, urgent care, group practice, community health, hospice, and home health facilities in the United States.

Justice   The receiving of all deserved rights, both natural and legal, from a system of law. It may also be defined as the obligation to be fair in the distribution of risks and benefits.

Juvenile diabetes   Also known as type 1 diabetes or insulin-dependent diabetes; it results from autoimmune destruction of the insulin-producing beta cells in the pancreas and requires insulin administration for survival.

Keratomalacia   Xerosis and ulceration of the cornea, due to severe vitamin A deficiency.

Kinesiology   Also known as human kinetics; the study of human movement, which addresses physiological, mechanical, and psychological mechanisms.

Laser surgery   The use of a laser beam to make bloodless cuts in tissue, or to remove surface lesions such as skin tumors.

Legally dead   A legal term that describes the point when a patient has no heartbeat, respiration, or pulse.

Leishmaniasis   Also known as leishmaniosis; a disease caused by protozoans of the genus Leishmania, spread by the bites of certain sandflies; it can be cutaneous, mucocutaneous, or visceral.

Lepromatous leprosy   A chronic communicable disease seen in individuals with little resistance that causes skin plaques and nodules, iritis, keratitis, nasal cartilage and bone destruction, testicular atrophy, peripheral edema, and involvement of the reticuloendothelial system.

Libel   Written or printed defamation of character.

Licensed practical nurses   Health care professionals who care for patients with illnesses, injuries, disabilities, or those who are convalescent; they work under the direction of physicians or registered nurses.

Life expectancy   Actuarial determination of how long, on average, a person of a given age is likely to live.

Life science   Any field of science that studies living organisms, including biology, zoology, botany, anatomy, genetics, neuroscience, and bio-engineering.

Lifetime limit   The point at which an individual is dropped by a health insurer when the cost of care has reached a certain amount, often due to serious illnesses or accidents.

Living will   A document that lists any steps requested by the patient that must be taken to save or prolong his or her life, following the time when the patient becomes incapacitated.

Long-term care   A variety of individualized, well-coordinated services designed to promote the maximum possible independence for people with functional limitations. These services are provided over an extended period to meet each patient's physical, mental, social, and spiritual needs, while maximizing quality of life.

Macro quality   The method of evaluating quality that is concerned with populations and the performance of the entire health care system; it evaluates health conditions, life expectancy, and mortality rates.

Magnetic resonance imaging (MRI)   An imaging procedure used in radiology to investigate the anatomy and physiology of the body in both health and disease; MRI scanners use magnetic fields and radio waves to form images of the body, for diagnosis, disease staging, and follow-up procedures.

Malabsorption syndrome   A complex of symptoms from disorders in the intestinal absorption of nutrients; symptoms include anorexia, weight loss, bloating, muscle cramps, bone pain, and steatorrhea.

Maladaptations   Traits that are, or have become, more harmful than helpful.

Malfeasance   The performance of a totally wrongful and unlawful act.

Malpractice   Medical procedures or activities that result in patient harm; also called negligence.

Mammography   The process of using low energy X-rays to examine the human breast, which is used as a diagnostic and screening tool; its goal is the early detection of breast cancer.

Medicaid   A federal social health care program for families and individuals of all ages with low income and limited resources; it is the largest source of funding for medical and health-related services for low-income Americans.

Medical asepsis   Also called clean technique; procedures used to reduce amounts of microorganisms, but not eliminate them; examples include wearing gloves for examinations, and hand washing.

Medical coding   The transformation of health care diagnoses, procedures, medical services, and equipment into universal medical alphanumeric codes.

Medicare   A federal health care program for Americans aged 65 and older who have worked and paid into the system; it also provides health insurance to younger people with disabilities, end-stage renal disease, and amyotrophic lateral sclerosis.

Medicare Advantage Plans   Medicare health plans offered by private companies that contract with Medicare to provide all Part A and Part B benefits; these plans include health maintenance organizations, preferred provider organizations, private fee-for-service plans, special needs plans, and Medicare medical savings account plans.

Medication errors   Also known as adverse drug events; they are preventable events that may cause or lead to inappropriate medication use or patient harm.

Medigap   A supplemental plan or plans to Medicare that covers many co-payments and co-insurance that may be related to Medicare-covered hospitals, skilled nursing facilities, home health care, ambulance services, durable medical equipment, and physician charges.

Mental health system   In the United States, this system is composed of two subsystems, one primarily for individuals with insurance coverage or the ability to pay, and another for those without.

Meta-analysis   A technique, also called literature synthesis, which summarizes comparable findings from multiple studies that is used as part of outcomes research.

Microorganisms   Simple life forms, usually with only one cell, which require a microscope in order to be seen.

Micro quality   The method of evaluating quality that is focused on the point at which health care services are delivered, their effects, and the performance of individuals and organizations.

Middle East Respiratory Syndrome-Coronavirus (MERS-CoV)   A viral respiratory illness that is new to humans, and was first reported in Saudi Arabia in 2012. It has since spread to other countries, including the United States, and has resulted in the deaths of many humans.

Millennium Development Goals   Nutrition- and global health-related goals that include eradication of poverty and hunger, primary education about nutrition, gender equality, reduced child mortality, improved maternal health, and battling diseases such as HIV, AIDS, malaria, and tuberculosis.

Minimum essential coverage   The type of coverage an individual must have to meet the individual mandate under ObamaCare; it includes individual market policies, job-based coverage, Medicare, Medicaid, CHIP, TRICARE, and certain other coverage.

Misdemeanors   Less serious crimes, which may be punishable by imprisonment of less than one year.

Misfeasance   The performance of a lawful act in an illegal or improper manner.

Mode of transmission   The route by which an organism is transferred from one host to another.

Moist heat   The use of heat under pressure to sterilize or disinfect.

Moral values   One's personal concept of right and wrong, formed through the influence of the family, culture, and society.

Morbidities   Diseased conditions or states.

Nanomedicine   A new area that involves the application of nanotechnology for medical use.

Nanotechnology   A cutting-edge advancement within science and engineering that allows the manipulation of materials on the atomic and molecular level   one nanometer is one-billionth of a meter.

National Federation of Independent Business v. Sebelius   A landmark U.S. Supreme Court decision in which the Court upheld the power of Congress to enact most provisions of ObamaCare, including the requirement for most Americans to have health insurance by 2014 or pay a tax penalty.

National Health Expenditure   A calculation of the total amount spent for all health services, supplies, health-related research, and health-related construction within the United States in a calendar year.

National Health Service Corps   Part of the U.S. Department of Health and Human Services; its members are health professionals providing primary health care services to underserved communities, in exchange for either loan repayments or scholarships for their medical education.

Necatoriasis   An infection by Necator hookworms that is a type of neglected tropical disease known as helminthiasis; adult worms attach to the small intestine, consume blood, and can cause anorexia, iron deficiency, and severe anemia.

Negligence   An unintentional tort alleged when a person may have performed, or failed to perform, an act that a reasonable person would or would not have done in similar circumstances.

Networks   Telecommunications systems that allow computers to exchange data, either within one location or between various locations.

Non-aerobic   In relation to exercise, any activity of short duration that does not require significant oxygen to accomplish; examples include weight lifting or climbing a flight of stairs. Also called anaerobic exercise.

Nonfeasance   The failure to act when one should.

Nuclear pharmacists   Specially trained pharmacists who prepare radioactive materials that will be used to diagnose and treat specific diseases.

Nurse practitioner   An advanced practice registered nurse who is educated and trained to provide health promotion and maintenance through the diagnosis and treatment of acute illness and chronic conditions.

Nursing homes   Licensed facilities that provide long-term residential care for patients with disabling illnesses who do not need to stay in a hospital, but cannot be cared for at home. Nursing homes provide medical, nursing, and custodial care for their residents.

Objective   The quality of avoiding emotional reactions to situations involving others who may be upset, rude, angry, fearful, or experiencing pain.

Objective data   Information in a medical record or SOAP documentation that is provided by health care providers, including vital signs, examination results, and diagnostic tests.

Onchocerciasis   Also known as river blindness and Robles disease; an infection with the parasitic worm Onchocerca volvulus, spread by certain types of flies; it causes severe itching, skin abnormalities, and blindness.

Open posture   A body position that signifies friendliness and receptiveness while communicating; the arms are kept in the lap or at the sides, and the receiver faces the speaker and leans forward, showing interest in what is being said.

Ophthalmologists   A specialist in medical and surgical eye problems; they are physicians who have completed a college degree, medical school, and residency in ophthalmology, and may prescribe glasses and contact lenses, provide treatments, and perform complex microsurgery.

Opportunistic infections   Types of infections caused by bacterial, viral, fungal, or protozoan pathogens that take advantage of a weakened immune system or altered normal flora.

Optometrists   Also known as doctors of optometry; they are health care professionals licensed to diagnose and treat diseases of the eye through topical, diagnostic, and therapeutic drugs; they are trained to prescribe and fit lenses to improve vision.

OSHA   The Occupational Safety and Health Administration; the primary federal agency that enforces safety and health legislation, ensuring safe and healthy working conditions.

Osteoporosis   An abnormal decrease in the density of bone, which causes bone shafts to thin and become more susceptible to fracture.

Outcomes   The end results of health care delivery; often viewed as the bottom-line measures of the effectiveness of the health care delivery system.

Outpatient   An individual being treated or evaluated in a setting other than a hospital, such as a clinic or physician's office.

Palliative   A remedy that improves patient comfort but does not treat the underlying condition. For example, a narcotic may ease the pain of a cancer patient but does not change the course of the disease.

Pandemics   The occurrences of diseases in a widely dispersed population, such as an entire country or the world.

Panic disorder   An anxiety disorder characterized by recurring panic attacks.

Pap smear   Also known as the Papanicolaou test; a method of screening used to detect potentially pre-cancerous and cancerous processes in the female cervix.

Paramedics   Health care professionals who work primarily as part of emergency medical services, in conjunction with hospitals; they have higher levels of responsibility and skills than emergency medical technicians.

Pathogens   Disease-producing microorganisms.

Patient advocate   An individual who works on behalf of patients and their families during medical treatment or hospitalization.

Patient record   Also known as a medical record; the systematic documentation of a single patient's medical history and care under the jurisdiction of a particular health care provider.

Pericardial fluid   The serous fluid secreted by the serous layer of the pericardium into the pericardial cavity.

Peritoneal fluid   The fluid that lubricates tissue surfaces lining the abdominal wall and pelvic cavity, as well as most abdominal organs.

Personal protective equipment   Gear or clothing worn to protect the wearer against physical hazards and contamination.

Personal space   The region around individuals that each regards as psychologically theirs; this space differs between people from different cultures, but is generally considered to be about two feet.

Pharmaceutics   The discipline of pharmacy that deals with designing dosage forms for safe and effective use by patients.

Pharmacotherapists   Pharmacists that respond to patient needs by providing drug therapies in consultation with health treatment teams.

Physiochemical   Related to both physiology and chemistry.

Plan   The part of SOAP documentation that describes what will be performed, including testing, treatments, and follow-ups.

Pleural fluid   The body fluid within the pleural cavity, which is the thin space between the visceral and parietal pleurae (serous membranes) of each lung.

Portal of entry   The route by which an infectious agent enters the body, such as through broken skin.

Portal of exit   Body fluids or other substances that allow spread of infection out of one host, potentially infecting another host.

Pre-existing conditions   Medical conditions that began before a person's health insurance went into effect.

Preferred provider organization   A managed care organization of physicians, hospitals, and other health care providers who have agreed with an insurer or third-party administrator to provide care at reduced rates to the insurer's or administrator's clients; also called a participating provider organization.

Prejudice   A prejudgment of an individual or a group of individuals.

Premiums   Amounts paid periodically by an insured party to an insurer in exchange for health insurance coverage to continue.

Prepaid health plan   A contract between an insurer and a subscriber or a group of subscribers in which specific health benefits are provided in return for the payment of periodic premiums; an example is BlueCross–BlueShield.

Preventive medicine   The branch of medicine aimed at preventing disease and promoting health in individuals, communities, and specific populations. Its goal is to protect, promote, and maintain health while preventing disease, disability, and death.

Primary care provider   A health care provider who acts as the first contact and primary point of continuing care for patients; examples include physicians, nurse practitioners, physician assistants, registered nurses, and pharmacists.

Privacy officer   As required under HIPAA, an individual in any facility that deals with private health information, who must maintain the security of all electronic medical records.

Processing   Collection and manipulation of data to provide meaningful information.

Professional distance   The amount of physical or social interaction that is considered appropriate between a professional and the people he or she serves.

Professionalism   The skill, good judgment, and polite behavior that is expected from a person who is trained to do a job well.

Programs   Collections of instructions that perform specific tasks when executed by computers; programs are required by computers in order to function.

Prospective utilization review   A review or authorization for elective procedures or services before they are rendered.

Prostate-specific antigen (PSA)   A glycoprotein enzyme secreted by the epithelial cells of the prostate gland that functions to liquefy semen, allowing sperm to swim freely; it is often elevated in the presence of prostate cancer or other prostate disorders.

Protected health information   Any information about an individual's health status, provision of health care, or payment for health care that is created or collected by a "covered entity," or a business associate of a covered entity.

Protocols   Guidelines for medical treatments, methods used in clinical trials or medical research studies, or rules followed by health care providers.

Protozoa   Simple microorganisms containing one cell, or sometimes no cells, found in moist soil or water; they usually act as parasites.

Prudent layperson standard   A requirement for a non-medical person of average knowledge to assist an injured person in order to avoid further harm or damage.

Psychiatric hospitals   Institutions that care for and treat patients affected with acute or chronic mental illnesses, in both inpatient and outpatient capacities.

Psychophysiologic   Pertaining to physical symptoms, usually controlled by the autonomic nervous system, with emotional origins and involving a single organ system; also known as psychosomatic.

Qualified Health Plans   Insurance plans certified by the Health Insurance Marketplace that provide essential health benefits, follow established limits on cost-sharing, and meet other requirements.

Quality   The degree to which health services for individuals and populations increase the likelihood of desired health outcomes and are consistent with current professional knowledge.

Quality assessment   The measurement of quality against an established standard.

Quality assurance   The process of institutionalizing quality through ongoing assessment and using the results of assessment for continuous quality improvement.

Quality control   A program that monitors all phases of business activities to ensure high quality.

Quality improvement   Improving or preserving quality of care while decreasing costs.

Quality improvement organizations   Private and usually non-profit organizations that assess whether care is provided and if it is necessary and reasonable, focusing on Medicaid and Medicare; they are usually run by physicians and other health care professionals.

Quality of care   The level of a patient's treatment in relationship to the best possible outcome, lowest possible costs, and overall satisfaction; it involves quality assurance, quality control, and continued quality improvement.

Quantitative method   The procedure used as part of quantitative research, the systematic investigation of observable phenomena, using statistical, mathematical, or computational techniques.

Radiopharmaceuticals   Radioactive pharmaceuticals, nuclides, or other chemicals used for diagnostic purposes, or for radiation therapy.

Reciprocity   The recognition by one jurisdiction, such as a state, of the validity of certificates and licenses issued by other jurisdictions.

Recissions   The "unmaking" of contracts between parties with the goal of bringing them, as much as possible, back to the positions they held prior to entering into the contracts.

Records management system The professional practice of managing the records of an organization throughout their life cycle, from the time they are created to their eventual disposal; also called records and information management.

Refugees People who are outside their country of citizenship because of fear of persecution and who are unable to obtain sanctuary from their home country; also people who do not have a nationality.

Registered nurses Graduate nurses who are registered and licensed to practice by a state board or other state authority.

Rehabilitation hospital An institution that specializes in providing restorative services to rehabilitate chronically ill and disabled individuals to their maximum level of functioning.

Religious Freedom Restoration Act of 1993 The Act that ensures religious freedom protection; as in U.S. Supreme Court cases concerning "Hobby Lobby" and others, where it was ruled that these businesses did not have to provide contraception as part of employee health care programs, based on religious beliefs of the company owners.

Reservoir A person, other living creature, or structure that is susceptible to the growth of pathogens.

Residency The period during which a physician receives specialized clinical training, which is required for board certification in medical or surgical specialties.

Res ipsa loquitur Literally, "the thing speaks for itself"; a situation that is so obviously negligent that no expert witnesses need be called. Also known as the doctrine of common knowledge.

Retail clinics Health clinics operated at retail sites such as pharmacies and supermarkets under consumer-friendly names such as Take Care®. They are staffed by nurse practitioners or physician assistants.

Retrospective utilization review A review of services after they have been rendered, usually based on medical charts.

Rickettsia A genus of rod-shaped gram-negative bacteria carried by parasites such as certain insects; examples of related diseases include typhus and Rocky Mountain spotted fever.

Rickettsiae More than one rickettsia.

Robotic surgery Also known as robot-assisted surgery or computer-assisted surgery; the use of automated systems to aid in surgical procedures. Either the surgeon uses direct telemanipulating instruments or the computer controls the manipulation of the surgical instruments.

Rotation A clinical assignment for medical students in a specific area of practice; clinical rotations may include internal medicine, general surgery, pediatrics, psychiatry, obstetrics, gynecology, and others.

Safety data sheet A listing of details concerning a hazardous chemical stored in a workplace; this includes trade and chemical names, chemical family, manufacturer, emergency, ingredient, physical data, fire and explosion data, and other information.

Salmonella A genus of rod-shaped gram-negative Enterobacteriaceae that is linked to typhoid fever, paratyphoid fever, and food poisoning.

Sanitization The reduction of microorganisms on a surface or object to a safer level.

Scarification Production in the skin of many superficial scratches or punctures, as for introduction of vaccine; formerly, this term meant "scarring."

Schistosoma A genus of blood flukes that may cause urinary, gastrointestinal, or liver disease; transmitted through fecal contamination of water and freshwater snails as intermediate hosts.

Schistosomiasis Also called bilharziasis or snail fever; a mostly tropical parasitic disease caused by larvae of various flatworms or blood flukes characterized as schistosomes.

Schizophrenia A mental disorder often characterized by abnormal social behavior and failure to recognize what is real; symptoms include altered thoughts, hallucinations, reduced social interaction, and lack of motivation.

Sedentary Characterized by sitting or resting for a great deal of time and having little to no regular exercise.

Seizures Changes in the electrical activity of the brain that may cause a wide range of symptoms, including violent convulsions, loss of muscular control, varying levels of consciousness, confusion, staring, and psychic symptoms.

Self-actualization The fulfillment of a person's own potential; this was defined by Abraham Maslow as the ultimate in his "hierarchy of needs" theorem.

Self-confidence The state of self-belief in one's own abilities, which aids in effective communications and interactions with others; it is demonstrated by calmness, smiling, and making eye contact when communicating.

Severe Acute Respiratory Syndrome (SARS) An infectious respiratory illness first reported in Asia, characterized by fever, dry cough, breathing difficulties, headache, and body aches; spread by contact or close contact with infected individuals, droplets, or body fluids. It ranges from mild illness to fatal.

Shock A medical emergency in which the organs and tissues do not receive adequate blood flow, potentially resulting serious damage or death.

Silicon nanotechnology A technique that uses microscopic pieces of silicon for blood filtering, as part of artificial kidney technology.

Skilled nursing facilities Institutions primarily engaged in providing skilled nursing care and related services for patients requiring medical or nursing care, or rehabilitation services.

Slander Oral defamation of character.

Sleeping sickness Also known as trypanosomiasis; an infection caused by Trypanosoma protozoa, passed to humans (in Africa only) through the bite of the tsetse fly; it leads to changes in mental processes or prolonged sleeping, and is fatal if not treated.

Smallpox An infection caused by the variola virus that has caused large epidemics worldwide, but today is relatively eradicated; primary symptoms include fever, chills, muscle aches, pus-filled papules, and skin scarring.

SOAP documentation Also known as SOAP notes, it is a method of documentation that contains subjective data, objective data, an assessment, and a plan; it is commonly used by providers of various health care areas.

Social Security Administration The federally run agency that administers social security, which consists of retirement, disability, and survivors' benefits.

Society A nation, community, or large group of people with certain goals, beliefs, or standards of living and conduct.

Socioeconomic Related to social and economic factors.

Soft skills Also called people skills; the things brought to a person's job that enhances performance, including integrity, dependability, respect, patients, good attitude, and ethics.

Software Computer programs containing sets of instructions that direct a computer's "hardware" to perform specific tasks or operations.

Somatostatin Growth hormone-inhibiting hormone (GHIH); a peptide hormone that regulates the endocrine system and affects neurotransmission and cell proliferation.

Specificity The quality or state of being specific, precise, explicit, clear, or detailed.

Spina bifida   A serious birth abnormality in which the spinal cord is malformed and lacks its normal protective skeletal and soft tissue coverings; it is linked to genetic conditions, insufficiency of folic acid, maternal diabetes, and prenatal exposure to certain anticonvulsant drugs.

Spirilla   Spiral-shaped bacteria.

Spores   Resistant forms of certain bacterial species.

Sporicidal   Able to kill spores.

Spreadsheet   An interactive computer application for organization, analysis, and storage of data in the form of tables, with rows and columns; a spreadsheet simulates a paper accounting worksheet.

Sputum   Thick mucus produced in the lungs and related airways.

Staphylococci   Non-motile sphere-shaped gram-positive bacteria capable of causing many types of infections, including impetigo, pneumonia, and septicemia.

State-based marketplaces   Also called state health insurance marketplaces; they are state-run exchanges where people can purchase health insurance coverage.

Stem cells   Cells that have the potential to develop into many different or specialized cell types; often used to replace damaged or injured cells in the treatment of disease.

Sterile field   An area that is free of microorganisms, which is used as a work area during surgery.

Sterilization   Elimination of all living microorganisms.

Stillbirth   Also known as intrauterine fetal death; the death of a fetus at any time after the 20th week of pregnancy.

Streptococci   Sphere-shaped anaerobic bacteria that occur in pairs or chains; an example of a related disease is strep throat.

Stress   A state of mental or emotional strain or tension resulting from adverse or very demanding circumstances.

Stunted   Shortened or retarded, commonly affecting growth.

Subjective data   The information in a medical record or SOAP documentation provided by the patient, which includes routine information, past medical or personal history, family history, and chief complaint.

Subpoena   A legal document requiring the recipient to appear as a witness in court or to give a deposition.

Subsidies   Amounts usually paid by a government to keep prices of products or services low, or to help businesses or organizations to continue to function.

Supplemental Security Income   A federal program that provides stipends to low-income individuals who are either elderly, blind, or disabled; it is administered by the Social Security Administration but funded by the U.S. treasury.

Surf   To explore the World Wide Web or Internet.

Surgical asepsis   Also called sterile technique; the elimination of all microorganisms from working areas or objects.

Surgical errors   Mistakes during surgery that may result in patient harm or even death; the most common surgical errors include leaving objects inside patients, performing incorrect procedures, and operating on the wrong side of the body.

Susceptible host   An individual who has little to no immunity against infection by a certain microorganism.

Swedish massage   A system of therapeutic massage and exercise for the muscles and joints; it was developed in Sweden in the 19th century; it is generally performed in the direction of the heart, for relaxation, relief of muscular tension, and to improve circulation and range of motion.

Symptomatology   The branch of medicine dealing with symptoms of disease.

Synovial fluid   A thick liquid found in the body's joints, bursae (joint sacs), and tendon sheaths.

Taboos   Negative traditions, objects, or behaviors that are thought to harm society and are therefore prohibited, restricted, or considered forbidden.

Targeted drug therapy   One of the major areas of pharmacotherapy for cancer, along with hormonal therapy and cytotoxic chemotherapy. Targeted drug therapy blocks the growth of cancer cells by interfering with specific targeted molecules needed for carcinogenesis and tumor grown, instead of interfering with all rapidly dividing cells.

Teaching hospital   An institution with an approved residency program for physicians.

Teamwork   Cooperation between individuals, which involves assisting each other, increasing patient satisfaction and job satisfaction, and increasing the likelihood of achieving the ultimate goal of excellent patient care.

Telemedicine   The provision of consultant services by off-site health care professionals to local professionals, using various methods of telecommunication such as videoconferencing.

Telemonitoring   The use of computer technology with the Internet or a phone line to monitor patient data between the patient's own home and a health care facility; it utilizes patient interaction, medication reminders, and wireless monitoring devices.

Telepharmacy   The delivery of pharmaceutical care via telecommunications to patients in locations where there is not direct contact with a pharmacist.

Telomeres   Protective caps on the ends of chromosomes that prevent DNA damage.

Teratogenic   Able to cause birth defects; examples of teratogenic substances (also called teratogens) include radiation, certain metals, thalidomide, diethylstilbestrol, ethanol, and cocaine.

Tort   A civil wrong committed against a person or property, excluding breach of contract.

Total quality management   An approach to the improvement of provision of services based on the idea that most quality failures are caused by flaws in processes, and that quality can be improved by controlling these processes.

Tourniquets   Tight bands placed around an arm or leg to stop bleeding from an injury below it, or during venipuncture.

Toxoplasmosis   A common infection with the protozoan intracellular parasite Toxoplasma gondii. The acquired form is characterized by rash, lymphadenopathy, fever, malaise, central nervous system disorders, myocarditis, and pneumonitis.

Trachoma   A chronic infectious disease of the eye caused by the bacterium *Chlamydia trachomatis*. It is characterized initially by inflammation, pain, photophobia, and lacrimation. It affects more than 40 million people worldwide.

Triage   The process of determining which patients require treatment more urgently than others.

TRICARE   A health care program of the U.S. Department of Defense Military Health System, which provides civilian health benefits for military personnel and retirees, and their dependents, including certain members of the Reserve Component; formerly known as CHAMPUS.

Trichomonas vaginitis   An infection caused by the protozoan Trichomonas vaginalis, with symptoms including burning, redness, itching, and discharge.

Trichuriasis   Infestation with the roundworm *Tricuris trichiura*. The condition is usually asymptomatic, but heavy infestation may cause abdominal pain, nausea, bloody diarrhea, and anemia. The worms may live 15 to 20 years. This condition affects over 700 million people worldwide.

Tuberculoid leprosy A chronic communicable disease seen in individuals with high resistance; it causes thickening of cutaneous nerves and painless, saucer-shaped skin lesions.

Tularemia A bacterial illness, caused by Francisella tularensis, which results in fever, rash, and greatly enlarged lymph nodes; it may be transmitted to humans through the bites of infected ticks or flies, as well as through contaminated food or water.

Typhoons Mature tropical cyclones developing in the Western Pacific Ocean.

Ultraviolet (UV) radiation Invisible light rays that may be used to kill microorganisms; also, the radiation emitted by the sun.

Uncompensated care Health care or services provided by hospitals or health care providers that are not reimbursed; this often occurs because of lack of insurance or inability to afford health care costs.

Underprivileged Lacking the standard of living and opportunities enjoyed by most people in a society.

Underwriting To sign and accept liability and guaranteeing payment in case loss or damage occurs; in insurance, this is provided by a large financial service provider such as a bank, insurer, or investment firm.

Universal coverage Health insurance coverage for all citizens.

Universal precautions Methods used to control infection, in which it should be assumed that all blood and most body fluids are infectious for certain pathogens (such as HIV and HBV); these methods are also used when dealing with broken skin and all mucous membranes.

Upcoding A fraudulent practice in which provider services are billed for higher CPT procedure codes than were actually performed, resulting in higher payments by Medicare or third-party payers.

Urgent care Health care that is not as severe as emergency department care, but is defined in relation to an illness, injury, or condition that is serious enough for a reasonable person to seek care right away.

Utilization The quantity of services used by patients, such as hospital days, physician visits, or prescriptions.

Utilization review A set of techniques used by or on behalf of purchasers of health care benefits to manage costs by influencing patient care decision-making through case-by-case assessments of appropriateness of care before it is provided.

Vector-borne transmission Indirect transfer of an infectious agent, occurring when a vector (such as an insect) bites an individual; an example of a related disease is malaria, transmitted to humans by mosquitos.

Vectors Carriers, such as animals or insects, that transfer infective agents from one host to another.

Vehicle transmission Also called vehicle-borne transmission; the indirect transfer of an infectious agent from a vehicle (fomite) that touches an individual or is ingested by the individual.

Veracity Truth-telling.

Viral hemorrhagic fevers Epidemic viral diseases carried by insects, such as Ebola virus disease, that cause fever, muscular pain, vomiting, diarrhea, internal and external hemorrhaging, and often death.

Virions Complete viral particles, consisting of DNA or RNA, surrounded by protein coats; they constitute the infective forms of viruses.

Viruses The smallest pathogenic agents, which can only live and grow inside living cells of other organisms; they consist of nucleic acid surrounded by a protein coat.

Wasted   Also called emaciated; it describes gradual deterioration, loss of strength and muscle mass, weakness, and sometimes loss of appetite.

Western medical paradigm   Also known as Western medicine; the management of pathology by studying disease, but ignoring energy and mind-related changes.

Word processing   Composing, editing, formatting, and printing of documents via the use of a computer and specially designed software.

Workers' compensation   A form of insurance providing wage replacement and medical benefits to employees injured during employment, in exchange for the employee giving up his or her right to sue the employer for negligence.

Xerophthalmia   A condition of dry, lusterless corneas and conjunctival areas, usually due to vitamin A deficiency; it is associated with night blindness.

Index

Page numbers in *italics* denote tables, those in **bold** denote figures.

9/11 terrorist attacks 259

abortion 38, 69–70
access to health care 4, 25–6, 410
accountability 175
Accountable Care Organizations (ACOs)
   36, 47
Accreditation Council for Occupational
   Therapy Education (ACOTE) 134
Accreditation Council on Optometric
   Education 136
Accreditation Council for Pharmacy
   Education 139
Accrediting Bureau of Health Education
   Schools 153
acting out, as defense mechanism *352*
acute care 13, 413, 414
acute disease 4
acute infective hepatitis (hepatitis A) 306,
   307, 308
addiction rehabilitation 20, *20*
Administration on Aging (AoA) 12, 198
administrative law 57
adolescents: alcohol consumption *250*;
   obesity in 242; smoking among *249*
adult day care 11
adult family care 19
adult foster care 18–19
Advance Payment ACO Model 47
advance practice nurses (APNs) 122
Advance Premium Tax Credit 42
advanced care directives 71
Advisory Committee for Women's Services
   192

aerobic bacteria 284
aerobic exercise 179
Aetna 49
Affordable Care Act *see* Patient Protection
   and Affordable Care Act (ACA)
Africa: HIV/AIDS 305; malaria 236;
   tuberculosis 235; *see also* sub-Saharan
   Africa
African Americans *see* blacks
age, and immunity 293
Agency for Health Care Policy and Research
   (AHCPR) 400
Agency for Healthcare Research and
   Quality (AHRQ) *108*, 393, 401
aging population 5, 10–11, 215, 412; *see
   also* elderly people
AIDS *see* HIV/AIDS
air pollution 214, 219
airborne transmission 291
Alaska, and Medicaid expansion 46
Alaska Natives 86, 191, *193*, 195, *201*
alcohol consumption 4, 24, 25, 26, 27, 202,
   247; adolescents *250*; effects of 250;
   Hispanics 194; moderate 243; Native
   Hawaiians 196; women 191
alcoholism/alcohol addiction 20, *20*, 26,
   202
alcohols, as antiseptics/disinfectants 296
alternative medicine 145
altruism 167
Alzheimer's disease 4, 11, 149, 191, 196,
   403
ambulatory care 257, 412
ambulatory centers 15–17

ambulatory surgical units/centers 15
amebic dysentery 287
American Association of Bioanalysts 154
American Association for Long-Term Care Insurance 18
American Association of Medical Assistants (AAMA) 67, 126
American Board of Medical Specialties 26–7, 121
American Board of Ophthalmology 138
American Board of Professional Psychology 149
American Certification for Healthcare Professionals (ACA) 156
American College of Preventive Medicine 26–7
American Dental Association 129, 131
American Dietetic Association 141–2
American Health Information Management Association (AHIMA) 382
American Heart Association 264
American Indians 37, 86, 191, *193*, 195, *201*
American Medical Association (AMA) 8, 59
American Medical Technologists (AMT) 126, 154, 156
American Optometric Association 136
American Osteopathic Association 120, 121
American Physical Therapy Association (APTA) 144
American Psychological Association (APA) 147
American Public Health Association 211
American Recovery and Reinvestment Act (ARRA) (2009) 66, 398, 401
American Red Cross 264, 266
American Registry for Diagnostic Medical Sonographers 152
American Registry of Radiologic Technologists (ARRT) 151
American Society for Clinical Pathology (ASCP) 153, 156
American Speech-Language-Hearing Association (ASHA) 139
amputation 19–20, 271
anaerobic bacteria 284
analytical studies 398
ancylostomiasis 238
anthrax 259, 291

antibiotics 4, 232; misuse/overuse 404; resistance to 26, 397, 404
antimicrobial resistance 231, 232
antiretroviral therapy 201, 305
antisepsis *295*, 296, 297
antiseptics *295*, 296, 297
anxiety disorders 247, 248, 417
apathy, as defense mechanism *352*
arbitration 62
Argentina, adolescent smokers *249*
Arizona, health insurance 50
ARRA *see* American Recovery and Reinvestment Act
arthritis 196
artifiial intelligence 368
ascariasis (roundworm) 237
ascaris lumbricoides **237**
Asian Americans *193*, 194–5, *201*, *204*, *224*, 414
assault and battery 58
assertiveness skills 345
assisted suicide 71–2
assisted-living facilities (ALFs) 19
Association of American Medical Colleges 6
ATHENA (expert system) 368
attention deficit hyperactivity disorder 248
attitude 166, 167
audiologists 138–9
autoclaves 298
automatic external defibrillators (AEDs) 165–6
autonomy, patient 67, 68, 168

baby boomers 11, 414
bacilli 284, **285**
bacteria 231, 284, **285**, 404
bacterial diseases 284
bacterial genetics 404
barrier precautions 318; *see also* personal protective equipment (PPE)
Basic Health Plans 42
BCG vaccine *235*
behavioral disorders 247
behavioral habits, as risk factors for disease 4, 24–5, 27, 202, 214, 241
belongingness 180, 338
beneficence 67
bioethics 67
biohazard labels 314, 315, 316

bioinformatics 369, 403–4
biomedical model of illness 218
biomedicine/biomedical research 68–9, 394, 402
biotechnology 398, 404
bioterror 258–9
bipolar disorder 247, 248
blacks (African Americans) 191, *193*, 195, 200, 201, *204*, 224, 414, 415
bladder cancer 411
bleach, household 298, 297
bleeding 273–5; arterial 274; internal 274–5; venous 274
Bloodborne Pathogens Standard 204; exposure incidents 313–14; labeling requirements 314; record-keeping 313, 314; universal precautions 311–12; written exposure control plan 312–14
BlueCross–BlueShield 87, 88, 92, 93
body language 339, 340, 341–3, 346
body mass index (BMI) 214, 220, 221, 243, 417
Body Substance Isolation (BSI) guidelines 311
botulinum toxin 259
brain death 72
brain-injured patients 15, 19–20
breast cancer 191, 192, 222, 243, 244, 403
breastfeeding 192, 214, 217, 219, 220, 224, 236
Britain, health system 94
bubonic plague 259
Budget Control Act (2011) 398
burnout 347
burns 271, **272**, 273
buruli ulcer 240

CAAHEP *see* Commission on Accreditation of Allied Health Education Programs
California, Medicaid expansion 47
Canada, health system 94
cancer 4, 202, 211, 213, 241, 243–5; in Black Americans 192; bladder 411; breast 191, 192, 222, 243, 244, 403; cervical 243, 244; colorectal 244; diagnostic tests 411; in the elderly 196; and genetics 403; liver 244; lung 213, 241, 244, 411; most common *244*; most prevalent cancer deaths *244*; in Native

Hawaiians and other Pacific Islanders 195; and obesity 222, 223, *245*, 415, 416; prostate 244, 411; risk factors for 244, *245*; screening 44, 245; smoking and 241, 244, 249; stomach *244*; therapies 245, 411
candida albicans 287
capitation 82, 88, 94
carbapenem-resistant Enterobacteriaceae 404
cardiac care units (CCUs) 16
cardiopulmonary resuscitation (CPR) 264
Cardiovascular Credentialing International (CCI) administration 152
cardiovascular disease 4, 20, 24, 211, 241, 242–3, 249; *see also* heart disease; hypertension; stroke
cardiovascular technologists and technicians 151–2
careers in health care profession *see* diagnostic divisions of the health care system; health care education; health care management; therapeutic divisions of the health care system
caring 62
caring competence 165, 167
carriers (of infectious agents) 289
case law 57
case-control studies 405
causation 396
Center for Medicare and Medicaid Innovation 43, 44, 45, 82
Center for Surgery and Public Health (Harvard University) 397
Centers for Disease Control and Prevention (CDC) 17, 24, 25, 212, 257, 397, 415
Centers for Medicare and Medicaid Services (CMS) 43, 87, 106, 386
Central Asia: alcohol consumption 250; cardiovascular disease 242; smoking 249
cerebrovascular disease 194, 414; *see also* stroke
Certficate of Clinical Competence in Audiology (CCC-a) 139
certification: clinical laboratory technologists 153–4; dietitians 141, 142; emergency medical technicians and paramedics 135, 136; health educators 157; massage therapists 146; medical

certification *continued*
    assistants 126; medical social workers
    149; pathologists 156; pathology
    assistants 156; pharmacy technicians
    141; phlebotomists 156; physician
    assistants 124; physicians 121;
    psychologists 148–9; radiologic
    technologists 150–1; respiratory
    therapists 134; school health educators
    158; surgical technologists 126
Certified Surgical Technologist (CST)
    credential 126
cervical cancer 243, 244
Chagas disease 239
chain of infection 288–93, **289**; causative
    agent 289; mode of transmission 290–2;
    portal of entry 292–3; portal of exit 290;
    reservoir 289; susceptible host 293
challenges facing health care systems: access
    to health care 23–4; habits and social
    conditions 24–5; lifestyle choices 26;
    maintaining quality of care 25; public
    health issues 25–6
CHAMPUS (Civilian Health and Medical
    Program of the Uniformed Services) 18,
    82, *see also* TRICARE
CHAMPVA (Civilian Health and Medical
    Program of the Department of Veterans
    Affairs) 85
charting 62
CHEDDAR format 381
chemical burns 273
chemical hazards and safety 322–4
chemical safety data sheets 322, 422–6
chemotherapy 295, 328
child/infant mortality 5, 26, 215, 220
children 21, 190–1; communicable diseases
    in 231, 234, 236; dependency 190;
    developmental vulnerability 190; disabled
    190, *200*; hepatitis B vaccination 309,
    310; HIV-infected 305; malnutrition 215;
    mental disorders in 248; new morbidities
    affecting 190; nutritional needs 224; oral
    health care 190; overweight/obese 27,
    221, 224; programs of health care 190–1,
    211; stunted 224; underweight 214, 219,
    220; uninsured 191; *see also* adolescents
Children's Health Insurance Program
    (CHIP) 37–8, 39, 42, 46, 47, 87, 203

Children's Health Insurance Program
    Reauthorization Act (2009) 87
China: HIV/AIDS 305; tuberculosis 235
chiropractors 143
chlamydia 231
cholesterol 24, 26, 27, 214, 218, 225, 243
chronic illness/disease 4, 11, 25, 196, 202,
    215, 414
chronic obstructive pulmonary disease
    (COPD) 213, 219
CINHAL (Cumulative Index to Nursing and
    Allied Health Literature) 369
circulating tumor DNA 403
civil law 57, 58, 62
clinical e-mail 348
Clinical Laboratory Improvement Act
    (CLIA) 153
clinical laboratory technologists and
    technicians 152–4
clinical nurse specialists 122
clinical practice guidelines 104, 400, 401
clinical research 395–6; control groups 395;
    double-blind studies 395, 396;
    institutional review boards (IRBs) 395;
    overview of advances due to 395;
    participants 395; peer-review committees
    395; subject bias in 395
Clostridium difficile 404
clothing: as form of communication 342;
    see also dress codes; personal protective
    equipment
co-payments 36, 92
CoARC (Committee on Accreditation for
    Respiratory Care) 134
cocaine use 24
cocci 284, **285**
coccobacilli 284
codes of ethics 67
cognitive impairment 18
cohort studies 398, 405
colorectal cancer 244
Commission on Accreditation of Allied
    Health Education Programs (CAAHEP)
    126, 152, 153
Committee on Accreditation for Respiratory
    Care (CoARC) 134
communicable disease (infectious disease) 4,
    211, 216, 230, 231–41; deaths 231, 232,
    233, 234; and disability 231; emerging

195; methods of controlling *233*; process 288; transmission of 231

communication 62, 167–8, 169, 172–3, 337–57; barriers to 349–50; dealing with conflict 353; defense mechanisms 351, *352–3*; feedback 340; five Cs of 340; interprofessional 347; methods of 347–9; negative 346–7; non-verbal (body language) 339, 340, 341–3, 346; and patient needs 339; positive 346; process 339–40; skills improvement 343–5; therapeutic 345–7; types of 340–3; verbal 340, 341; written 350–1

communities, disease prevention and health promotion in 211, 212

community health services: for children 191; for the elderly 413

community quality collaboratives *108*

community residential care 19

comparative effectiveness research 401

compartmentalization, as defense mechanism *352*

compensation, as defense mechanism *352*

competence 62; caring 165, 167; culturally competent care 193, 414

complementary and alternative medicine 145

complex humanitarian emergency (CHE) 259

comprehension (understanding), patient and personal 168, 345

compromised host 293

computed (axial) tomography (CT) 6, 36, 150, 366, 369

computer viruses 348, 371

computers in health care 348, 362–71; benefits of *363*; computer security concerns 358, 371; diagnostic imaging 367–70; electronic medical records (EMRs) 44, 348, 365; information management 363–4; patient monitoring 362–3; research 369; spreadsheets 365; telemedicine 123, 370; telepharmacy 370; treatment 368–9; types used in 359, **360**, **361**, 361

concurrent utilization review, managed health care 92

Conestoga Wood Specialties case 41

confidentiality 59, 65, 66, 168, 349, 381, 382, 401

conflict, dealing with 353

Congressional Budget Office 36

consent: expressed 62; implied 62; informed 61–2, 394, 401; obtaining, in emergency situations 263; for use/release of medical records 381

Consolidated Omnibus Budget Reconciliation Act of 1985 (COBRA) 86

constitutional law 57

constructive input/criticism 110, 170

Consumer-Patient Radiation Health and Safety Act 130

contact transmission 290, *291*

continuing care communities 18–19

continuing education 170, 410

continuous quality improvement 106

contraception 41, 44, 192

contract law 59–61; breach of contract 60; contractual capacity 60; expressed contracts 60, 61; implied contracts 60, 61; and informed consent 61–2; and termination of treatment 61

control groups, clinical research 395

cost-efficiency (effectiveness) 104

costs *see* health care costs

Council on Academic Accreditation 139

Council on Social Work Education 149

CPR (cardiopulmonary resuscitation) 264

creosols 296

criminal law 57–8

critical care nurses 122

critical pathways 104

critical thinking 170–1

Cubans 194

cultural diversity, respect for 168, 172–3, 193

cultural relativism 217

culturally competent care 193, 414

culture and health 217–20; health behaviors 219; health beliefs and practices 217–19; health care providers *219*

Cumulative Index to Nursing and Allied Health Literature (CINAHL) 369

customer satisfaction 107, 109–10; methods to provide better *110*; *see also* patient satisfaction

customer service 100–15

customers: external 100; internal 100, 110

damages 59, 62

Data Services Hub 39

death and dying: alcohol-related 250; communicable diseases 231, 232, *233*, 234; determination of death 67; ethical issues 71; leading causes of 4, 20, 213, 219, 242–3, 246; legal death 73; medical error and 102; smoking-related 249; stages of grief 71; *see also* mortality rates

deductibles 36

defamation of character 59

defense mechanisms 351, *352–3*

defensive medicine 9

defibrillators 265–6

degenerative diseases 4, 11

dementia 196; *see also* Alzheimer's disease

denial, as defense mechanism *352*

Dental Admissions Test (DAT) 129

dental assistants 132–3

Dental Assisting National Board 133

dental hygienists 130–2

dentists 127–30

Department of Agriculture, Supplemental Food Program for Women, Infants, and Children 191

Department of Defense 42

Department of Education 191

Department of Health and Human Services (DHHS) 57, 82, 86, 198, 400

Department of Veterans Affairs 203, 397

depersonalization, as defense mechanism *352*

depression 243, 247, 248, 417

dereliction 59

descriptive studies 398

diabetes mellitus 4, 202, 215, 219, 246–7, 397, 414, 416; in Black Americans 194; complications 246, 247; deaths from 246; emergencies 268; in Asian Americans 194; in Native American women 191; in Native Hawaiians and other Pacific Islanders 195–6; and overweight/obesity 218, 222, 223, 246; screening 211; and smoking 249; type 1 246; type 2 218, 222, 246, 415, 418

diagnostic divisions of the health care system: cardiovascular technologists and technicians 151–2; clinical laboratory technologists and technicians 152–4; pathologists 156; pathology assistants 156; phlebotomists 154–6; radiologic technologists 150–1; radiologists 150

diagnostic errors 63, 102

diagnostic imaging 6, 36, 150, 365–8, 379

diagnostic tests: for cancer 411; health insurer denials for 105

diarrheal diseases 219, 231, 232, 236–7, 404

dietitians 141–3

digital X-Rays 366

diplococci 284

diptheria 231

direct cause 59

disability 190, 198, 199–200, 202, 215; and communicable diseases 231, *241*; levels of *200*; mental disorders contribution to 202, 247, 248; and non-communicable diseases *241*; physical 202; social 202

disability-adjusted life years (DALYs) 213, 214, 231

disaster preparedness plans 259–61

disaster tags 258

disasters 258; man-made 258–9, *260*; natural 258, 259, *260*, 261–2

disciplinary research 396

discrimination, as barrier to communication 350

disease 216; culture and perceptions of 218

disinfectants/disinfection *295*, 295, 296, 297, 299, 312

disposable gloves 296

dissociation, as defense mechanism *352*

distress 176

DNA research 403

do-not-rescitate (DNR) orders 73

doctors of osteopathic medicine (DOs) 120, 121, 150

domestic violence 25, 192, 203

domiciliary care 19

Domiciliary Care for Homeless Veterans Program 203

double-blind studies 395, 396

dress codes 175, 180

drug testing/trials 395

drug therapy *see* medication

drug use/addiction 20, *20*, 24, 25, 26, 214, 247

drug utilization review, managed health care 92

dry heat sterilization *295*, 298

dual-eligibles 43

durable power of attorney 71

duty 59

duty of care 64

e-mail communications 348

Early Periodic Screening, Diagnosis, and Treatment program 191

East Asia: cancer 243; cardiovascular disease 242–3; communicable diseases *233*; diabetes deaths *246*; smoking 249

Eastern Europe: alcohol use disorders 250; cardiovascular disease 242

Ebola virus 25–6, 102, 216, 230, 259

echocardiography 151

ecological perspective of health behaviors 220

education: and alcohol consumption 250; health 25, 215; level of 24, 203, 249

Educational Resources Information Center (ERIC) 369

efficacy research 400

efficiency 39, 104

EKG technicians 151

elder abuse 198

elder abuse forensic centers 198

elderly people 196–9, 410, 413, 414; old-old population 413; young-old population 413; *see also* aging population

elderly support ratio 215

electrical impedance tomography (EIT) 366

electromagnetic radiation 328

electronic medical records (EMRs) 44, 348, 365, 378, 381–2, *383*, 384

elephantiasis (filariasis) 238

emergencies 256–62; emergency and urgent care 257–8; liability in 63, 264; natural and man-made disasters 258–61; triage process 257, 258; *see also* emergency procedures

emergency departments 14, 23

Emergency Medical Services (EMS) 263

emergency medical technicians (EMTs) 135, 136

Emergency Medical Treatment & Labor Act (1986) 257

emergency procedures 263–75; automatic external defibrillators (AEDs) 265–6; bleeding 273–5; burns 271, **272**, 273; cardiopulmonary resuscitation (CPR) 264; diabetic emergencies 268; fainting 268–9; first aid 266–7; fractures 269, *270*; hyperthermia 275; hypothermia 275; seizures 267; shock 267–8; sprains 270; strains 271; wounds 271

emergency severity index (ESI) 257

emergent patients 258

emerging infectious diseases 295

empathy 173, 344

employer organizations *108*

Employer Shared Responsibility Payment 41, 44

employers *108*; and health insurance coverage 36, 37–8, 40, 41, 43, 44, 47, 50, 86, 87, 88–90; maintenance of employee medical records 384

Employment Retirement Income Security Act (ERISA) 86

end-of-life issues 71–2

enthusiasm, professional 174

environmental barriers to communication 349

environmental factors, and risk of disease/illness 4, 27, 214

Environmental Protection Agency (EPA) 315

epidemiology 212, 398–7, 404; experimental studies 398; observational studies 398, 399; qualitative methods in 399; quantitative methods in 398–9

epidermal growth factor receptor 411

equitability 104

ergonomics 325–7

Essential Health Benefits 44, *45*, 47

esteem needs 180, 338–9

ethanol 296

ethical issues 56, 66–73; abortion 69–70; biomedical concerns 68–9; codes of ethics 67; death and dying 71; end-of-life issues 71–2; and global health 216; health care rationing 70; organ transplantation 70; patient's rights and responsibilities 68; professional ethics 68; in research 395, 398, 401–2; stem-cell research 69; values 66, 67

ethnic minorities 191, 193–4, 203, 414; *see also* Alaska Natives; American Indians; Asian Americans; blacks; Hispanics; Latinos; Native Hawaiians and other Pacific Islanders
ethyl alcohols 297
ethylene oxide 298
Europe: alcohol consumption 250; cardiovascular disease 242; communicable diseases 233; female smokers 249; iodine deficiency 221; mental health costs 247; obesity 223, 224; *see also* Eastern Europe
eustress 175–6
euthanasia 71–2
examination gloves 296
executive branch of government 57
experimental medicine (biomedical research) 394, 402
expert systems 368
exposure control plan 312–14
external customers 100
eye contact 341, 346
eyewash stations 323, 324

facial expressions, and communication 341
facultative bacteria 284
failure mode and effects analysis 102
failure to diagnose 63
fainting 268–9
fat intake 202, 223, 225, 243
fax transmission 348
Federal Employees' Compensation Act (FECA) program 89
Federal Employment Liability Act (FELA) 89
Federal Poverty Level (FPL) 37, 42, 44, 45, 84, 193
federal workers' compensation programs 89, 90
Federally-Facilitated Marketplace 48
Federation of State Massage Therapy Boards (FSMTB) 145, 146
fee-for-service (indemnity) plans/payments 82, 88, 414
feedback: about feedback 340; negative (closed) styles of 340; patient 345; positive (open) styles of 340
fertility rates 215

fetal alcohol syndrome 250
fiber optics 368
fidelity 67
filariasis 238
financing and payment for services 81–99; government-funding 82–7; private-funding 87–94; reimbursement 82; *see also* health insurance
fire extinguishers 319, **320**
fire safety and emergency plan 318–21; R-A-C-E procedure 321
first aid 266–7
Florida, and Medicaid 47
fluoroscopy 150
folk illnesses 218
fomites 289
food, processed/fast 222, 223, 416
food cultures 222–3
Food and Drug Administration 41, 192, 328, 402
fractures 269, *270*
France, health system 94
fraud 9, 59
friendliness 344
fungi 231, 287

gas sterilization *295*, 298
gastroenteritis 287
GEMS (expert system) 368
gene therapy 6, 369
general anesthesia 63
general care units (GCUs) 14
general hospitals 13–14
generic drugs 36
genetic risk factors 4, 29, 403
genomics 404
genuineness 345
Georgia, and Medicaid 46
geriatrics 410, 414
GIDEON (expert system) 368
global health issues 210–29; communicable diseases 230, 231–41; culture and health 217–20; ethical and human rights concerns 216; health and education 215; life expectancy 213–14; non-communicable diseases 230, 241–50; nutrition 220–5; obesity 221–4; population growth and aging 215; poverty and the economy 215; risk

factors for disease 214; smallpox eradication 212; universal health coverage 216–17

gloves 296, 312, 318; disposable 296; latex 325; utility 296

gonorrhea 284, 404

Good Samaritan laws 63, 263

government-sponsored health services research 397

grooming 341

gross domestic product (GDP): effects of alcohol use on 250; health care costs share of 39

habits *see* behavioral habits

hand gestures 342

hand hygiene 293–4, 312

Hansen's disease (leprosy) 239–40

hard skills 166

hazard labels 314, 315

hazardous waste disposal 316, **317**; double-bagging technique 316; personal protective equipment 316

hazardous waste management 315–16

Health Administration Center 85

health behaviors 219–20, 241; ecological perspective 220; *see also* behavioral habits

health beliefs and practices 217–19

health calculators 368

health care administrators 157

health care costs 5, 9, 37–8, 39, 40, 215; *see also* National Health Expenditure

health care education 157–8

Health Care and Education Reconciliation Act (2010) 39

Health Care for the Homeless program 203

health care industry 5

health care management 157

health care rationing 70

health care reform 35–6, 37–8, 410

health care services 12–22; ambulatory centers 15–17; financing and payment for *see* financing and payment for services; home health care 17–18, 83, 412, 413; hospice care 21–2, 413; hospitals 13–14; long-term care facilities 18–19, 197–6, 413, 414; mental health services 13, 20–1, 248, 413; overutilization of 104, 106, 10, 401; post-acute brain injury

facilities 15; provider-induced demand 93; quality of *see* quality; rehabilitation hospitals 19–20, 413; reimbursement for 81; research *see* health services/systems research; underutilization of 104, 106, 401; utilization of 93

health care students, scholarships and loan repayments for 43, 44

health education 25, 215

health educators 157

health exchanges 37–8, 42, 43, 44, 46, 47

health information technicians 157

Health Information Technology for Economic and Clinical Health (HITECH) Act 66

health insurance 4, 5, 81, 216–17, 410; adult children (under 26) 44, 47, *48*; cancelations *48*, 88; contraception-related coverage 42, 192; cost of premiums 43, 47, *48*, 50; dual-eligibles 43; employers and 36, 37–8, 40, 41, 43, 44, 47, 50, 86, 87, 88–90; Essential Health Benefits 44, *45*; exemptions 37–8; funding, distribution of **9**; health exchanges 37–8, 42, 43, 44, 46, 47; indemnity (fee-for-service) 82, 88, 414; individual mandate 40, 44; lifetime limit 410; managed care 91–3; and pre-existing conditions 44, 201; premium and cost-sharing subsidies 37–8, 40, 41, 42, 43, 46; prepaid 88–9; shared responsibility 42, 44; workers' compensation 89–90; *see also* Medicaid; Medicare; privately funded health care; uninsured people

Health Insurance Marketplace 42

Health Insurance Portability and Accountability Act (HIPAA) (1996) 66, 371, 378, 384–6; complaint form 427; notice of privacy practices 384–5; security rule 385

health insurance reviewers 104–5; denials for diagnostic tests 105; preauthorization of procedures 105

health literacy 414

Health Maintenance Organization Assistance Act (1973) 91

health maintenance organizations (HMOs) 86, 87, 88–9, 91–2

health outcomes: and patient–caregiver interactions 102; *see also* outcomes research
health of professionals 178–80
health promotion 211, 212
Health Resources and Services Administration (HRSA) 195, 205
health services/systems research 396–7, 399–400, 404
health and wellness programs 19
health-adjusted life expectancy 213
HealthCare.gov 39, 40–1, 47
Healthy People 2020 27, 28
hearing impairment 11, 196, 199, 350
heart disease 4, 25, 143, 202, 213, 218, 219, 241, 242, 243; and alcohol consumption 250; in Black Americans 194; and diabetes 246, 247; in the elderly 196; and overweight/obesity 24, 223, 415, 416; women and 191, 192
heat stroke 275
hematuria 411
hepatitis 241, 287; hepatitis A (HAV) 306, *307*, 308, 311; hepatitis B (HBV) *286*, 306, *306*, 308–10, 311, 312, 313, 314; hepatitis C (HCV) 306, *307*, 308, 310, 314; hepatitis D (HDV) *307*, 310; hepatitis E (HEV) *308*, 310–11; hepatitis G (HGV) *308*, 311
heredity 23, 293, 369
high-deductible health plans 91
high-fasting plasma glucose 214
hip fracture 11, 196, 368
HIPAA *see* Health Insurance Portability and Accountability Act
Hispanics 193–4, 201, *204*, 224
histoplasmosis 287
histotechnicians 154
HIV/AIDS 25, 200–1, 204, 211, 216, 218, 219, 220, 230, 231, 232, 235, 304–6, 312, 314, 397; antiretroviral therapy 201, 305; methods of transmission 305; in Native Americans 195; numbers affected 305, 306; prevention efforts 305–6; and tuberculosis 235; in women 191, 201
Hobby Lobby case 41
holistic health care 18
home health agencies 17

home health aids 5
home health care 17–18, 83, 412, 413
home remedies 218, 219
homeless 202–3
Homeless Chronically Mentally Ill Veterans program 203
homeostasis 338
homophobia 201
hookworm disease 238
hospice care 21–2, 83, 413
Hospital Readmissions Reduction Program (HRRP) 36, 39, 44
hospital-acquired (nosocomial) infections 262, 283, 293, 404
hospitals 13–14; accreditation 13; bed occupancy rate 15; general 13–14; home health departments 17; psychiatric 13, 413; registered 13, *14*; rehabilitation 19–20, 413; teaching 13
"hot" and "cold", theories of 218
HRSA (Health Resources and Services Administration) 195, 205
human factors 103
Human Genome Project 369, 394
human papillomavirus (HPV) 192, 244
human rights 216
Humana 49
humor, as defense mechanism 351
hygiene 4, 211, 219; hand 293–4, 312; personal 175, 180
hyperglycemia 268
hyperlipidemia 222
hypertension 24, 26, 195, 196, 211, 214, 222, 242, 243, 414, 417
hyperthermia 275
hypoglycemia 268
hypothermia 275

IHI (Institute for Healthcare Improvement) *108*
illegal/undocumented immigrants 37, 42, 45, 204–5
Illinois, health insurance 50
illness 218; biomedical model of 218; culture and perceptions about 217, 218–19
immigrants, illegal/undocumented 37, 42, 45, 204–5
immigration 25
immunity 4; age and 293

immunization 25, 26, 44, 191, 211, 215, 232, 293; *see also* vaccination
immunotherapy 245
income, and Medicaid eligibility 84
indemnity (fee-for-service) plans 82, 88, 414
India, tuberculosis 235
Indian Health Care Improvement Act 195
Indian Health Service 42, 86, 195
individual responsibility for health 26
Individuals with Disabilities Education Act 191
Indonesia: adolescent smokers *249*; tuberculosis 235
infant/child mortality 5, 26, 215, 220
infection control 283–302; antiseptics/antisepsis 295, 296, 297; chain of infection 288–93; classification of microorganisms 284–7; disinfectants/disinfection *295*, 295, 296, 297, 299; hand hygiene 293–4; infectious disease process 288; medical asepsis 299; microorganism control *295*, 294–5, *295*; personal protective equipment (PPE) 295–6; sanitization 297, 299; sterilization *295*, 296, 298, 299; surgical asepsis 299
infectious disease *see* communicable disease
influenza 231, 234
influenza H1N1 (swine flu) 25
influenza H5N1 (bird flu) 25
influenza H7N9 25
information management 363–4
information sharing 102
information technology (IT) departments 362
informed consent 61–2, 395, 401
infrared technology 369
initiative 174
injuries 14, 16–17, 19–20, 25, 58, 63, 89, 195, 211; alcohol-related 250; mental illness-influenced 247; road 219, 232
inpatient hospital services 13
Institute for Healthcare Improvement (IHI) *108*
Institute for Healthcare Policy and Innovation (University of Michigan) 397
Institute of Medicine (IOM) 397, 401
institutional review boards (IRBs) 395
instrument nurses *see* surgical technologists

integrity 166, 174
intellectualization, as defense mechanism *352*
intensive care units (ICUs) 14
intentional torts 58–9
intermediate nursing care facilities 18
internal customers 100, 110
Internal Revenue Service (IRS) 39, 40, 41, 43
Internet 348, 371, 385; health care applications 40, 48
internship 120, 121, 138
interpersonal skills 344–5
invisible illness 202
iodine deficiency 221
IOM (Institute of Medicine) 397, 401
ioninzing radiation *295*, 328
IRBs (institutional review boards) 395
iron/iron deficiency 214, 221
irritable bowel syndrome 236
ischemic heart disease 213, 219, 223, 227, 241, 242
isopropanol 296
isopropyl 297
Italy, GDP and alcohol use 250

Jenner, Edward 212
Johnson, Lyndon B. 82
Joint Commission, The (TJC) 14, 64, 65
Joint Review Committee on Education in Radiologic Technology (JRCERT) 150, 151
judgment, professional 170–81
judicial branch of government 57, *108*
justice 67, 68

Kaiser Foundation Health Plan 88–9
Kaiser Permanente 88–9
keratomalacia 221
Kübler-Ross, Elisabeth 71

labeling, of hazardous materials 314, 315, 316
laboratory reports 379
laptop computers 359, 361, 362
laser surgery 6, 369
latex allergy 325
Latin America: cancer 243; communicable diseases *233*; diabetes deaths *246*

Latinos 193–4, 414; and health insurance 46, 193

law 57; classifications of 57–8; federal 57; state 57

lead/lead screening 191, 214

legal issues 56, 57–66; contract law 60–2; medical malpractice 59, 62–3; privacy 65–6; professional liability 63; provider's rights and responsibilities 65; *respondeat superior* (vicarious liability) 60; standard of care and duty of care 64; tort liability 58–9

legislative branch of government 57

leishmaniasis 239

leprosy 239–40

liability, professional 63

liability insurance 63

Liaison Council on Certification for the Surgical Technologist (LCCST) 126

Liason Committee on Medical Education (LCME) 120

licensed practical (vocational) nurses (LPNs) 122, 123

licensure: audiologists 139; cardiovascular technologists and technicians 152; clinical laboratory technologists and technicians 153, 154; dental hygienists 130, 131–2; dentists 129, 130; dietitians 141; massage therapists 145–6; medical social workers 149; nurses 123; occupational therapists 134; optometrists 137; pharmacists 139, 140; phlebotomists 155; physicians 121; radiologic technologists 150; rehabilitation counselors 150

life expectancy 4, 5, 10, *11*, 101, 191, 195, 213–14; at birth 213, 230; health-adjusted 213

life-sustaining treatments 71

lifestyle 4, 25, 26, 214, 222, 241, 293

listening skills 344, 346

liver cancer 244

living wills 71

long-term care 18–19, *49*, 197–8, 413, 414

love and belongingness 180, 338

lower respiratory infections 4, 219, 231, 232

lung cancer 213, 241, 244, 411

Lyme disease 292

macro quality 101

magnetic resonance imaging (MRI) 6, 36, 150, 366, 367

mainframe computers 359

malabsorption syndrome 236

maladaptations 218

malaria 211, 216, 217, 219, 220, 231, 232, 236, 287

malfeasance 59

malnutrition 210, 215, 220–1

mammography 4, 150, 245

man-made disasters 258–9, *260*

managed care health insurance 91–3; health maintenance organizations (HMOs) 86, 87, 88–9, 91–2; preferred provider organizations (PPOs) 93; utilization review 92, 107

marijuana use 24

Maslow, Abraham 180, 338–9

Massage and Bodywork Licensing Examination (MBLEx) 145–6

massage therapists 145–6

material safety data sheets (MSDS) 315

measles 230, 232

Medicaid 11, 13, 14, 18, 39, 43, 81, 82, 84, 85, 399; and adult foster care 19; children and 87, 190, 191; coverage gap 46; disabled people 198, 199; and the elderly 81, 196–7, 198; eligibility 84; enrollment and payouts *84*; expansion 37, 38, 39, 40, 41, 42, 44, 45–6, 46–7, *48*; and hospice care 22; and long-term care 18; spending 10, 36; and the uninsured 204; women and 192

medical asepsis 299

medical assistants *5*, 124, 126

medical coding 362

Medical College Admission Test 120

medical device manufacturers 394, 398, 402

medical doctors (MDs) 120, 121, 150

medical errors 101–2; methods to reduce deaths/adverse effects from 102

medical history 378

medical malpractice 59, 62–3, 384; lawsuits 9, 62

medical model of health care 9–10

medical records 362, 364, 377–90; charting by exception format 380; CHEDDAR format 381; chronological arrangement

379, 380; contents of 378–9; electronic (EMRs) 44, 348, 365, 378, 381–2, *383*, 385; guidelines for usage of 382; and HIPAA 378, 384–6; medical documentation 383–4; patient consent for use/release of 381; patients' rights regarding 385; personal health records 392–3; photocopying 349; privacy and confidentiality of 66, 349, 381; problem-oriented (POMR) 380; and research 384; SOAP documentation 380–1; source-oriented (SOMR) (conventional method) 379–80

medical schools 120

medical social workers 149

medical technologies 6, 7, 36, 410–11

medical writing 350–1, 382–3

medicals savings accounts (MSAs) 90–1; contributions 90; distributions 91

Medicare 6, 13, 14, 19, 42, 43, 47, 81, 82–3, 86, 198, 399; claim form (CMS-1500) 83; disabled people 198, 199; and home health care 17–18; and hospice care 22; Part A (Hospital Insurance) 83, 196; Part B (Medical Insurance) 83, 196; Part C (Medicare Advantage) 6, 43, 83, 196; Part D (Prescription Drug Plans) 83, 196; reimbursement 36, 39; spending 10, 36

Medicare Cost Plans 83

Medicare Medical Savings Account Plans 83

Medicare Modernization Act 83

Medicare Prescription Drug, Improvement, Modernization Act 91

Medicare Private Fee-For-Service Plans 83

Medicare Shared Savings Program 47

medication 383–4, 404; computers and administration/dispensing of 363, 370; errors 102; generic drugs 36; health risks 402

Medigap insurance 83

MEDLINE 369

mental disability 202

mental disorders 20–1, 191, 215, 241, 247–8

mental distress, infliction of 59

mental health costs 247

mental health services 13, 20–1, 248, 413

mental health system 21

meta-analysis research projects 400

Mexicans 194

micro quality 101

microorganisms 283–4; classification of 284–7

Middle East and North Africa: cardiovascular disease 243; communicable diseases *233*; diabetes deaths 246

Middle East Respiratory Syndrome-Cononavirus (MERS-CoV) 28

midwives 122

Migrant Health Program 205

migrant workers 204–5

military medical care *see* CHAMPVA; TRICARE

Millennium Development Goals 220

minerals *see* vitamins and minerals

minicomputers 359

Minnesota, health insurance 50

misfeasance 59

moist heat sterilization *295, 298*

molds 287

moral values 66

mortality rates 101; infant/child mortality 5, 26, 195, 220

Multistate Pharmacy Jurisprudence exams 140

My Healthy People application 28

nanomedicine 6

nanotechnology 6, 411

National Accrediting Agency for Clinical Laboratory Sciences (NAACLS) 153

National Alliance for Health Information Technology (NAHIT) 381

National Association of Boards of Pharmacy (NABP) 140

National Association of School Psychologists 147, 148

National Business Coalition on Health *108*

National Business group on Health *108*

National Center for Competency Testing (NCCT) 126, 156

National Center for Health Services Research and Health Care Technology 400

National Center for Health Statistics 24

National Certification Board of Therapeutic Massage & Bodywork (NCBTMB) 145, 146

National Commission on Certification of Physician Assistants (NCCPA) 124

National Committee for Quality Assurance (NCQA) *108*

National Council Licensure Examination (NCLEX-RN) 123

National Credentialing Agency for Laboratory Personnel 154

National Federation of Independent Business v. Sebelius 40, 41

National Health Expenditure (NHE) 10, 36–7

National Health Service Corps (NHSC) 43

National Health Service (NHS), Britain 94

National Healthcare Association (NHA) 126, 141

National Hospice and Palliative Care Organization 21–2

National Institutes of Health (NIH) *108,* 394, 396, 399, 401

National Library of Medicine 369

National Prevention, Health Promotion and Public Health Council 27

National Quality Forum (NQF) *108*

National Registry of Emergency Medical Technicians (NREMT) 135, 136

Nationally Certified School Psychologist (NCSP) designation 148–9

Native Americans *see* Alaska Natives; American Indians

Native Hawaiians and other Pacific Islanders *193*, 195–6, *201*

natural disasters 258, 259, *260*, 261–2

Nebraska, health insurance 450

needs, hierarchy of 180, 338–9

neglected tropical diseases (NTDs) 216, 237–41

negligence 59, 62, 384; four Ds of 59; *see also* medical malpractice

Neisseria gonorrhoeae 404

New Zealand, GDP and alcohol use 250

NIH *see* National Institutes of Health

non-communicable diseases 4, 211, 230, 241–50

non-English speakers 350

non-ionizing radiation *295*

non-verbal communication (body language) 339, 340, 341–3, 346

nonfeasance 59

North American Pharmacist Licensure Exam (NAPLEX) 140

nosocomial (hospital-acquired) infections 283, 293, 404

not-for-profit hospitals 13

notebook computers 359, 361

nuclear pharmacists 139

nurse practitioners 122

nurses 122–3

nutrition 4, 179, 202, 220–5; nutritional needs (during adulthood and old age 225; during infancy and childhood 224); and obesity 221–4; and pregnancy 224; undernutrition/malnutrition 210, 215, 220–1

nutritional status 293

nutritionists 141

Obama, Barack 38, 40, 53

obesity 28, 214, 219, 221–4, 243, 415–17; adolescent 242; in Asian Americans 194; childhood 28, 221, 224; and diabetes 218, 222, 223, 246; health outcomes linked to 24, 415, 416–17; legislation 417; in migrant workers 204–5; in Native Hawaiians and other Pacific Islanders 196; and susceptibility to illness 293; as treatable, reversible condition 417; vaccine research 403

observational studies in epidemiology 398, 399

obsessive-compulsive disorders 248

Occupational Safety and Health Act (1970) 303

Occupational Safety and Health Administration (OSHA) 68, 89, 127, 303–4, 384

Occupational Safety and Health Administration (OSHA) standards: chemical hazards and safety 322–4; employee responsibilities 328–9; ergonomics 325–7; fire safety and emergency plan 318–21; hazard communication 315–18; labeling requirements 314, 315; physical safety 324–5; radiation hazards 328; workplace violence 328; *see also* Bloodborne Pathogens Standard

occupational therapists 133–4

Odoreader 411

Office of Disease Prevention and Health
Promotion 29

Office of Elder Justice and Adult Protective
Services 198

Oklahoma, health insurance 50

old people *see* elderly people

Older Americans Act (1965) 198

onchocerciasis 239

online healthcare enrollments 40, 48

ontogeny 396

openness 345

operating room technicians 126

ophthalmologists 136, 138

optometrists 316–18

oral health care: in children 190; *see also*
dental assistants; dental hygienists;
dentists

organ transplantation 6, 70, 404

organizational cost control 93

osteoporosis 11, 13, 24, 192, 225, 269

out-of-network providers 93

outcomes research 400–11; comparative
effectiveness research 401

outpatient care 15–17, 412

overutilization of services 104, 106, 107,
401

overweight 24, 214, 221, 222, 223, 294,
416; *see also* obesity

oxygen hazards 319–20

palliative care 21–2

pandemics 25–6

panic disorder 247

Pap smears 4, 245

paramedics 135–6

parasitic infections 232

participating provider organizations *see*
preferred provider organizations (PPOs)

pathogens 283–4

pathologists 156

pathology assistants 156

patient advocacy 173

patient autonomy 67, 68, 168

patient care partnership 68

patient comprehension 168

patient education 102, 104

patient monitoring, using computer
technology 362–3

Patient Protection and Affordable Care Act
(ACA) 5, 27, 29, 35–53, 81–2, 82, 87,
190, 401, 410; advantages and
disadvantages of 47–50; cost of 46; goals
38, 39; health insurance (adult children
(under 26) 45, 48, *49*; cancelations *49*;
contraceptive coverage 42, 192; cost of
premiums 44, 48, *49*, 50; employer
provision 36, 37–8, 40, 41, 43, 44, 47,
50; Essential Health Benefits 44, *45*, 47;
health exchanges 37–8, 42, 43, 44, 45,
47; individual mandate 40, 44; and long-
term care *49*; minimum essential
coverage requirements 42; and pre-
existing conditions 44, 201; premium
and cost-sharing subsidies 37–8, 40, 41,
42, 43, 46, 86; preventive services 44, *49*;
shared responsibility provision 42, 44;
state Medicaid expansion 37, 37–8, 39,
40, 41, 42, 44, 45–6, 46–7, *48*); Hospital
Readmissions Reduction program
(HRRP) 36, 39, 44; implementation of
37–9, 44; legal challenges to 40–1;
payment reform 44; pharmaceutical fees
44; public support for/opposition to 46;
Supreme Court modifications 41

patient questionnaires, computerized 368

patient records *see* medical records

patient respect 67, 68, 168

patient satisfaction 107, 109–10, 400;
surveys 102, 107, 110, 403

patient self-governance 103

patient–caregiver interactions, and health
outcomes 102

Patient-Centered Outcomes Research
Institute (PCORI) 401

patient's rights and responsibilities 68

peer-review committees 395

Pennsylvania, health insurance 50

people skills (soft skills) 166

persistence, professional 171

personal computers 359, 361, 362

personal digital assistants (PDAs) 361

personal hygiene 175, 180

personal protective equipment (PPE) 295–6,
312, 313, 316, 318

personal space 342

personal well-being 400

pharmaceutical companies 394, 398, 402

pharmaceutical fees 45
pharmacists 139–40
pharmacoeconomics 140
pharmacotherapists 139
pharmacy informatics 140
Pharmacy Technician Certification Board (PTCB) 141
pharmacy technicians 140–1
phlebotomists 154–9
photocopying 348–9
phylogeny 396
physical examination forms 378–9
physical exercise 243, 417; and health care professionals 179; lack of 26, 202, 214, 222, 223
physical impairments to communication 349
physical safety, in the workplace 124–5
physical therapists and therapist assistants 5, 143–5
Physician Assistant National Certifying Exam (PANCE) 124
physician assistants 5, 123–4
physician orders 379
physicians 120–2
physiological needs 180, 338
Pioneer ACO Model 48
polio 211, 218
population growth 215
portal of entry 292–3
positron emission tomography (PET) 366
post-acute brain injury facilities 15
post-traumatic stress disorder 21, 248; in nurses 123
posture, as form of communication 342
poverty 25, 26, 196, 215, 220, *413*; Federal Poverty Level (FPL) 39, 43, 45, 46, 84, 193
pre-existing medical conditions 44, 104, 201
preauthorization of procedures 105
preferred provider organizations (PPOs) 93
pregnancy: alcohol consumption in 250; malaria and 236; and nutrition 224
prejudice, as barrier to communication 350
prenatal care 25, 26
prepaid health plans 88–9
prevention 4, 211, 212
preventive care services 44, *49*, 92
preventive medicine 26–7, 397, 402

primary care 8, 23
primary care physicians (PCPs) 122
primary care providers (PCPs) 91
privacy 65–6, 68, 168, 381, 382, 385, 401; invasion of 59
privately funded health care 36, 44, 47, 86, 87–93; BlueCross–BlueShield 87, 88, 92, 93; direct payments from patients 93–4; disabled people 199, 202; Kaiser Foundation Health Plan 88–9; managed care 91–3; medical savings accounts (MSAs) 90–1; self-insured plans 90; workers' compensation 89–90
problem solving, health care *171*
problem-oriented medical records (POMR) 380
procedural law 57
professional practice/professionalism 165–86; acceptance of constructive input 170; accountability 175; appearance and dress codes 175, 180; communication *see* communication; comprehension, patient and personal 168; continuing education 170, 410; cultural diversity, respect for 168, 172–3; empathy 173; enthusiasm 174; flexibility 173; good judgment 170–81; integrity and honesty 166, 174; persistence 171; personal health 178–80; personal hygiene 175, 180; professional distance 169; respect for patients 168; self-motivation 174; stress management 175–8; teamwork 171–82
Program of All-Inclusive Care for the Elderly (PACE) 198
progress notes 379
projection, as defense mechanism *352*
prospective utilization review, managed health care 92
prostate cancer 244, 411
prostate-specific antigen (PSA) levels 411
protozoa 287, **288**
provider's rights and responsibilities 65
prudent layperson standard 257
psychiatric hospitals 13, *413*
PsychINFO 369
psychologists 147–9
psychophysiologic malfunctions 218
public health 25–6, 210, 211–12
public health research 397, 404

Public Health Service, Office on Women's Health 191–2
PubMed 369
Puerto Ricans 194

Qualified Health Plans 43
qualitative research methods 399
quality: dimensions of 101–3, 104; macro 101; micro 101
quality assessment 101
quality assessment and performance improvement (QAPI) programs 106
quality assurance 103–5
quality of care 25, 39, 101, 104, 384; improvement of 106–7; maintenance of 104
quality control 103
quality improvement organizations 107, *108*
quality of life, health-related 103
quantitative research methods 398–9

radiation: ionizing *295*, 328; non-ionizing *295*, 328
radiation burns 273
radiation hazards 328
radio-pharmacists 139
radiologic technologists 150–1
radiologists 150
Rand Corporation Health Division 397
rationalization, as defense mechanism *352*
reaction formation, as defense mechanism *352*
recissions 88
recording-keeping *see* medical records
registered nurses (RNs) 122, 123
regression, as defense mechanism *352*
regulated medical waste 316
rehabilitation counselors 150
rehabilitation hospitals 19–20, 413
reimbursement for health care services 82, 384; capitation 82, 88, 94; fee-for-service payments 82, 88; through salaries 82
Religious Freedom Restoration Act (1993) 41
repression, as defense mechanism *353*
res ipsa loquitor 62
research 393–408; biomedical (experimental medicine) 394, 402; clinical *see* clinical research; computerized resources for 369;

conflicts of interest 402; disciplinary 396; epidemiological 398–9, 404; ethics 395, 398, 401–2; expenditures 398; future challenges 403–4; health services/systems *108*, 396–7, 399–400, 404; and medical record data 384; meta-analysis projects 400; outcomes 400–1; patient satisfaction 403; public health 397, 404; translational 394
residency (physicians) 120, 121, 138
resistance: antibiotic 26, 397, 404; antimicrobial 231, 232
respectfulness 168, 345
respiratory therapists and technicians 134–5
respondeat superior 60
retail clinics 16–17
retrospective utilization review, managed health care 92
rickettsial infections 231, 287
risk factors for disease 202, 214, 219, 241–2; *see also* behavioral habits; environmental factors; lifestyle
risk management 104
road injuries 219, 232
robotic surgery 6, 368–9
Roe v. Wade (1973) 70
root cause analysis, of medical errors 102
Russia, smoking in 249

safety 104
safety needs 180, 338
safety in the workplace *see* infection control; Occupational Safety and Health Administration (OSHA) standards
salaries *8*: cardiovascular technologists and technicians 152; chiropractors 143; clinical laboratory technologists and technicians 154; dental assistants 133; dental hygienists 132; dentists 130; dietitians 142; emergency medical technicians and paramedics 136; health care administrators 157; health educators 157; health information technicians 157; massage therapists 146; medical assistants 126; medical social workers 149; nurses 123; occupational therapists 134; ophthalmologists 138; pathologists 156; pathology assistants 156; pharmacists 140; pharmacy technicians

salaries *continued*
141; phlebotomists 156; physical
therapists and therapist assistants 144,
145; physician assistants 123; physicians
121; psychologists 149; radiologic
technologists 151; rehabilitation
counselors 150; reimbursement for health
care services through 82; respiratory
therapists and technicians 134, 135;
school health educators 158; surgical
technologists 126
saliva testing 411
salmonellosis 292
salt 223, 225, 243
sanitation 215, 219, 232, 236
sanitization 297, 299
sarcasm, as defense mechanism *353*
SARS (Severe Acute Respiratory Syndrome)
26, 216
scarification 218
schistosomiasis (snail fever) 217, 238
schizophrenia 247, 248
school health educators 157–8
screening programs 4, 44, 211, 245
scrubs 126
sedentary lifestyles 416
seizures 267
selective attention, as defense mechanism
353
self-actualization 180, 339
self-confidence 173
self-employed, health insurance 91, 410
self-motivation 174
senior centers 21
sensitivity to patient needs/situations 345
September 11, 202 terrorist attacks 259
serum hepatitis (hepatitis B) *286*, 306, *307*,
308–10
Severe Acute Respiratory Syndrome (SARS)
26, 216
sharps disposal 312
sharps injury log 314
shock 267–8
skilled nursing facilities 18
sleep 417; of health care professionals
179–80
Small Business Health Options program
(SHOP) 47
smallpox 259; eradication 212

smoking (tobacco use) 4, 24, 202, 214, 218,
219–20, 243, 249–50; adolescents *249*;
and cancer 241, 244, 249; cessation 27;
deaths related to 249; ethnic minorities
194, 196
Snyder Act (1921) 86
SOAP documentation 380–1
social conditions 25
social disability 202
Social Security Act 257; Title V (Maternal
and Child Health) 191
Social Security Administration 39
Social Security Disability Insurance (SSDI)
199, 201
society 217
Society of General Internal Medicine 397
socioeconomic status 4, 24, 222, 249; and
alcohol use 250
soft skills 166
somatostatin 403
source-oriented medical records (SOMR)
379–80
South Korea, GDP and alcohol use 250
South/Southeast Asia: adolescent alcohol
consumption *250*; communicable
diseases 231, *233*
specialization 6, 8
spirilla 284, **285**
spores 284, 287
sprains 270
spreadsheets 365
standard of care 64, 384
staphylococcus bacteria 404
state workers' compensation programs 89
State-Based Health Exchange Marketplace
39, 48
state-based marketplaces 39
statutory law 57
stem-cell research 69
sterile field creation 299
sterile gloves 296
sterilization *295*, 296, 298, 299; of water 297
stomach cancer *244*
strains 271
streptococci 284, 404
stress 293, 417; causes of 177; management
175–8
stroke 191, 192, 202, 213, 215, 219, 241,
242–3, 415

sub-Saharan Africa: cardiovascular disease 242; communicable diseases 231, *233*; HIV/AIDS 305

subcultures 217

subject bias in clinical research 395

sublimation, as defense mechanism 351, *353*

subnotebook personal computers 361

substance abuse 13, 25; *see also* alcohol use/addiction; drug use/addiction

Substance Abuse and Mental Health Services Administration 192

substantive law 57

sugar 222, 223, 225, 243

suicide 20, 195, 247, 248; assisted 71–2

supercomputers 359

Supplemental Security Income (SSI) 84, 199, 201

suppression, as defense mechanism 351, *353*

Supreme Court 57; modification of Affordable Care Act 41

surgery: laser 6, 369; robotic 6, 368–9; same-day 412

surgical asepsis 299

surgical errors 102

surgical scrubs 294, 299

surgical technologists 126

susceptible host 293

Swedish massage 145

system knowledge 396

tablet PCs 361

target knowledge 396

targeted drug therapy 6

tax credits 37–8, 42, 43

teaching hospitals 13

teamwork 171–82

Tech in Surgery-Certified (TS-c) credential 126

technological advancements 6, 9, 410–12

telecommunication 348

telemedicine 123, 370, 417

telemonitoring 362

telepharmacy 370–1

telephone skills 348

Temporary Assistance for Needy Families (TANF) 84

Tennessee, health insurance 50

termination of treatment 61

Texas, and Medicaid 46

therapeutic divisions of the health care system: audiologists 139–9; chiropractors 143; dental assistants 132–43; dental hygienists 130–2; dentists 127–30; dietitians 141–3; emergency medical technicians and paramedics 135–6; massage therapists 145–7; medical assistants 5, 124, 126; medical social workers 149; nurses 122–3; occupational therapists 133–4; ophthalmologists 136, 138; optometrists 136–8; pharmacists 139–40; pharmacy technicians 140–1; physical therapists and therapist assistants 5, 143–5; physician assistants 5, 123–4; physicians 120–2; psychologists 147–9; rehabilitation counselors 150; respiratory therapists and technicians 134–5; surgical technologists 126

TherapyEdge HIV 368

think tanks 397

tinea pedis (athlete's foot) 287

tobacco use *see* smoking

tone of voice 342

tort liability 58–9

torts 62; intentional 58–9; unintentional 58, 59

total quality management 106

touch, as form of communication 342

tourniquets 274

trachoma 239

transformation knowledge 396

transitional care units (TCUs) 14

translational research 394

trauma centers 14

traumatic brain injuries 15

treatment: appropriateness studies 400; computerized 368–9; outcomes research 400–1; testing 395

triage 257, 258

TRICARE (formerly CHAMPUS) 18, 82, 85

trichomonas vaginitis 287

trichuriasis 238

Trump, Donald 37

trypanosomiasis 239

tuberculosis 4, 25, 27, 195, 201, 205, 211, 216, 219, 220, 231, 232, 235; and HIV 235

tularemia 259

Turkey, adolescent smokers *249*

ultrasound (ultrasonography) 69, 366, **367**
ultraviolet (UV) radiation 298
uncompensated care 37
undernutrition 220–1
underutilization of services 104, 106, 401
underweight children 214, 219, 220
underwriting 88
undocumented/illegl immigrants 37, 42, 45, 204–5
undoing, as defense mechanism *353*
Uniform Commercial Code 60
uninsured people 46, 47, *49*, 82, 203–4, 410; children 191; direct payments for services 93–4; homeless 203; Latinos and Hispanics 46, 194; Native Americans 195; women 192
unintentional torts *58*, 59
United States Medical Licensing Examination (USMLE) 121
United States Nuclear Regulatory Commission 328
United States Public Health Service 397
UnitedHealthGroup 49
universal health coverage 216–17
university health services research *108*, 397
unsafe sex practices 24, 26, 219, 250
upcoding 9–10
urbanization 222–3
urgent care 257
urgent care centers 16–17, 257, 258
urgent patients 258
Utah, and Medicaid expansion 46
utility gloves 296
utilization of health care services 93; overutilization 104, 106, 107, 401; underutilization 104, 106, 401
utilization management 107
utilization reviews 101, 106, 107; managed health care 92, 107; protocols for 106

vaccination 4, 232; BCG 235; hepatitis A 306, 311; hepatitis B 309–10, 311, 313; smallpox 212; status 293; *see also* immunization
values 66, 67
vascular technology 151
vector-borne transmission *291*, 292

vectors for disease 231
vehicle transmission *290*, 292
veracity 67
veterans, homeless 203
Veterans' Administration 18, 43
Veterans' Disability Pensions 199
vicarious liability 60
violence 25, 191, 192, 203; and alcohol consumption 250; workplace 328
viral hemorrhagic fevers 259; *see also* Ebola virus
viral hepatitis *see* hepatitis
viruses 231, 284, 287
visual impairment 11, 196, 199
vitamins and minerals 221, 224, 225; calcium 225; iodine deficiency 221; iron/iron deficiency 214, 221; vitamin A deficiency 221; vitamin D 225; zinc deficiency 221

Washington, D. C., and Medicaid expansion 45, 47
water 4, 214, 215, 219, 231, 232, 236, 237, 238, 251; sterilization of 297
wellness centers 18
Wennberg, John 399
Western medical paradigm 218
women 191–2, 201, 202–3; alcohol-related deaths 191; cancer deaths 243; education of 215; and HIV/AIDS 305; obesity rates 223; and smoking 249; *see also* breast cancer; breastfeeding; pregnancy; prenatal care
Women's Health Initiative 192
work hours: audiologists 138; cardiovascular technologists 151; clinical laboratory technologists 152; dietitians 141; emergency medical technicians and paramedics 135; medical assistants 124; medical social workers 149; nurses 123; occupational therapists 134; pharmacists 139; pharmacy technicians 141; physical therapists and therapist assistants 144, 145; physicians 120; respiratory therapists 134; surgical technologists 126
Workers' Boards (Workers' Compensation Committee) 89

workers' compensation 89–90
workplace safety *see* infection control;
     Occupational Safety and Health
     Administration (OSHA) standards
World Health Organization (WHO) 212,
     216, 235, 248, 250, 309, 397
wounds 271
written communication 350–1

X-Rays 366
xerophthalmia 221
xylenols 296

yeasts 287

Zika virus 234
zinc deficiency 221